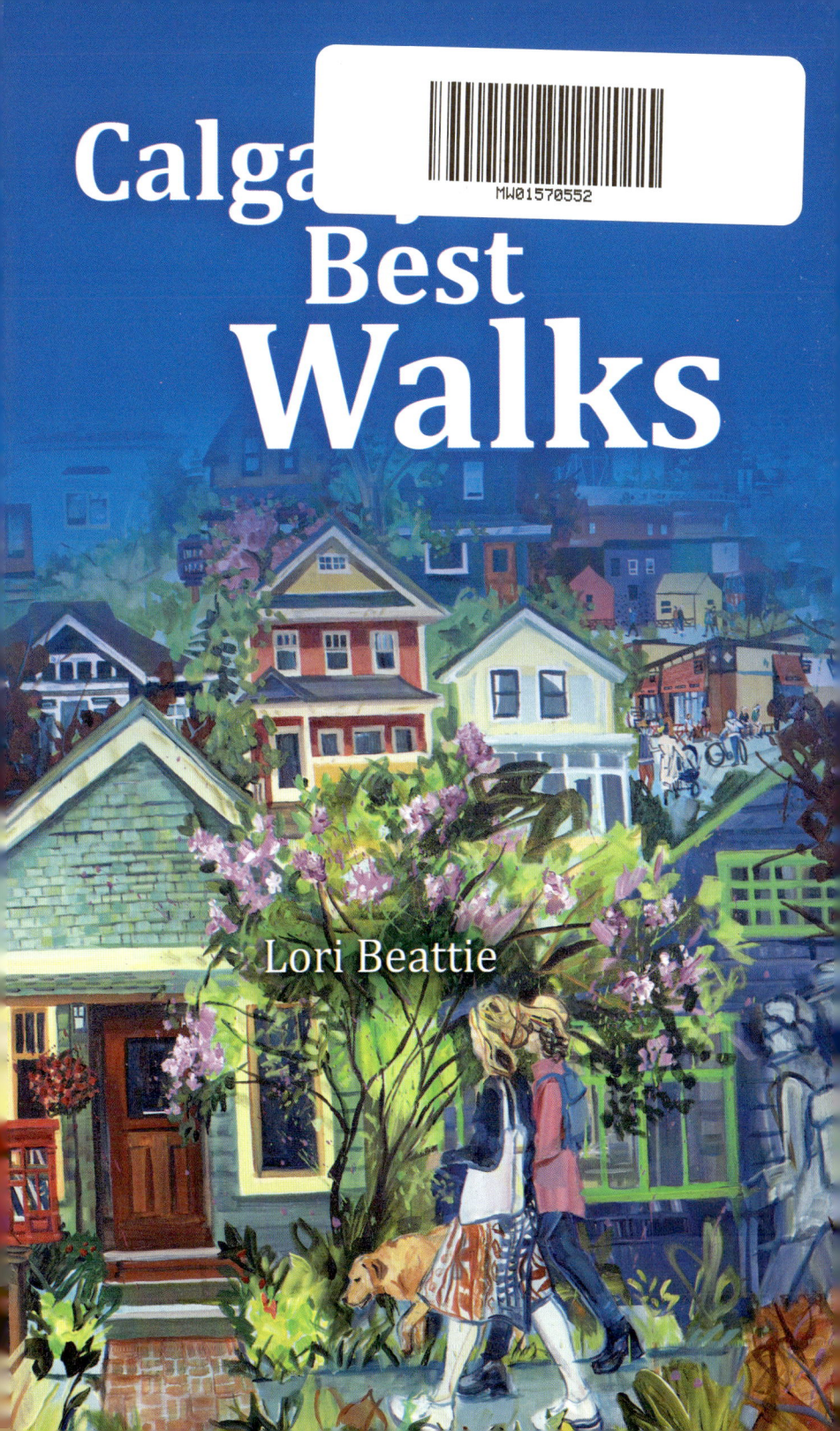

Calgary's Best Walks

Lori Beattie

Calgary's Best Walks
Expanded 3rd Edition 2025

copyright © 2015, 2020, 2025 Lori Beattie

All rights reserved. No part of this publication may be reproduced, stored in a retrieval system or transmitted, in any form or by any means, electronic, mechanical, recording, or otherwise, without prior written permission of the publisher, except in the case of a reviewer, who may quote brief passages in a review to print in a magazine or newspaper, or broadcast on radio or television. In the case of photocopying or other reprographic copying, users must obtain a license from Access Copyright, the Canadian Copyright Licensing Agency.

Published by: **Fit Frog Adventures**
Calgary, AB
www.fitfrog.ca
Instagram & Facebook: @lorifitfrog
lorib@fitfrog.ca

Connect with the author on Instagram and Facebook @lorifitfrog or at www.fitfrog.ca

Order books!
Retailers and individuals can contact Fit Frog Adventures by email at lorib@fitfrog.ca and learn more at www.fitfrog.ca/guidebooks. Combine orders of Calgary's Best Walks with Calgary's Best Bike Rides. Standard industry discounts apply.

For permissions to reproduce the works of art in this volume, grateful acknowledgement is made to the copyright holders thereof.

Maps, book design, book cover, layout and photo-retouch by **Sergio Gaytán**

Front cover artwork and interior artwork, as marked, copyright **Jill Thomson**, www.jillthomson.ca

Interior artwork, as marked, copyright **Pam Weber**, www.pamweber.com

Photographs, as marked, copyright **Sara Tehranian**, Instagram @sara.tehranian

Photographs as marked, copyright **Cody Stuart**, Instagram @betamanic

All other photographs copyright **Lori Beattie**

1 2 3 4 5

Library and Archives Canada Cataloguing in Publication
Title: Calgary's best walks: 95 urban jaunts and nature strolls and tasty coffee shops / Lori Beattie.

Names: Beattie, Lori, 1970- author

Description: Expanded 3rd edition.

Identifiers: Canadiana 20250101769 | ISBN 9780993953545 (softcover)

Subjects: LCSH: Walking—Alberta—Calgary—Guidebooks. | LCSH: Hiking—Alberta—Calgary—Guidebooks. | LCSH: Nature trails—Alberta—Calgary—Guidebooks. | LCSH: Coffee shops—Alberta—Calgary—Guidebooks. | LCSH: Calgary (Alta.)—Guidebooks. | LCGFT: Guidebooks.

Classification: LCC GV199.44.C22 C335 2025 | DDC 917.123/38044—dc23

Printed in Canada

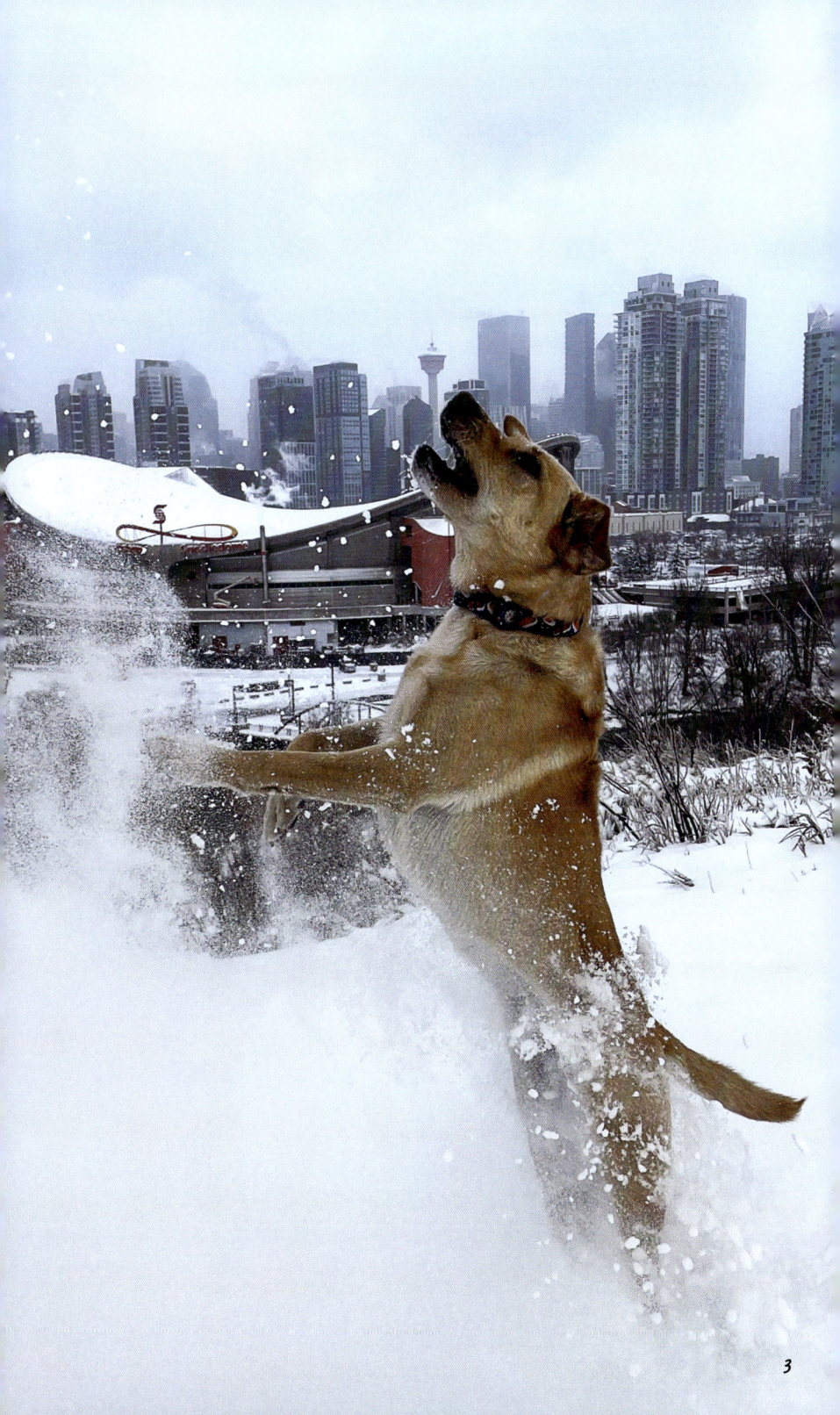

All of the walks in this book are situated on the traditional territories of the peoples of the Treaty 7 region in Southern Alberta, which includes the Stoney (Îyârhe) Nakoda Nations (Chiniki, Bearspaw, Wesley), the Tsuut'ina, the nations of the Blackfoot Confederacy (Siksika, Piikuni, Kainai) and the Otipemisiwak Métis Government of the Métis Nation within Alberta District 5 and 6 as well as everyone who makes their homes in the Treaty 7 region of Southern Alberta.

You will come across Indigenous history and knowledge throughout the book as it is an interesting and integral part of Calgary's story. To broaden your cultural understanding, or to discover where to experience the culture of the Treaty 7 nations go to Calgary Tourism at www.visitcalgary.com or the Calgary Library at www.calgarylibrary.ca and search for Indigenous experiences.

Phonetic pronunciation
   Piikuni – Pee-kah-nee
   Siksika – Seeg-see-kah (emphasis on kah) (g/k almost sound the same)
   Kainai – G-ai-nah (g and k almost sound the same)
   Tsuut'ina – Soot-tenna
   Chiniki – Chin-ick-ee

Siksikaitsitapi Medicine Wheel, Nose Hill Park

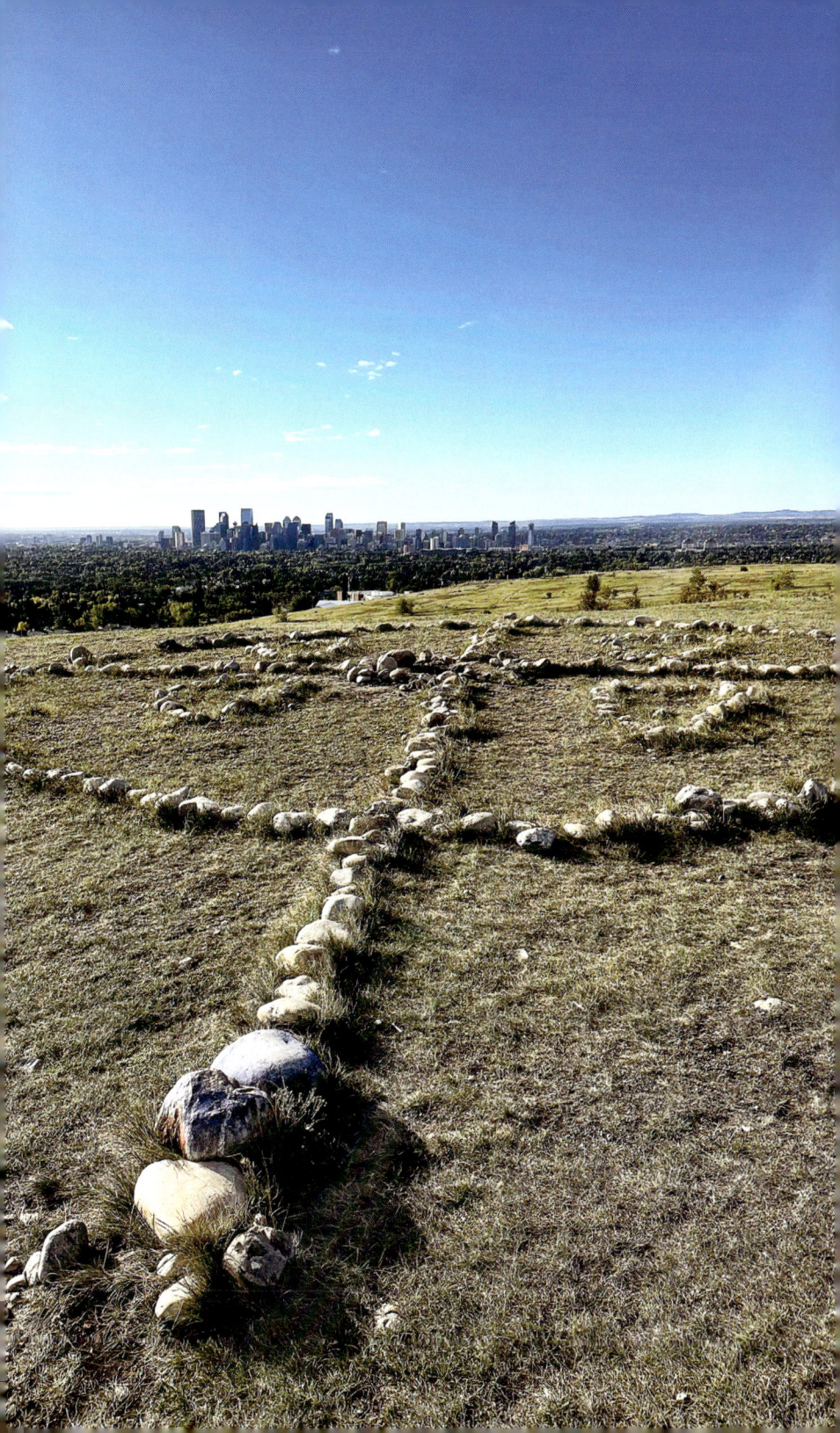

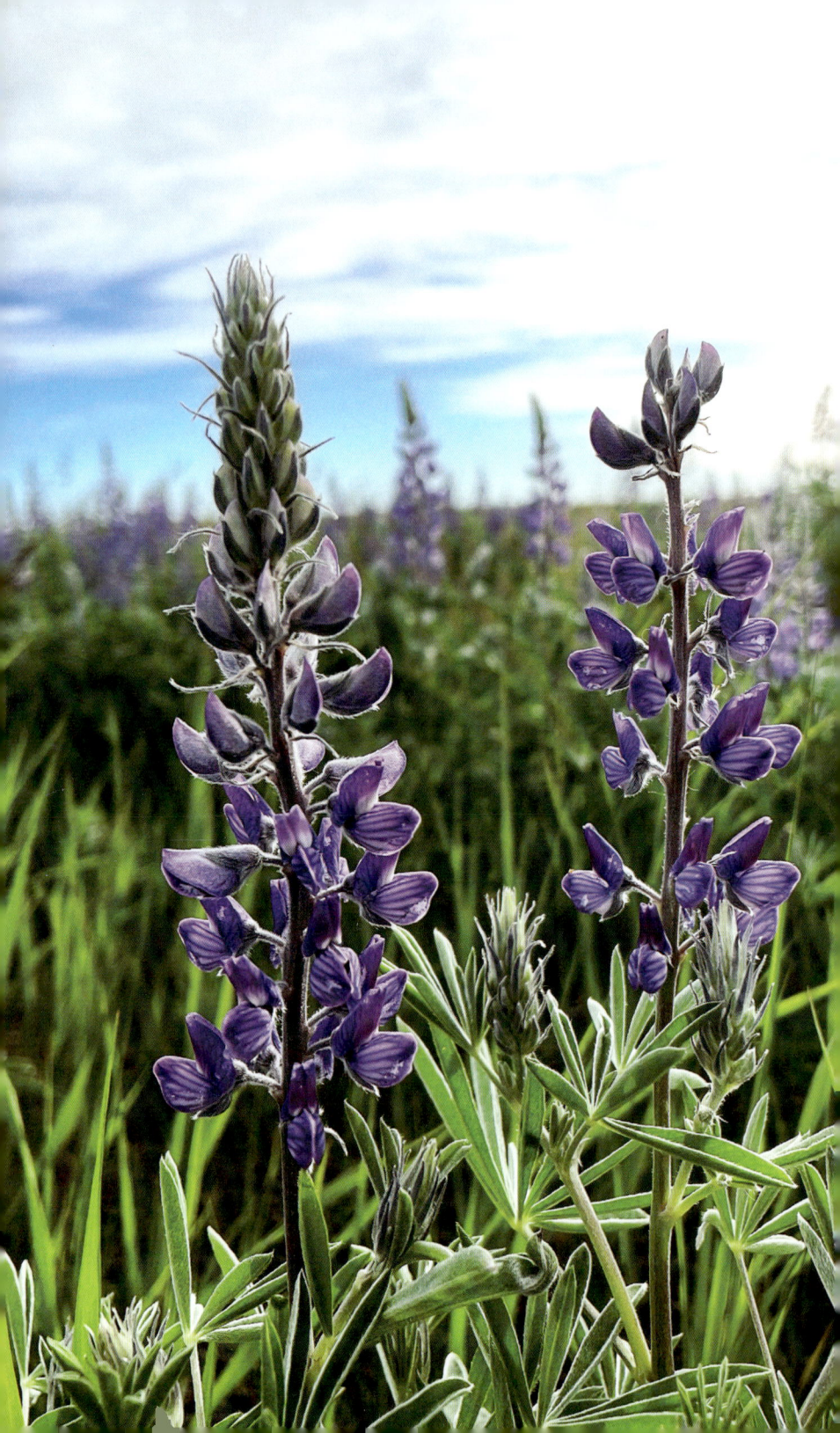

Other books by Lori Beattie

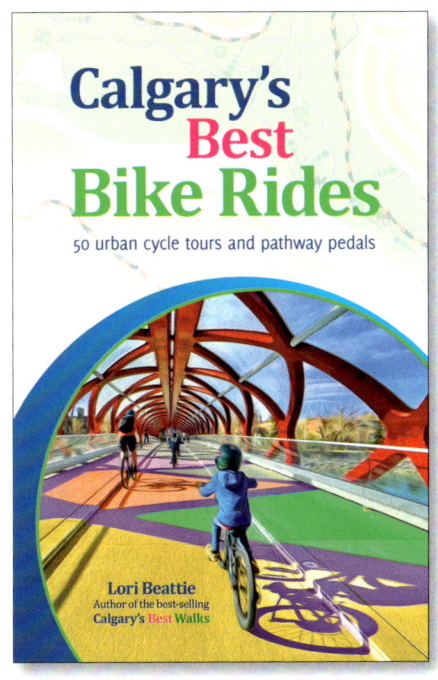

Calgary's Best Bike Rides
(Fit Frog Adventures, 2022)

Calgary's Best Walks:
45 Urban Jaunts and Nature Strolls
(Fit Frog Adventures, 2020)

Calgary's Best Walks:
35 Urban Jaunts and Nature Strolls
(Fit Frog Adventures, 2015)

Calgary's Best Bike Rides and Trails
(Fifth House Publishers, 2004)

Calgary's Best Hikes and Walks
(Fifth House Publishers, 2002)

Lupins, Nose Hill

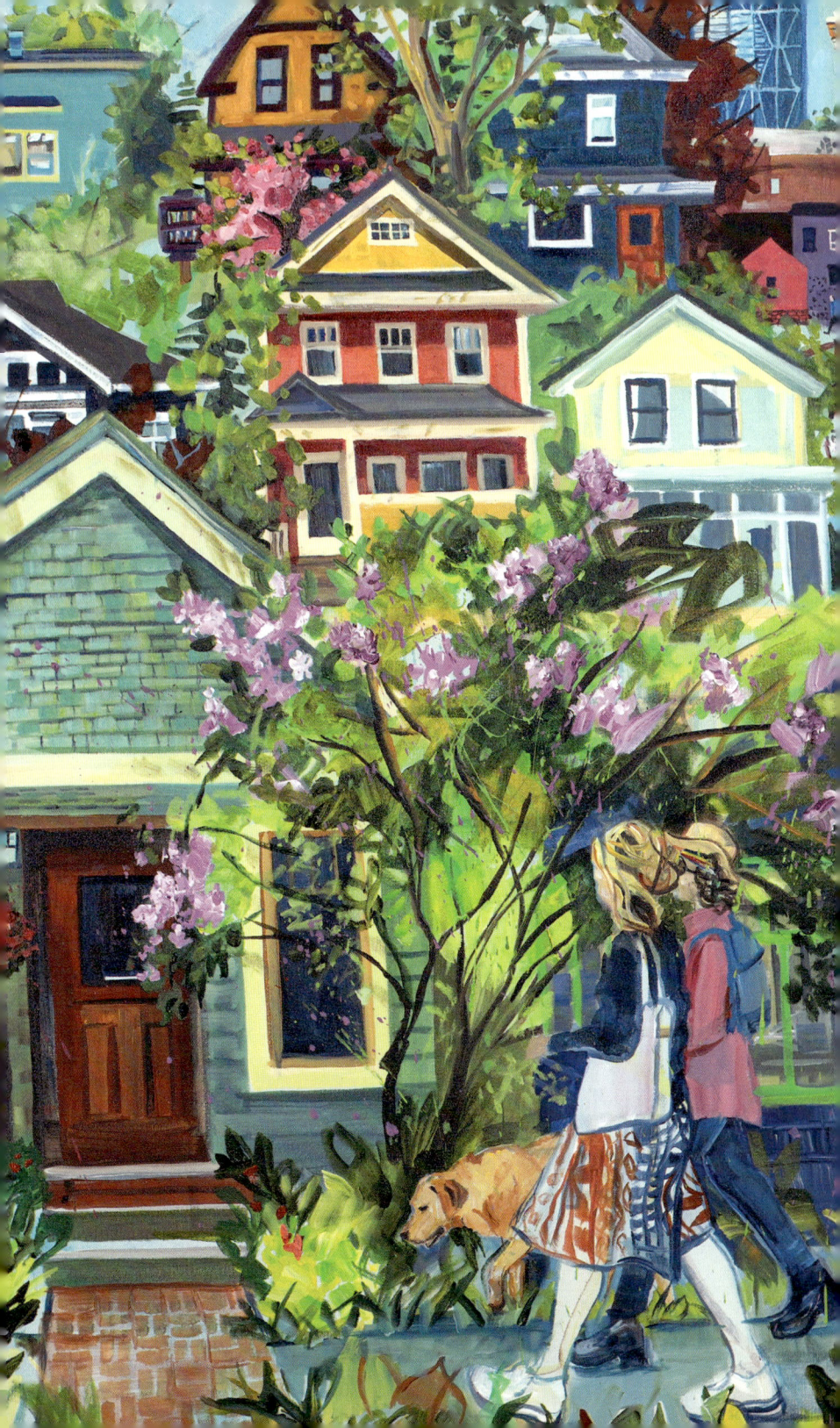

Calgary's Best Walks

Lori Beattie

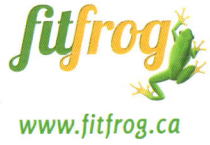

www.fitfrog.ca

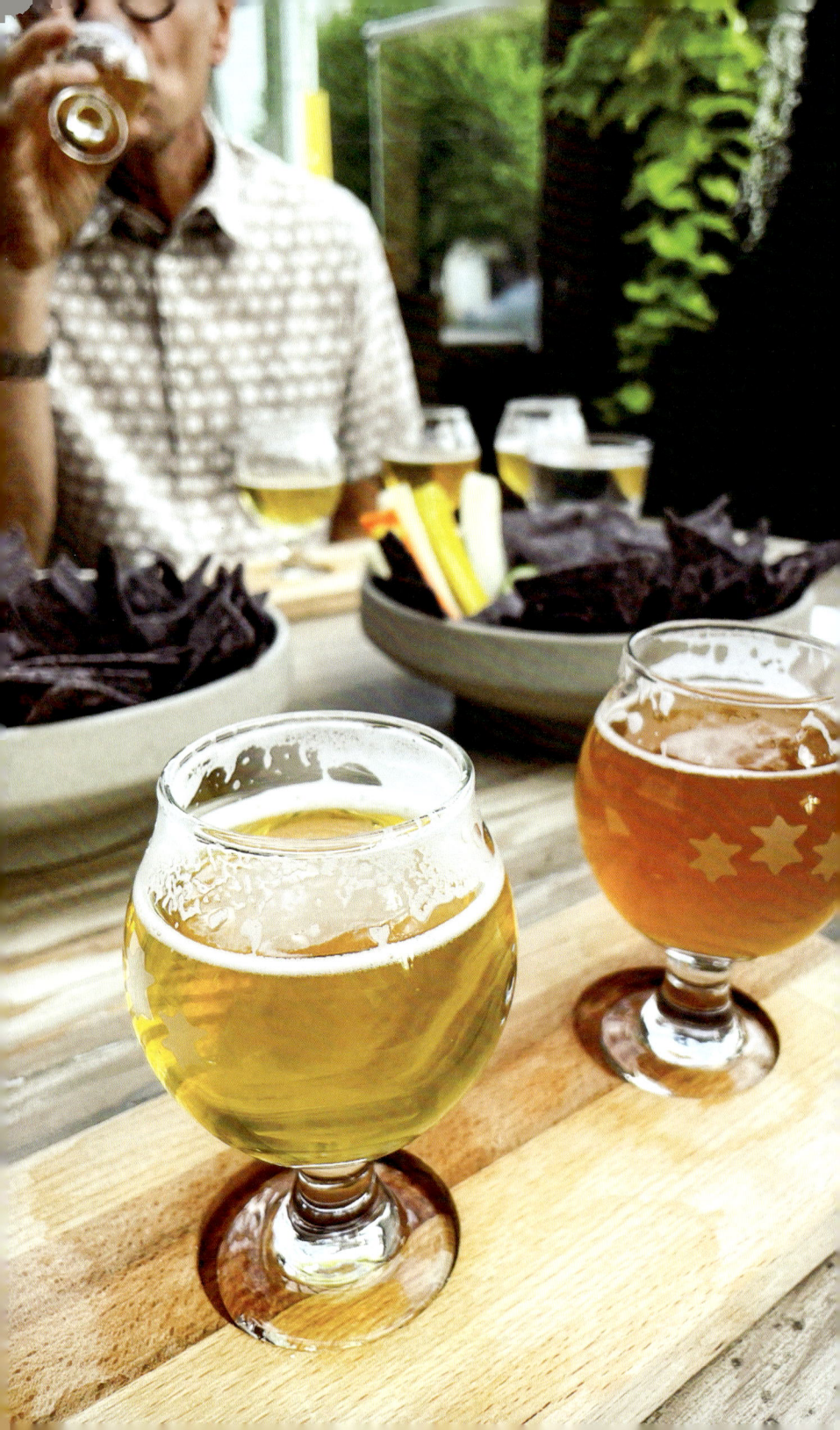

Contents

Introduction 13

How to Use this Book. 14

Map Legend 16

Category Descriptions 18

Category Descriptions Chart 20

Walks Overview. 23

The Walks. 29

Best of Calgary's Best Walks 304

Best Hikes and Walks Beyond Calgary 306

Contributors 316

Author 318

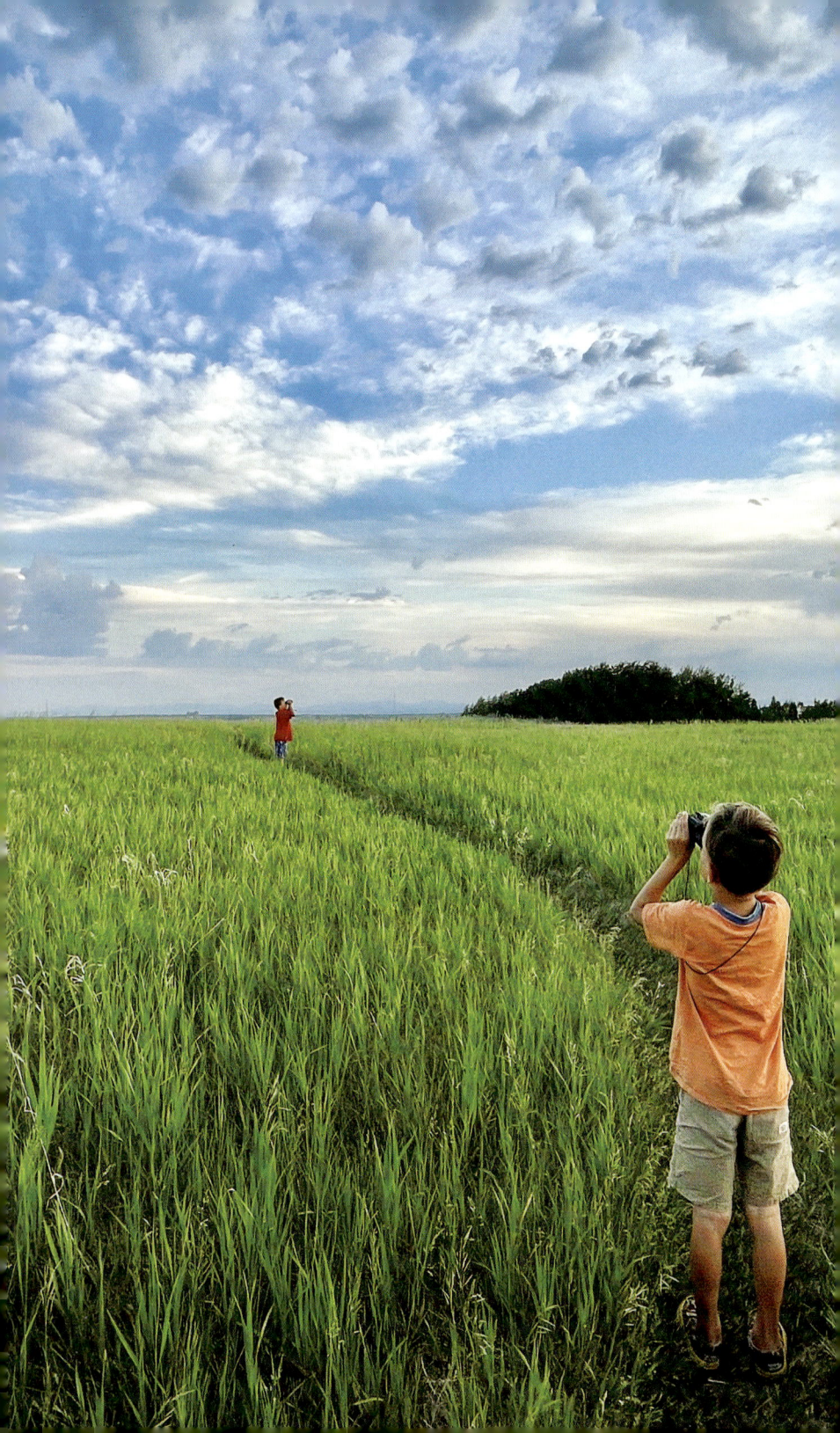

Introduction

Walking makes me happy! It helps me clear my head, sparks my creativity, and gives me new perspectives. Stepping out into the great outdoors has always been my go-to, whether it was in the wilds of New Brunswick where I grew up or through the neighbourhoods and parks of Calgary that I now call home. Changing my route mid stride, turning down an alley to check out a mural or taking a cut through path or set of stairs just to see where it goes, that is the joy of urban exploring. And all that fresh air and sunshine does wonders for my mood.

"Walking works like a drug, bringing happiness to those who choose to take the first step!" This is a quote from the book Happy City, and I put this to the ultimate test when life threw me a curve ball in the summer of 2024. While going through chemotherapy all fall, I kept on walking, every day. Research shows that walking like a happy person, head up, shoulders back and a smile at the ready, makes you feel happier. It works! Cancer is a challenge of epic proportions and walking helped me keep my mental game strong. Walking and surrounding myself with upbeat people; my family, friends and fellow Fit Frog (& dog) walkers who stepped out with me through it all.

When you step out on the walks in my book, be sure to get lost sometimes. I mean, not really lost, but also, maybe not completely sure of where you are. The routes are meant as a guide, but there is a lot more to see and people to meet on the next street over. Just like when you travel to other cities or countries for a change of pace, urban exploring in Calgary gets you out of a rut. It refreshes and invigorates, and it helps you feel more connected to your city. Have fun and I hope to run into you on walkabout!

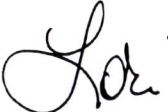

Nose Hill by Cody Stuart

How to Use this Book

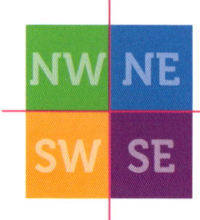

Walks are colour-coded by quadrant.

Walk Details

All the walk's details are included in this section. You'll find information on route categories, public transit options, parking, and the locations of public bathrooms. For current trail updates, including closures, check the City of Calgary website. (www.calgary.ca)

I provide route distances measured in kilometres. A person who walks regularly has an average pace of 5 km per hour. If the route is hilly, generally speaking, for every 100 m gained in elevation, you should add 10 minutes to your walk-time estimate. You gain between 35 and 50 metres in elevation when you climb from the river valley to the top of Calgary's escarpments. For those of you who enjoy counting steps as part of the 10,000/day step challenge, take note that with an average step length of 80 cm, you will walk 1,312 steps/km. If you complete a route that is 7.5 km or more, you will walk at least 10,000 steps.

See Category Descriptions (page 20) for information on the walk categories.

Highlights, Detours & Destinations

This section provides extra information specific features in along the walk or ways for the urban explorer to extend or expand their walks.

Walk at a Glance

The Walk at a Glance is a route description that provides you with an overview of the walk, as well as information on items of note relative to the area the walk covers.

Map

1. Each route is marked by a specific colour and route number — arrows denote suggested directions.

2. Line widths correlate to pathways and roadways. The widest line is a road, the narrow solid line is a paved pathway, and the dashed narrow line is a dirt, shale, or grass pathway.

3. The maps in this book also show hills. The largest dots denote uphill portions. A route line that extends from a small dot to a large one indicates an uphill climb.

Continuity-marks help you find where a map intersects as you move from one page to the next.

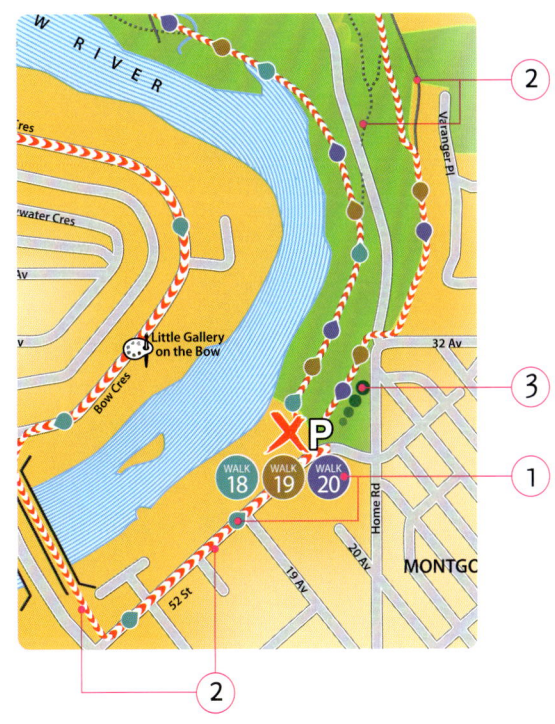

Map Legend

Main Route

Paved - one direction
 Road
 Pathway

Gravel - one direction
 Pathway

Paved - both directions
Road
Pathway

Gravel - both directions
Pathway

Alternate Route

Paved - one direction
 Road
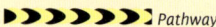 Pathway

Gravel - one direction
 Pathway

Paved - both directions
Road
Pathway

Gravel - both directions
Pathway

Nearby pathway

Paved road

Paved path

Unpaved path

Continuity

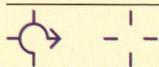

Continuity-marks show map's overlapping points from one page to the next in a spread

Symbols

Walk start	LRT start	LRT station	 Parking	North	Restrooms
 Commercial Area	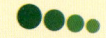 Uphill/Downhill	 Foot bridge	 Traffic bridge	 LRT	Railroad
Artwork	Viewpoint	On-leash area	Off-leash area	Playground	Powerline
Coffee shop	Ice cream parlor	Brewery	Restaurant	Convenience store	Picnic area
Stairs	Library	Firehouse	 Sign	Interpretative sign	Park Office
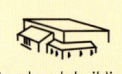 Landmark building	School	Church/Temple	House	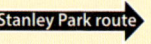 Connection to another route, should you want a longer walk	

Walk number · Title · Quadrant · Walk Details · Map layout on pages · Finder tab

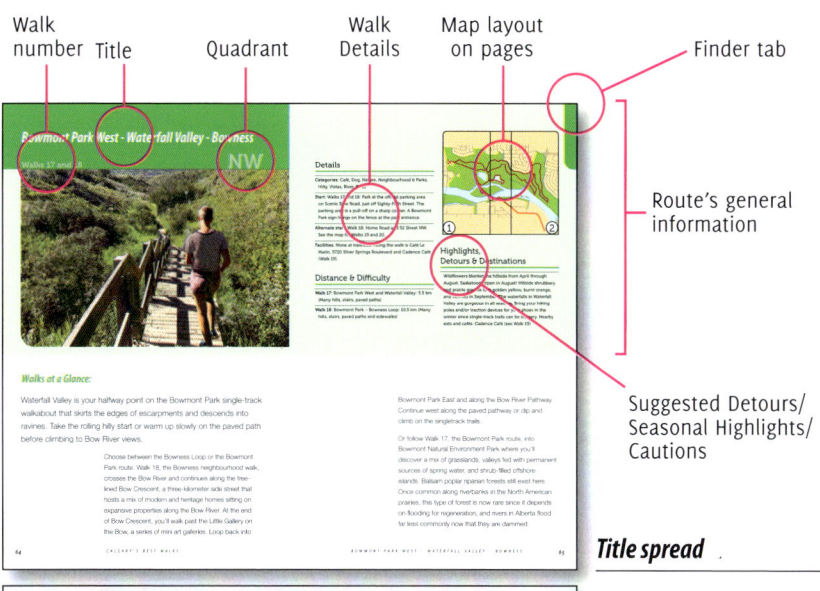

Route's general information

Suggested Detours / Seasonal Highlights / Cautions

Title spread

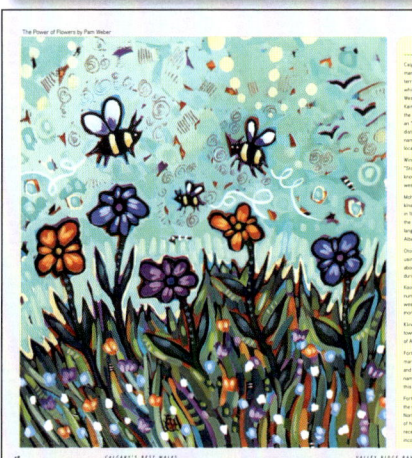

Sidebar

Content spread

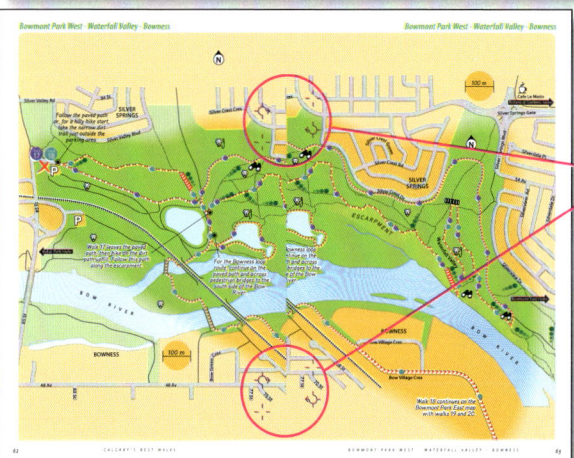

Map

Continuity-marks show map's overlapping points from one page to the next

Map spread

Category Descriptions

Families and Children

All of the routes in the book are great for kids, which is why I have not added a "kids" category. The varied terrain and the sights make all of the walks interesting. Make the walk more fun for kids by stopping for a picnic lunch, taking the single-track trail with the chickadees, or enjoying a playground. Of course, a post-walk ice cream guarantees success!

LRT

If "LRT" is included in the category description, a LRT stop is along the route or close to it.

Café

If I include "café" in my description, you can be sure that a recommended, independent, coffee shop is along the route or close by.

Dog

My dog loves it! The routes are mostly on-leash with the occasional off-leash park. Dogs are welcome on all routes except those in the Sandy Cross Conservation Area, Leighton Art Centre, Weaselhead Flats, the Jackrabbit Trail, and Inglewood Bird Sanctuary.

Nature

The word "Nature" indicates that most of or the entire walk is in the wilderness.

Neighbourhoods and Parks

This description tells you that the route will take you through natural area parks and green spaces, as well as along sidewalks through residential communities with canopies of trees, as well as varied landscaping, architecture, and colourful gardens from spring through fall.

People Watch and Shop

The route passes by or travels along a pedestrian-friendly shopping street with independent shops, restaurants, and cafés.

Hilly

If I use the word "hilly" in the category description, know that there is more than one significant hill climb.

Stroller

This category description is one to watch out for if you are walking with a toddler or baby. Big-wheeled strollers can easily manage "Stroller" routes. Small-wheeled strollers should stick to the neighbourhood walks, not the natural areas with gravel pathways.

Historic

Inner-city community walks are always historic. The route travels through residential communities with canopies of trees, as well as varied landscaping, architecture, and colourful gardens from spring through fall.

Vistas

If you want to see the Rocky Mountains, river valley or downtown views, choose a route with "Vista" in the category description.

River

You'll enjoy flowing water when walking "River" routes.

Birds

Many species of feathered friends are your walking companions on the wetlands and river sections of these routes.

Category Descriptions Chart

	Walk #	
NW	1-5	Glenbow Ranch Provincial Park and Haskayne Park
	6-9	Cochrane
	10	Royal Oak Wetlands and Ravines
	11	Arbour lake - Royal Oak-Scenic Acres - Twelve Mile Coulee
	12	Twelve Mile Coulee - Tuscany
	13	Bowness Park - Baker Park- Douglas Fir Trail
	14	Romeo & Juliet - Greenwood - Farmer's Market - Bowness
	15-16	Valley Ridge Ravines and Bearspaw Dam Trail
	17-18	Bowmont Park West - Waterfall Valley - Bowness
	19-20	Dale Hodges Park - Bowmont Park East - Botanical Gardens
	21	Botanical Gardens of Silver Springs
	22-27	Varsity, Dalhousie and Edgemont Ravines
	28-30	Nose Hill Park
NE	31-32	Huntington Hills-Nose Creek-Thorncliffe-Highland Park-Queens Park
	33	West Nose Creek / Confluence Park
	34	Winston Heights- Renfrew- Tuxedo Park- Nose Creek- Vista Heights
	35	Bridgeland-Bow River-Nose Creek
NW	36-39	Confederation Park-Capitol Hill-Mount Pleasant-Crescent Heights-SAIT
	40-42	Kensington- Sunnyside Garage Art- McHugh Bluff-Princes Island-Bow River
	43	Briar Hill - Hounsfield Heights - West Hillhurst -Westmount
	44-46	Parkdale- St. Andrews Heights- University District- Montgomery
SW	47-48	Douglas Fir Trail- Wildwood- Quarry Road Trail- Edworthy West
	49	Patterson - Coach Hill - Paskapoo Slopes
	50-52	Strathcona and Aspen Ravines, Springbank Hill and Signal Hill
	53-55	Sunalta- Beltline- Mount Royal- Bankview- Scarboro- Kilarney
	56-57	Downtown and Beltline Murals and Art
	58	Roxboro-Erlton-Ramsay
	59	Stanley Park- Roxboro- Mount Royal- East Elbow
	60	Sandy Beach-Elbow Park-Britannia
	61-62	Elbow River to Bow River
	63-64	Garrison- Currie- North Glenmore- Altadore- Glenmore Dam
	65-66	Weaselhead Flats Park & Jackrabbit Trail
	67-68	Glenmore Reservoir - Bel-Aire - Mayfair - Kingsland - Haysboro
	69	Griffith Woods Park
	70-72	Ann & Sandy Cross Conservation Area
	73-74	Leighton Art Centre loop-Bird Box Walk
	75	Brown Lowery Provincial Park
SE	76-81	Fish Creek Provincial Park
	82	Legacy Environmental Reserve
	83-84	Sue Higgins-Carburn- Beaverdam Flats Parks - Ogden- Lynnwood
	85-86	Southview-Dover-Irrigation Canal
	87-89	Elliston Park- Forest Lawn- International Avenue- Southview- Inglewood
	90-93	Pearce Estate Park- Inglewood Bird Sanctuary- Ramsay- St. Patrick's Island
NW-NE-SW-SE	94-95	Tour de Calgary, South and North Calgary Pathways

LRT	Café	Dog	Nature	Neighbourhoods & Parks	People watch & shop	Hilly	Stroller	Historic	Vistas	River	Birds	Walk #
		✔	✔			✔	✔		✔	✔	✔	1-5
	✔	✔	✔	✔		✔	✔		✔	✔	✔	6-9
✔		✔	✔	✔					✔		✔	10
✔	✔	✔	✔	✔		✔			✔		✔	11
✔		✔	✔			✔			✔		✔	12
	✔	✔	✔	✔		✔	✔	✔		✔	✔	13
	✔	✔	✔	✔		✔	✔	✔	✔	✔	✔	14
		✔	✔	✔		✔				✔	✔	15-16
	✔	✔	✔	✔		✔			✔	✔	✔	17-18
	✔	✔	✔	✔		✔			✔		✔	19-20
		✔	✔				✔				✔	21
✔	✔	✔	✔	✔		✔	✔		✔		✔	22-27
	✔	✔	✔			✔			✔		✔	28-30
	✔	✔	✔	✔		✔	✔		✔			31-32
		✔	✔			✔			✔	✔	✔	33
	✔	✔	✔	✔		✔			✔	✔	✔	34
✔	✔	✔	✔	✔	✔	✔	✔		✔	✔	✔	35
	✔	✔	✔	✔	✔	✔	✔	✔	✔		✔	36-39
✔	✔	✔	✔	✔	✔	✔	✔	✔	✔	✔	✔	40-42
✔	✔	✔	✔	✔	✔	✔			✔	✔		43
✔	✔	✔	✔	✔	✔	✔	✔		✔	✔		44-46
	✔	✔	✔	✔		✔			✔	✔	✔	47-48
	✔	✔	✔	✔					✔		✔	49
✔	✔	✔	✔	✔		✔			✔		✔	50-52
✔	✔	✔	✔	✔	✔	✔	✔	✔	✔	✔		53-55
✔	✔	✔	✔	✔	✔		✔	✔		✔	✔	56-57
✔	✔	✔	✔	✔	✔	✔		✔	✔	✔		58
✔	✔	✔	✔	✔	✔	✔	✔		✔	✔		59
	✔	✔	✔	✔		✔	✔		✔	✔	✔	60
✔	✔	✔	✔	✔	✔	✔	✔	✔	✔	✔	✔	61-62
	✔	✔	✔	✔	✔	✔	✔	✔	✔	✔	✔	63-64
	✔		✔			✔			✔	✔	✔	65-66
	✔	✔	✔	✔		✔	✔		✔	✔	✔	67-68
			✔	✔			✔			✔	✔	69
			✔			✔			✔		✔	70-72
			✔			✔			✔		✔	73-74
		✔	✔			✔			✔	✔	✔	75
✔	✔	✔	✔	✔		✔	✔		✔	✔	✔	76-81
	✔	✔	✔			✔			✔		✔	82
	✔	✔	✔	✔		✔	✔	✔	✔	✔	✔	83-84
	✔	✔	✔	✔	✔	✔			✔	✔	✔	85-86
✔	✔	✔	✔	✔		✔			✔		✔	87-89
✔	✔	✔	✔	✔	✔	✔	✔	✔	✔	✔	✔	90-93
✔	✔	✔	✔	✔	✔	✔	✔	✔	✔	✔	✔	94-95

CATEGORY DESCRIPTIONS CHART

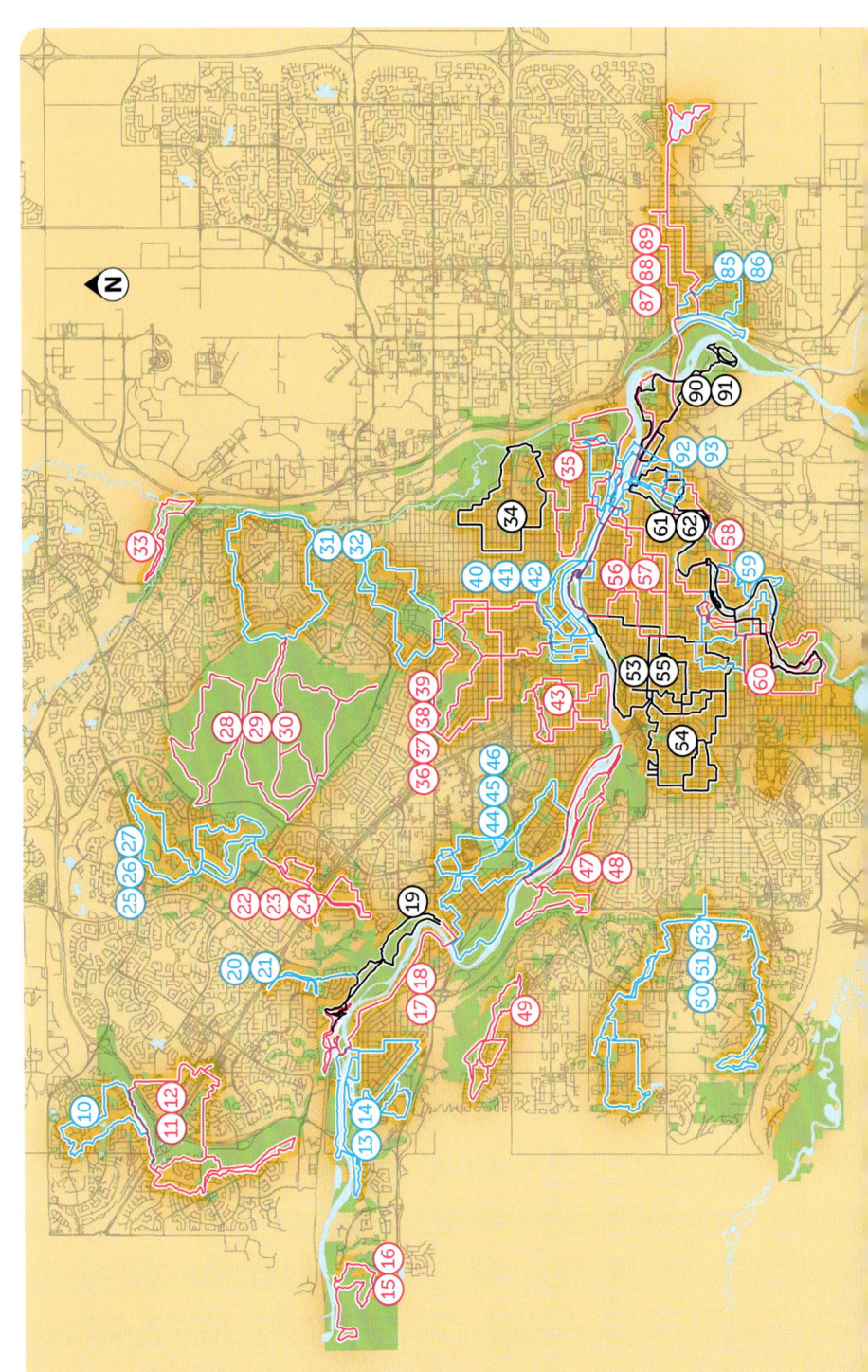

Walks Overview - Map 1 of 3

	Walk #		Page
NW	10	Royal Oak Wetlands and Ravines	42
	11	Arbour lake - Royal Oak-Scenic Acres - Twelve Mile Coulee	46
	12	Twelve Mile Coulee - Tuscany	46
	13	Bowness Park - Baker Park- Douglas Fir Trail	52
	14	Romeo & Juliet - Greenwood - Farmer's Market - Bowness	52
	15-16	Valley Ridge Ravines and Bearspaw Dam Trail	58
	17-18	Bowmont Park West - Waterfall Valley - Bowness	64
	19-20	Dale Hodges Park - Bowmont Park East - Botanical Gardens	70
	21	Botanical Gardens of Silver Springs	76
	22-27	Varsity, Dalhousie and Edgemont Ravines	82
	28-30	Nose Hill Park	92
NE	31-32	Huntington Hills-Nose Creek-Thorncliffe-Highland Park-Queens Park	100
	33	West Nose Creek / Confluence Park	106
	34	Winston Heights- Renfrew- Tuxedo Park- Nose Creek- Vista Heights	110
	35	Bridgeland-Bow River-Nose Creek	114
NW	36-39	Confederation Park-Capitol Hill-Mount Pleasant-Crescent Heights-SAIT	120
	40-42	Kensington- Sunnyside Garage Art- McHugh Bluff-Princes Island-Bow River	128
	43	Briar Hill - Hounsfield Heights - West Hillhurst -Westmount	136
	44-46	Parkdale- St. Andrews Heights- University District- Montgomery	142
SW	47-48	Douglas Fir Trail- Wildwood- Quarry Road Trail- Edworthy West	148
	49	Patterson - Coach Hill - Paskapoo Slopes	154
	50-52	Strathcona and Aspen Ravines, Springbank Hill and Signal Hill	158
	53-55	Sunalta- Beltline- Mount Royal- Bankview- Scarboro- Kilarney	166
	56-57	Downtown and Beltline Murals and Art	174
	58	Roxboro-Erlton-Ramsay	182
	59	Stanley Park- Roxboro- Mount Royal- East Elbow	190
	60	Sandy Beach-Elbow Park-Britannia	196
	61-62	Elbow River to Bow River	202
SE	85-86	Southview-Dover-Irrigation Canal	272
	87-89	Elliston Park- Forest Lawn- International Avenue- Southview- Inglewood	272
	90-93	Pearce Estate Park- Inglewood Bird Sanctuary- Ramsay- St. Patrick's Island	282

Walks Overview - Map 2 of 3

	Walk #		Page
SW	63-64	Garrison- Currie- North Glenmore- Altadore- Glenmore Dam	208
	65-66	Weaselhead Flats Park & Jackrabbit Trail	216
	67-68	Glenmore Reservoir - Bel-Aire - Mayfair - Kingsland - Haysboro	222
	69	Griffith Woods Park	230
	76-81	Fish Creek Provincial Park	244
SE	83-84	Sue Higgins-Carburn- Beaverdam Flats Parks - Ogden- Lynnwood	262

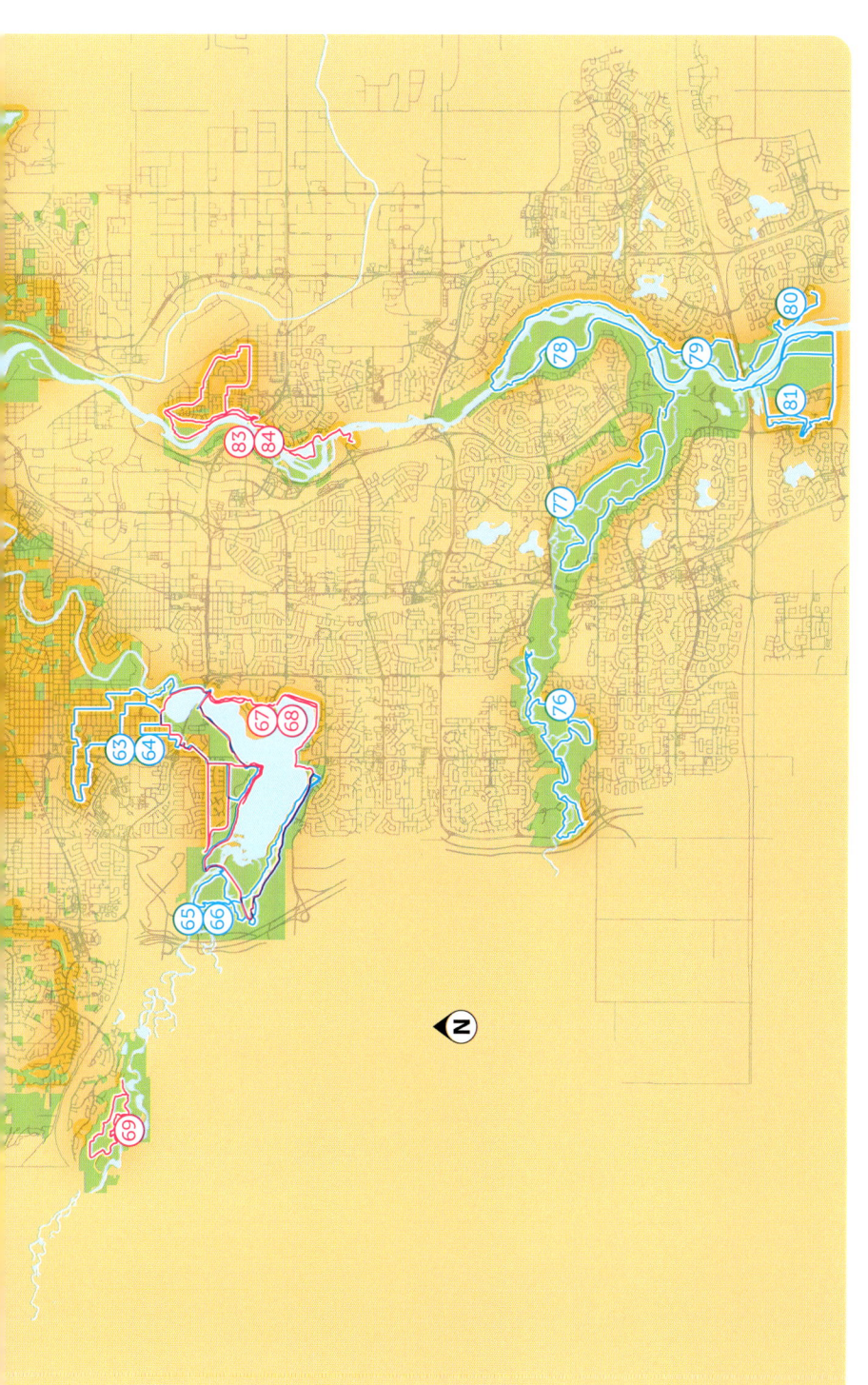

OVERVIEW MAPS

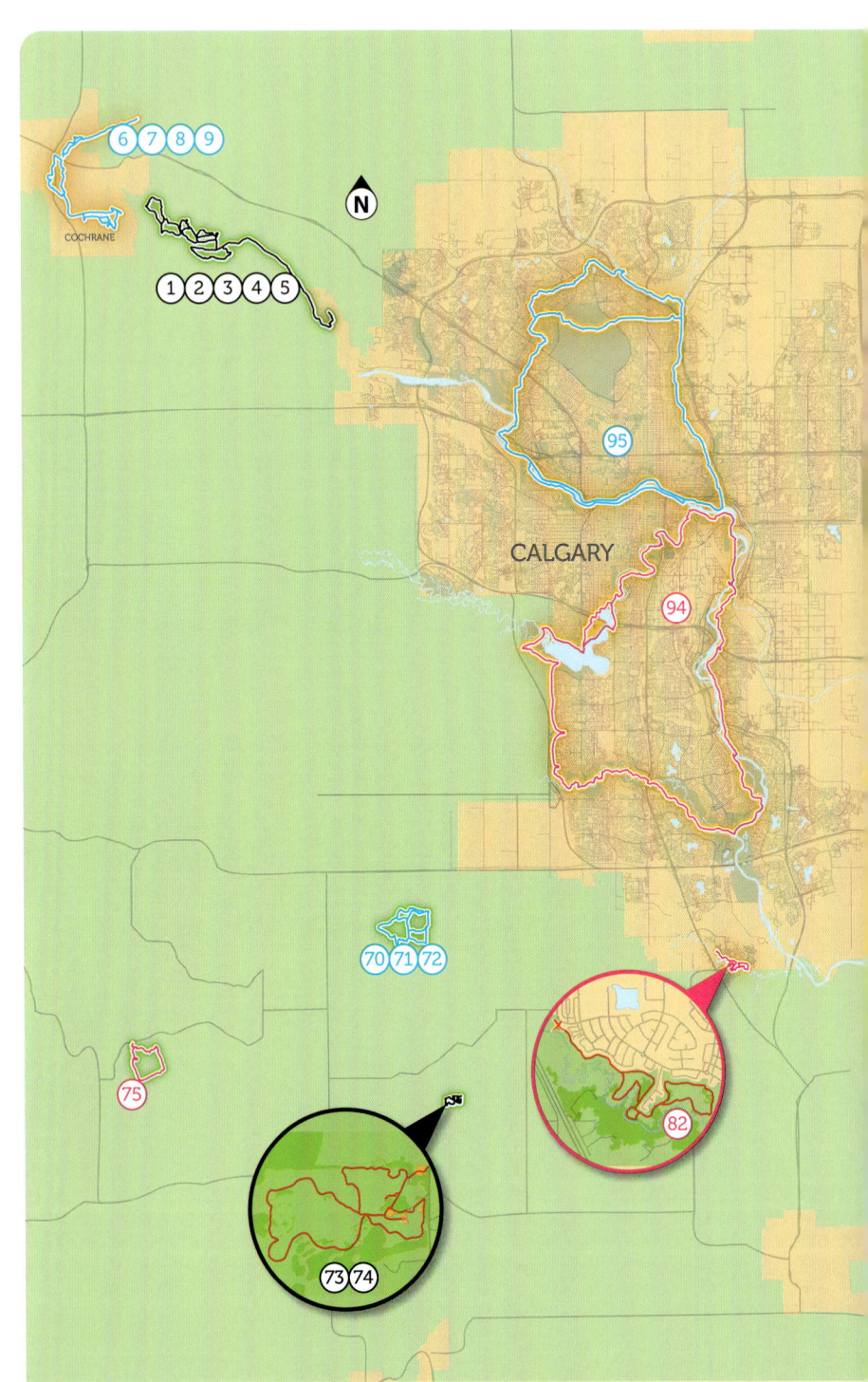

Walks Overview - Map 3 of 3

	Walk #		Page
NW	1-5	Glenbow Ranch Provincial Park and Haskayne Park	32
	6-9	Cochrane	32
SW	70-72	Ann & Sandy Cross Conservation Area	236
	73-74	Leighton Art Centre loop-Bird Box Walk	236
	75	Brown Lowery Provincial Park	236
SE	82	Legacy Environmental Reserve	256
NW-NE-SW-SE	94-95	Tour de Calgary, South and North Calgary Pathways	294

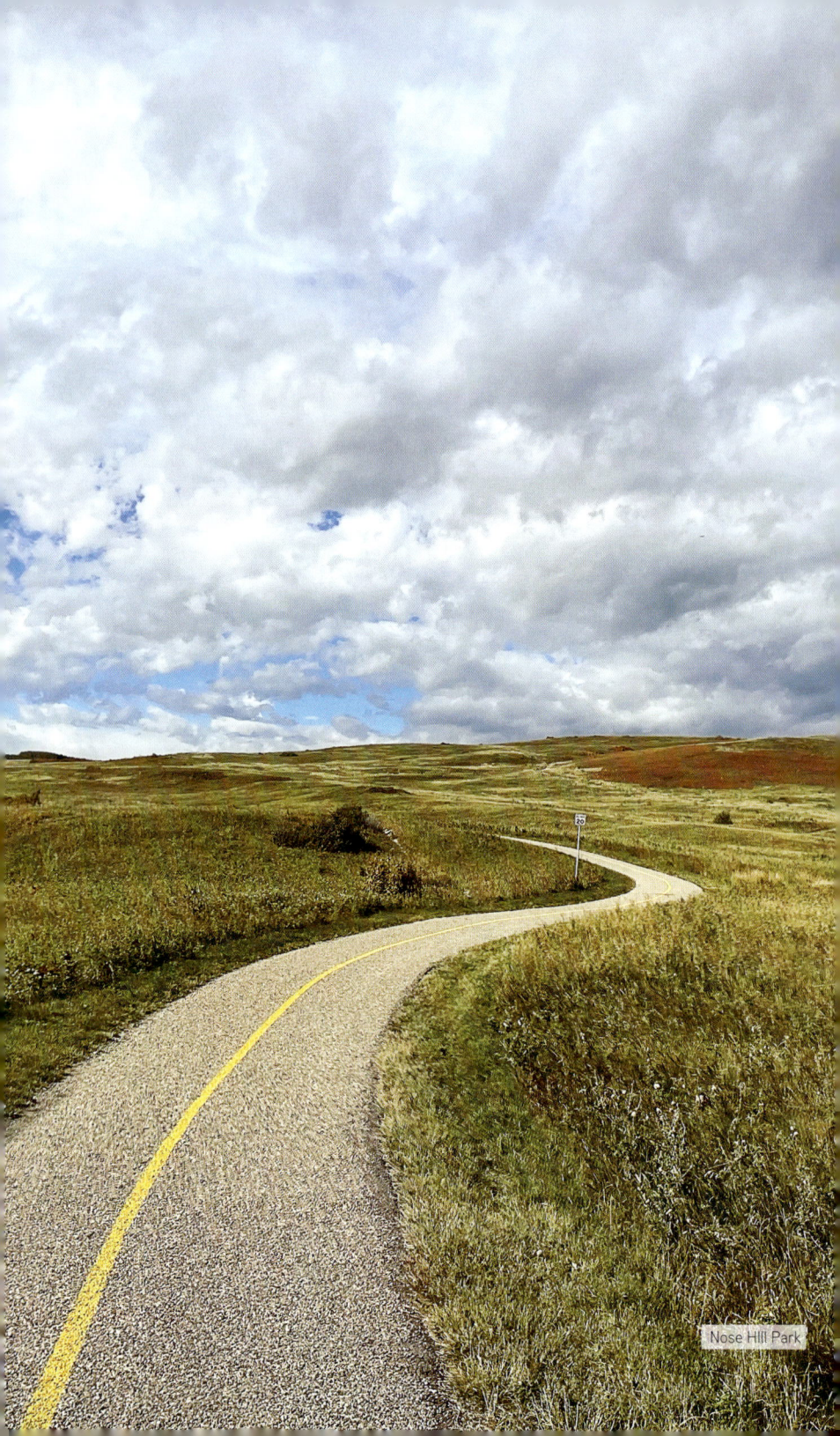

The Walks

	Walk #		Page
NW	1-5	Glenbow Ranch Provincial Park and Haskayne Park	32
	6-9	Cochrane	32
	10	Royal Oak Wetlands and Ravines	42
	11	Arbour lake - Royal Oak-Scenic Acres - Twelve Mile Coulee	46
	12	Twelve Mile Coulee - Tuscany	46
	13	Bowness Park - Baker Park- Douglas Fir Trail	52
	14	Romeo & Juliet - Greenwood - Farmer's Market - Bowness	52
	15-16	Valley Ridge Ravines and Bearspaw Dam Trail	58
	17-18	Bowmont Park West - Waterfall Valley - Bowness	64
	19-20	Dale Hodges Park - Bowmont Park East - Botanical Gardens	70
	21	Botanical Gardens of Silver Springs	76
	22-27	Varsity, Dalhousie and Edgemont Ravines	82
	28-30	Nose Hill Park	92
NE	31-32	Huntington Hills-Nose Creek-Thorncliffe-Highland Park-Queens Park	100
	33	West Nose Creek / Confluence Park	106
	34	Winston Heights- Renfrew- Tuxedo Park- Nose Creek- Vista Heights	110
	35	Bridgeland-Bow River-Nose Creek	114
NW	36-39	Confederation Park-Capitol Hill-Mount Pleasant-Crescent Heights-SAIT	120
	40-42	Kensington- Sunnyside Garage Art- McHugh Bluff-Princes Island-Bow River	128
	43	Briar Hill - Hounsfield Heights - West Hillwurst -Westmount	136
	44-46	Parkdale- St. Andrews Heights- University District- Montgomery	142
SW	47-48	Douglas Fir Trail- Wildwood- Quarry Road Trail- Edworthy West	148
	49	Patterson - Coach Hill - Paskapoo Slopes	154
	50-52	Strathcona and Aspen Ravines, Springbank Hill and Signal Hill	158
	53-55	Sunalta- Beltline- Mount Royal- Bankview- Scarboro- Kilarney	166
	56-57	Downtown and Beltline Murals and Art	174
	58	Roxboro-Erlton-Ramsay	182
	59	Stanley Park- Roxboro- Mount Royal- East Elbow	190
	60	Sandy Beach-Elbow Park-Britannia	196
	61-62	Elbow River to Bow River	202
	63-64	Garrison- Currie- North Glenmore- Altadore- Glenmore Dam	208
	65-66	Weaselhead Flats Park & Jackrabbit Trail	216
	67-68	Glenmore Reservoir - Bel-Aire - Mayfair - Kingsland - Haysboro	222
	69	Griffith Woods Park	230
	70-72	Ann & Sandy Cross Conservation Area	236
	73-74	Leighton Art Centre loop-Bird Box Walk	236
	75	Brown Lowery Provincial Park	236
SE	76-81	Fish Creek Provincial Park	244
	82	Legacy Environmental Reserve	256
	83-84	Sue Higgins-Carburn- Beaverdam Flats Parks - Ogden- Lynnwood	262
	85-86	Southview-Dover-Irrigation Canal	272
	87-89	Elliston Park- Forest Lawn- International Avenue- Southview- Inglewood	272
	90-93	Pearce Estate Park- Inglewood Bird Sanctuary- Ramsay- St. Patrick's Island	282
NW-NE-SW-SE	94-95	Tour de Calgary, South and North Calgary Pathways	294
		Best Hikes and Walks Beyond Calgary	306

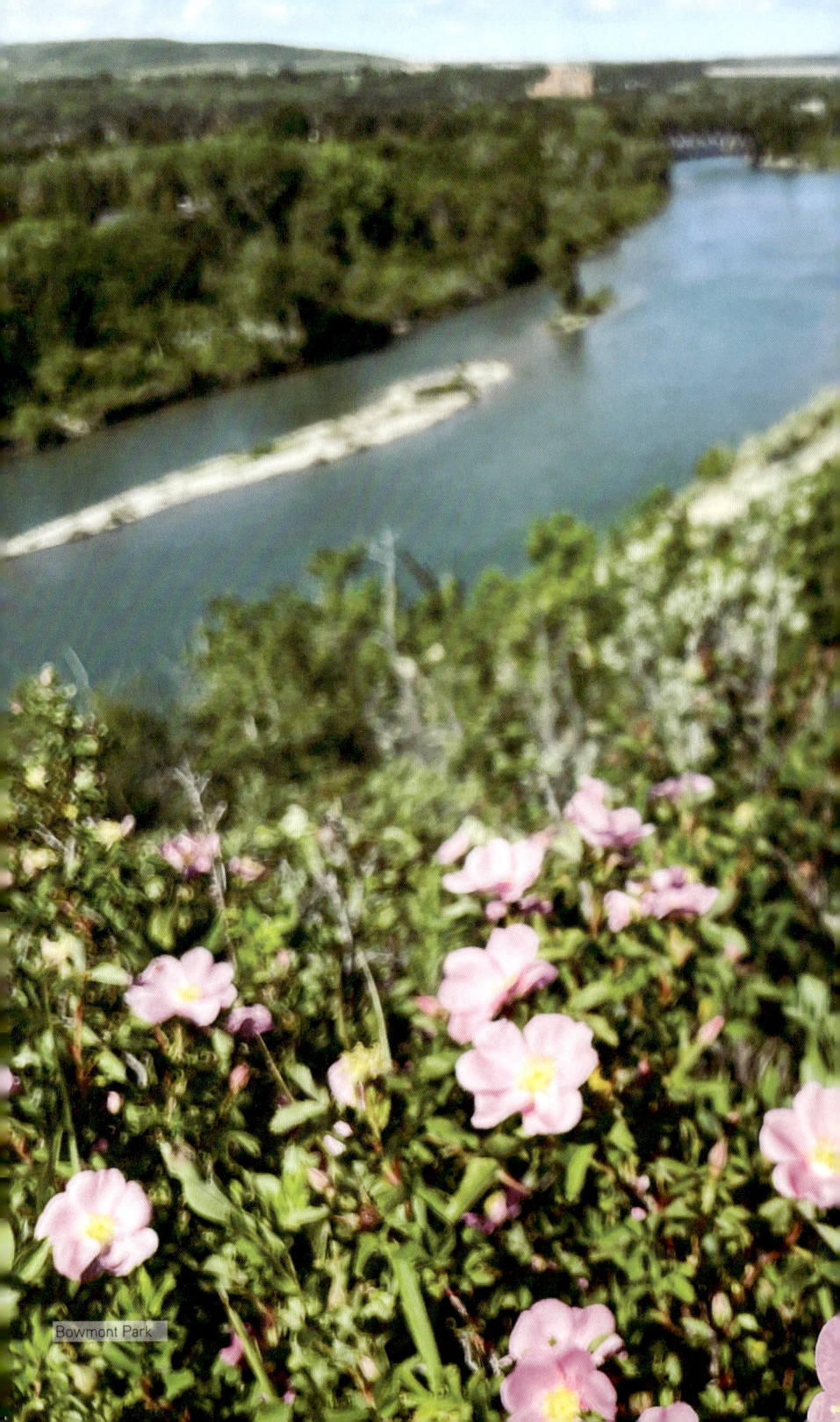
Bowmont Park

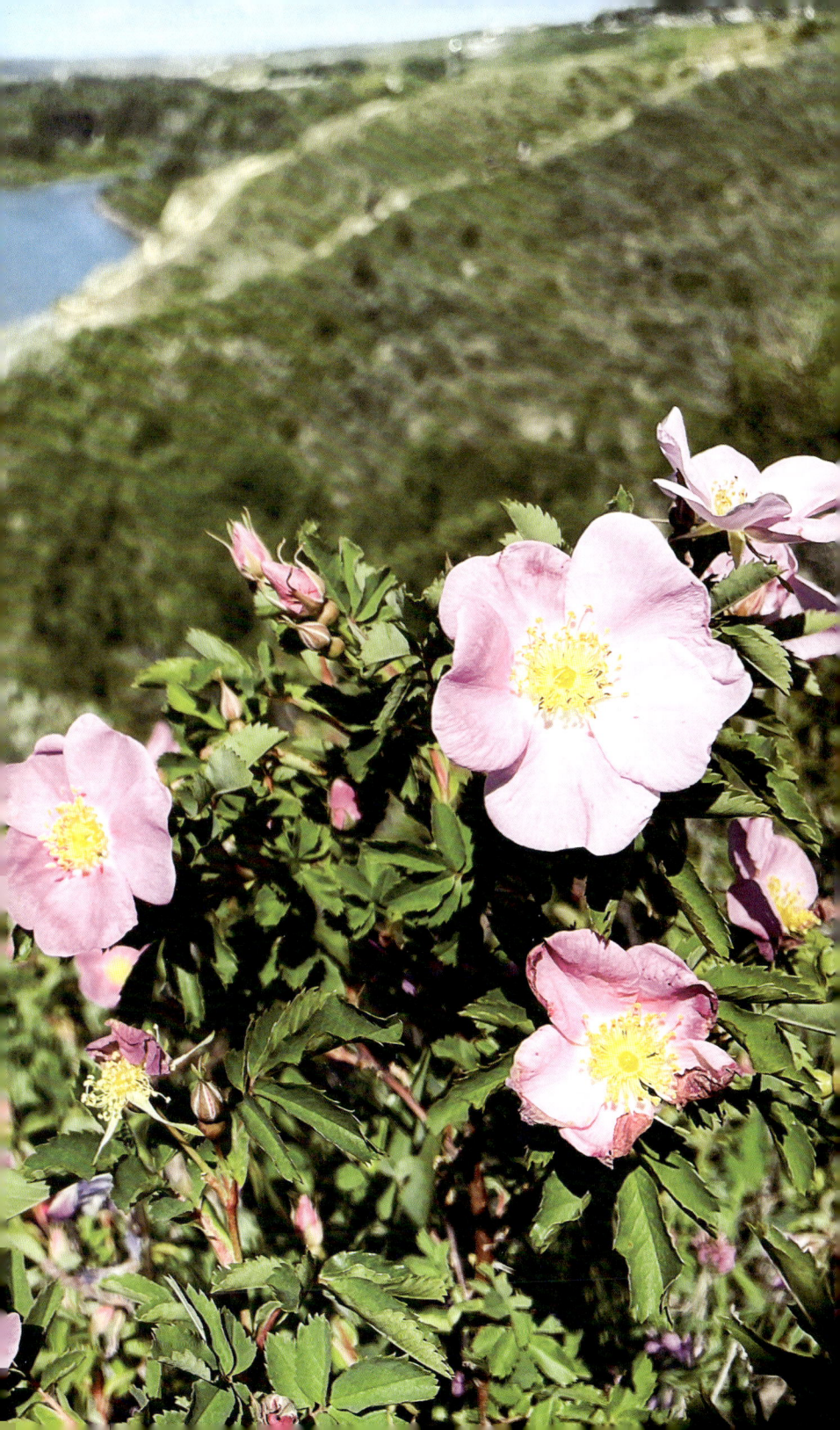

Cochrane, Glenbow Ranch Provincial Park and Haskayne Park

Walks 1-9

NW

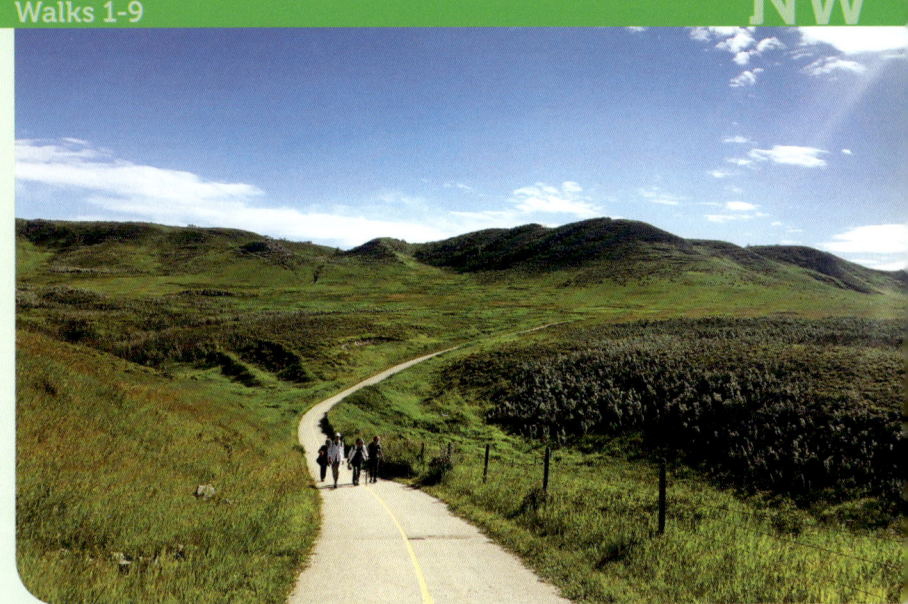

Walks at a Glance:

Alberta's trademark, big, blue skies are a constant companion on all these walks. And when the clouds roll in, the textures and patterns of the land juxtaposed to the blue backdrop draw your eyes high. The Chinook arch is especially impressive; its distinctive straight-line cloud formation and warm westerly winds provide welcome respite in mid-January. Be prepared: the winds can be fierce, especially pre-Chinook, when gusts foreshadow the rise in temperatures.

Vast and open, Glenbow Ranch Provincial Park is situated along the north bank of the Bow River between Calgary and Cochrane in Rocky View County and has 40 km of interconnecting paved and gravel pathways. And you will see trains. Since 1883 trains have travelled through this piece of prairie as part of their cross-

Details

Categories: Café, Dog, Nature, Neighbourhood & Parks, Hilly, Stroller, Vistas, River, Birds

Start: Walks 1-5: Glenbow Ranch: Glenbow Road, off Highway 1A, about 4 km east of the town of Cochrane. Walk 5: Haskayne Park: off Highway 1A, 9000, 149 Street, NW.
Walks 6, 7: Cochrane Ranche, Highway 22 and 1A;
Walks 8, 9: Riverfront Park, Griffin Road and Highway 22;
Walk 9: Jim Uffelmann Park: River Avenue at Bow River

Facilities: Glenbow Ranch: Bathrooms at trailhead and along the trails. Visitor Centre on site. Haskayne Park: Bathrooms and picnic tables; Cochrane Ranche: bathrooms

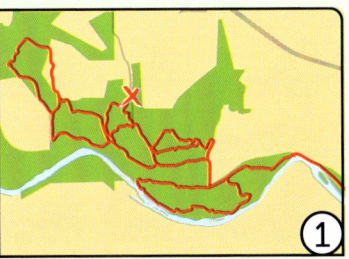

Glenbow Ranch Provincial Park and Haskayne Park

Distance & Difficulty

Walk 1: Mountain View Loop: 8.5 km (many hills, paved and gravel paths)

Walk 2: Mountain View short loop: 7 km (many hills, paved and gravel paths)

Walk 3: Bow River Loop: 11 km (hills, paved and gravel paths)

Walk 4: Yodel Loop: 4.5 km (hills, paved and gravel paths)

Walk 5: Glenbow to Haskayne Park return: 20 km return (mostly flat, paved path)

Walk 6: Cochrane Ranche Loop: 2 km (hills, gravel paths)

Walk 7: Cochrane Ranche- Big Hill Creek: 9 km (mostly flat, gravel paths)

Walk 8: Cochrane Mitford- Glenbow – Riverfront: 5 km (hills, paved and gravel paths)

Walk 9: Cochrane Riverfront - Riviera Loop: Riverfront park start: 10 km or Jim Ufflemann Park start: 6 km (hills, paved and gravel paths)

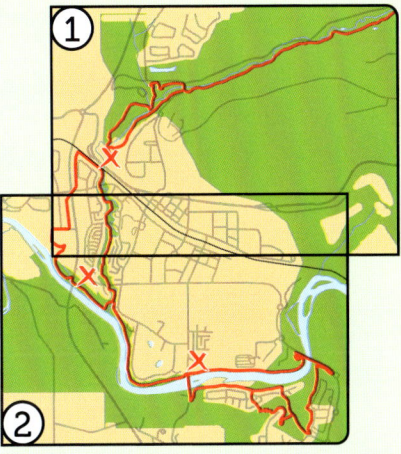

Cochrane

Highlights, Detours & Destinations

Glenbow Ranch trails are closed intermittently to allow cattle to graze the park's fescue grasslands. Animals in the park include everything from deer, elk, and moose, to badgers, coyotes, and ground squirrels, not to mention numerous species of birds and insects. During spring and fall migration migrating birds such as warblers, sparrows, and raptors frequent the park. The spring breeding season attracts Vesper Sparrow, Mountain Bluebird, and Western Meadowlark as well as riparian species like Baltimore Oriole and many swallows, sparrows, and flycatchers.

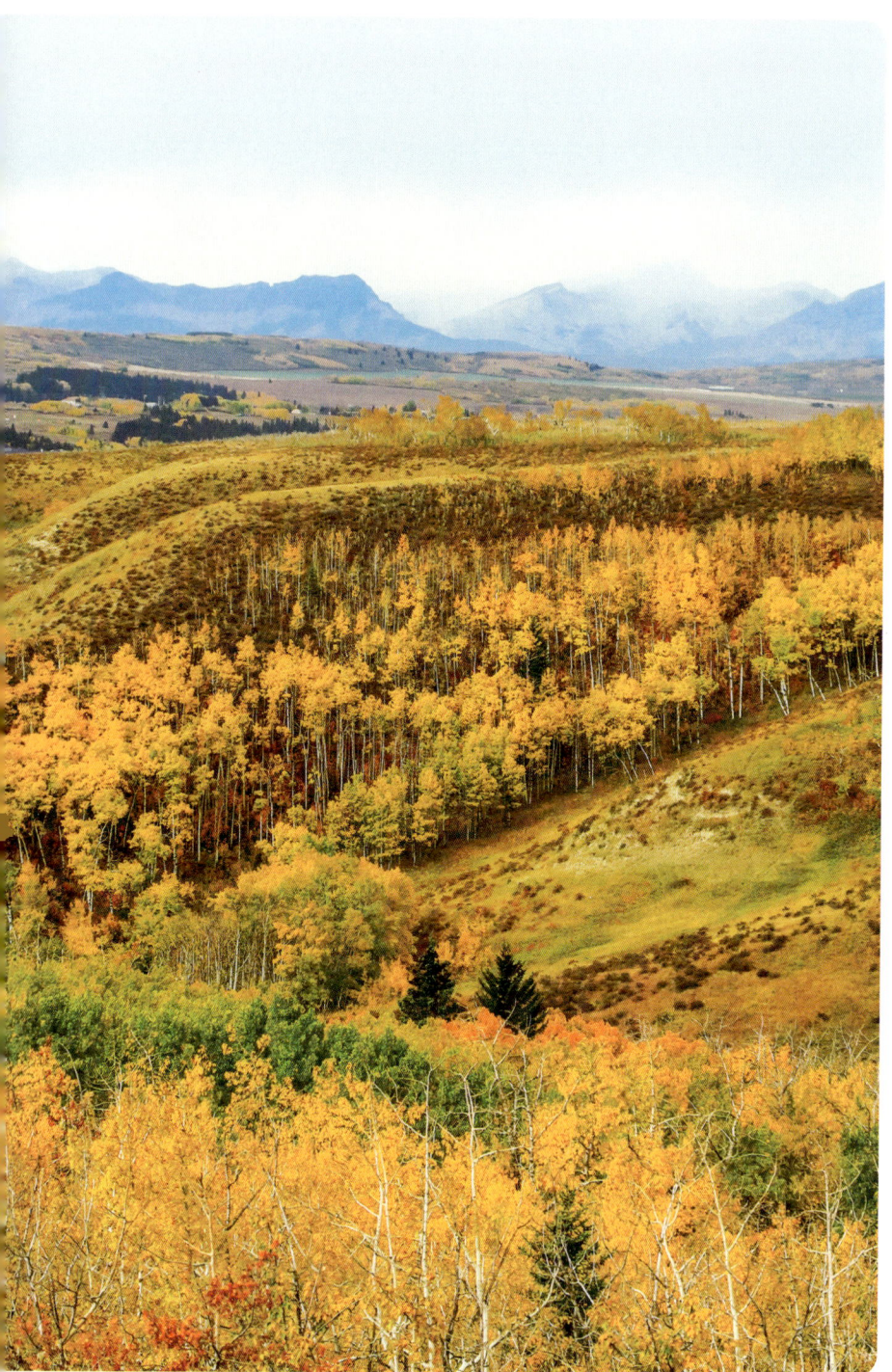
Glenbow Ranch by Sara Tehranian

Canada trek. The town of Cochrane has a multitude of pathways and wilderness trails that lead to superb views of the surrounding foothills and Rocky Mountains.

Walks one and two follow the hilly western section of Glenbow Ranch Park through rolling grasslands, past aspen-filled coulees to boundless views of the Bow River Valley and the Rockies beyond. Walks three through five follow Glenbow Ranch trails east towards the Bow River and to Haskayne Park. Interpretive signs along the route provide interesting background on Alberta's ranching heritage and geological history. Walks 6 and 7 explore the Historic Cochrane Ranche and Bighill Creek trail. These walks offer up wide-open vistas along with creek side shaded pathways that are also popular with moose and deer. Walks 8 and 9 follow ravine pathways to the Bow River, through off leash parks, past playgrounds and into surrounding neighbourhoods.

When you walk on this land just west of Calgary, you follow in the footsteps of the First Nations peoples who lived and hunted in the area up to four thousand years ago. Evidence of tipi rings, cairns, and bison kills have been found in the Cochrane area. In 1881 Glenbow Ranch was part of the Cochrane Ranche, Western Canada's first large scale cattle ranch. Here, ranchers discovered their cattle could not withstand the harsh winters as the bison had; a lesson that was critical to the success of future southern Alberta ranches.

Cattle still roam the fields at Glenbow Ranch, as the park remains a working ranch. Grazing helps maintain the health and vigour of the fescue grassland landscape. In the fall and winter, the cattle eat the tall, protein-rich grasses. Their cropping of the grasses allows sunlight to reach the roots, leading to healthy grass growth in the spring. The big open of these foothills walks calms the mind and refreshes the spirit.

Glenbow Ranch Provincial Park and Haskayne Park

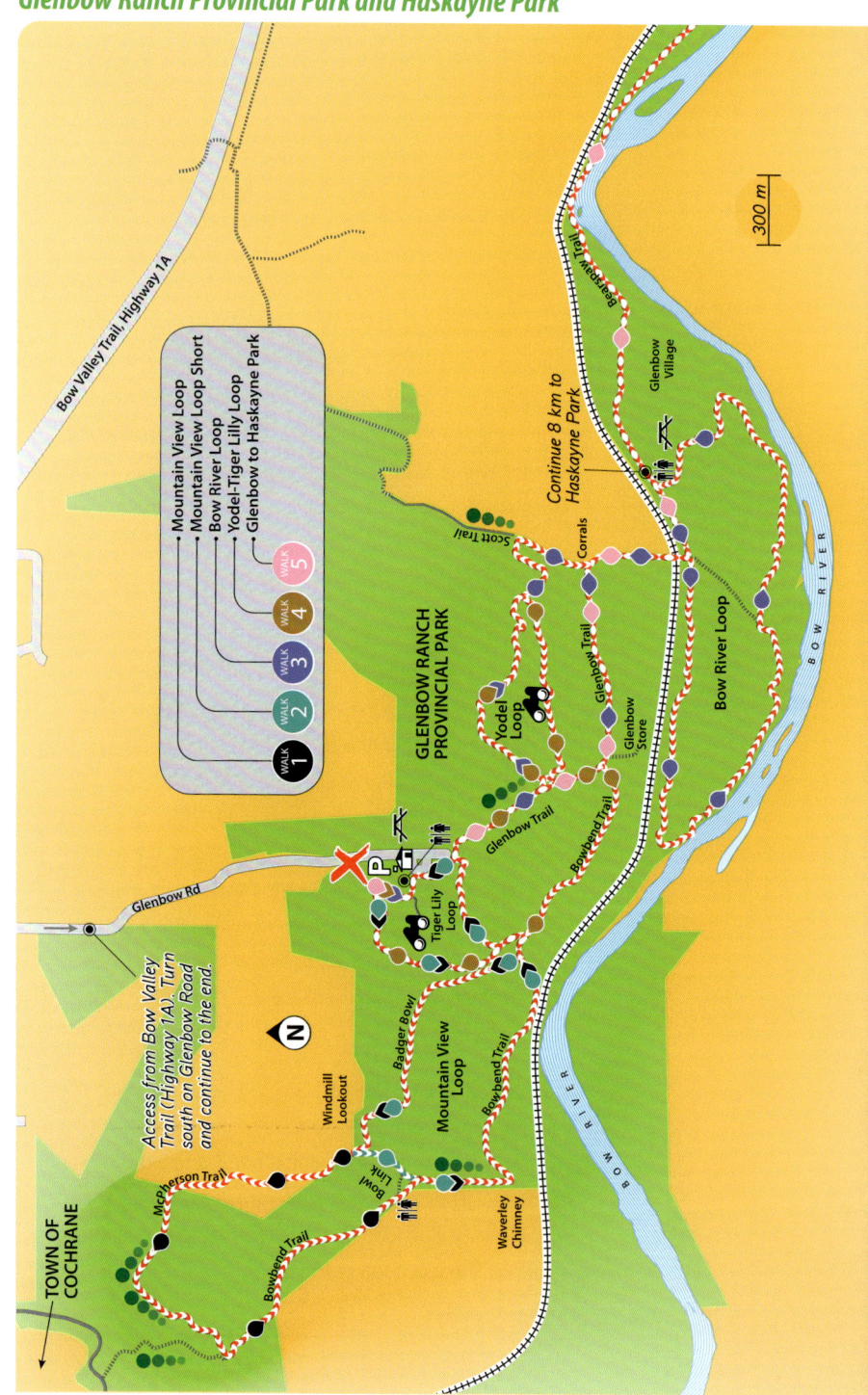

Glenbow Ranch: Sandstone and Bricks

In 1905, when Alberta officially became a province, there was an immediate demand for stone that could be used to build government buildings like the legislature, courts, and universities. Glenbow became one of many sandstone quarries around the province to supply building materials for these structures. A townsite was developed that included a store, a post office, a school, and a railway station. When building was complete, the quarry was shut down in 1912.

Shortly after a brick factory was established near the Glenbow store. Many former quarry workers were hired to make bricks. The Glenbow brick operation was strategically located between the quarry pit (source of clay) and the Bow River (water source), and quite close to the railway that provided effective transport of the finished bricks. However, the brick-making operation did not last long and was abandoned just prior to the First World War. The stone and brick productions made Glenbow very popular until 1920, when the once-vibrant community turned into a ghost town.

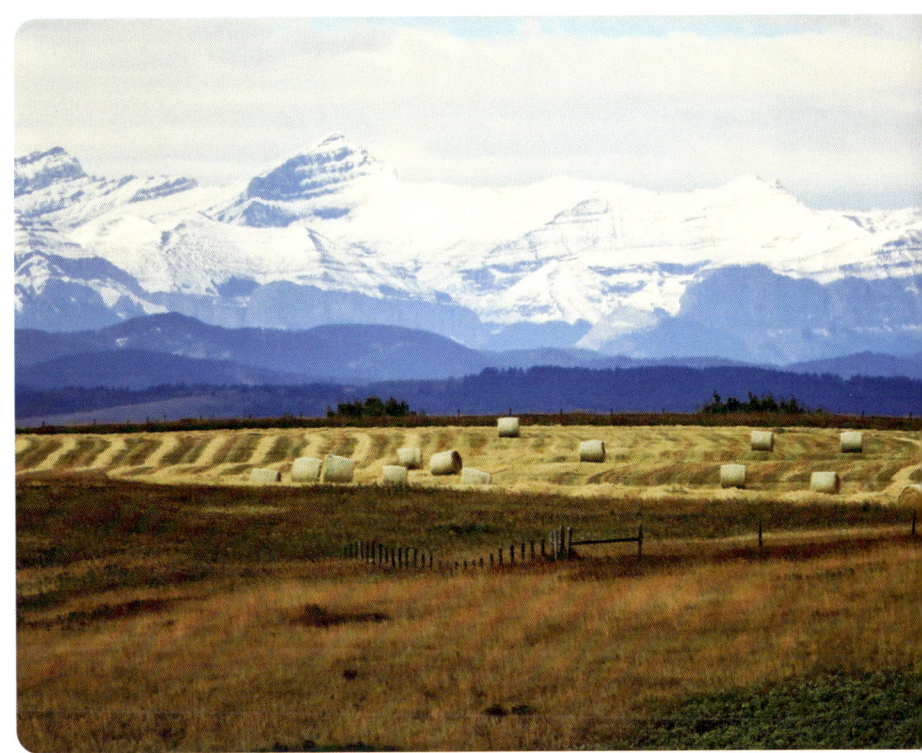

Mountain Landscape by Sara Tehranian

Cochrane

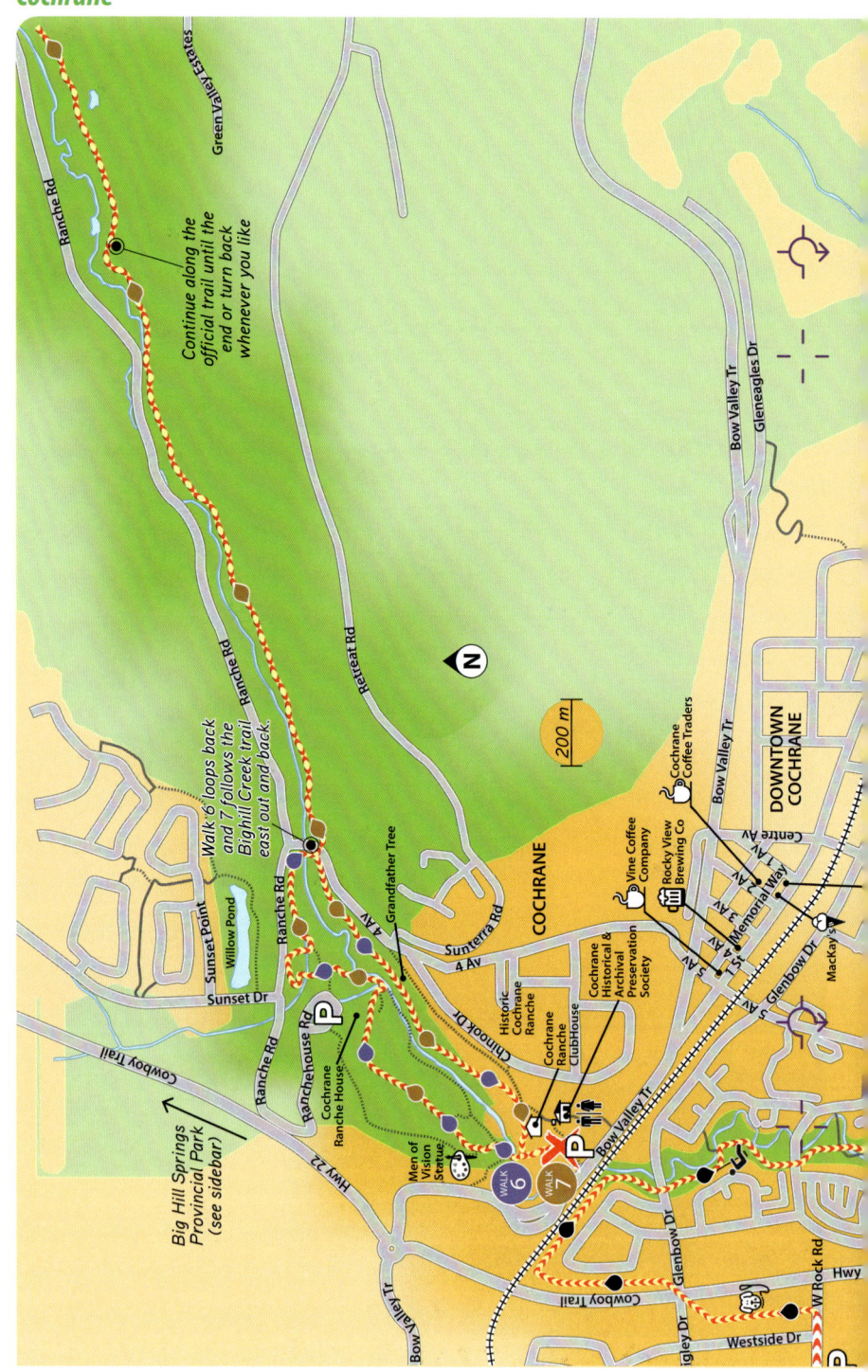

Cochrane

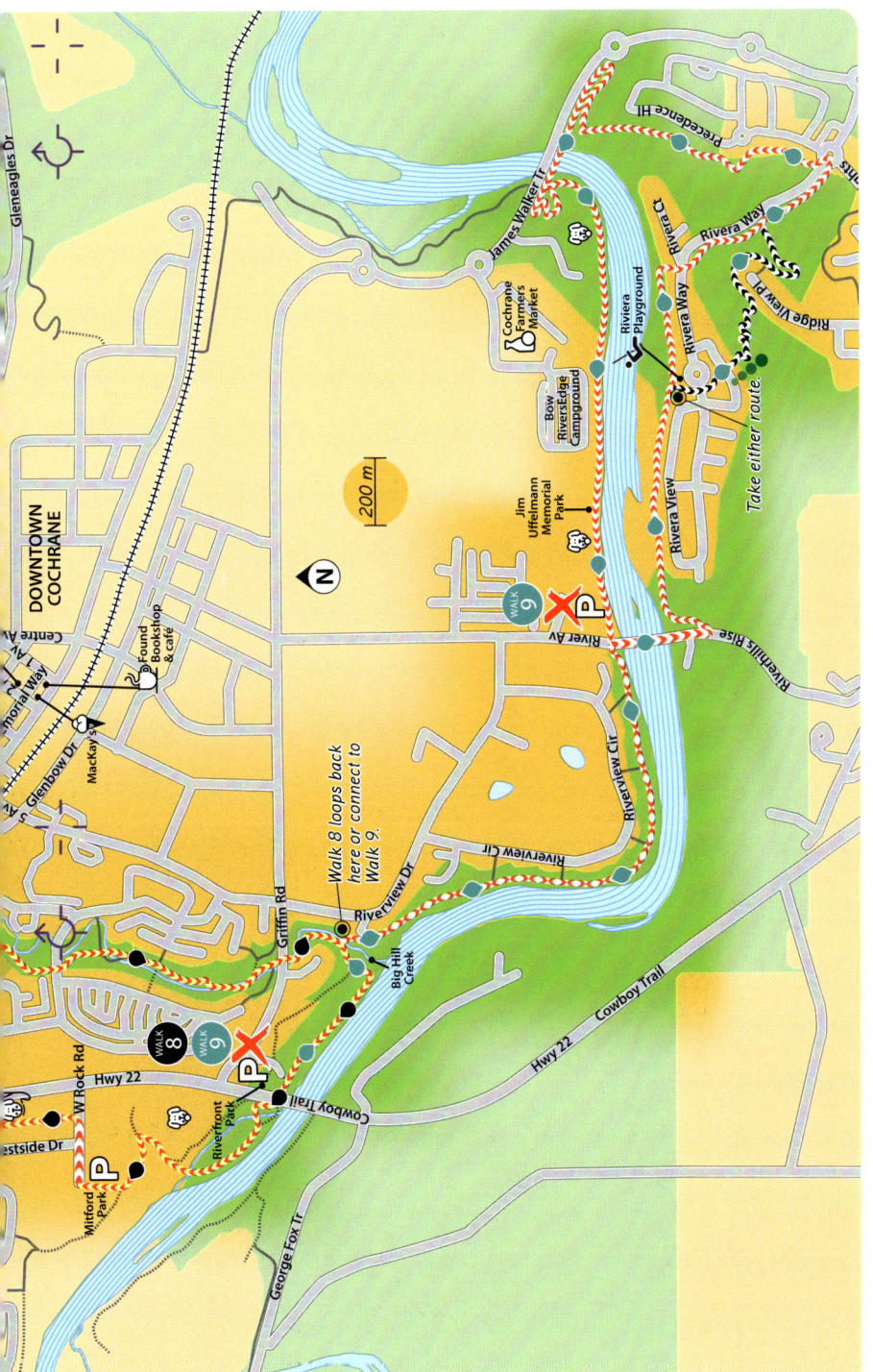

Big Hill Springs Provincial Park

Just 10 km north of Cochrane, this park is perfect for families with young children looking for a stroll and a picnic. The parks water features, waterfalls and a gentle creek, have made it an attraction for thousands of years, with the Blackfoot Plains Indians and Cree camping in the protection of the coulee and hunting bison using jumps on both sides. The 1880's brought ranchers, and again the springs were an attraction, with the first creamery in Alberta locating in 1891 on their reliable waters and lasting 30 years. Later, from 1951-1956 a fish hatchery was attracted for the same reason. The springs and water tumbling over ancient tufa formations attracted picnickers from the 1920's onward. Pack a lunch and plan a visit!

Location:
10 km north of Cochrane on Hwy. 22 & 7 km east on Hwy. 567

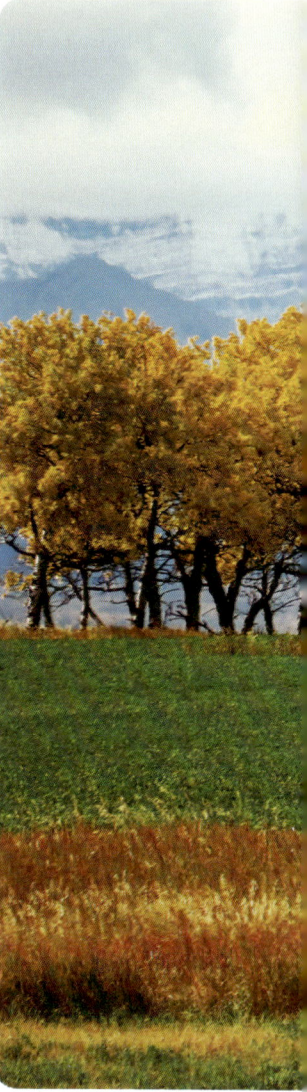

Tasty Pit Stops

If you didn't bring your lunch to the ranch, head to micro roaster Vine Coffee or to Cochrane Coffee Traders for a cuppa fresh-roasted coffee, hot and cold seasonal drinks and house-made lunches and baked goods. If it is a hot day and you feel the need for some ice cream, join the crowds at MacKay's ice cream shop. Serving house-made ice cream since 1948, MacKay's is a destination drive for Calgarians. Grab a cold one at the Rocky View Brewing microbrewery and drop in for food and drink specials daily and live music on Saturdays. And be sure to drop into Found Bookshop for a huge selection of used and new books plus a cozy café where you can settle in and curl up with that new book.

Location
Vine Coffee Company: 516, First Street West
Cochrane Coffee Traders: 114 Second Avenue West
MacKay's: 220 First Street West
Found Bookshop & café: 208, 1 Street
Rocky View Brewing: 420, 1 Street West

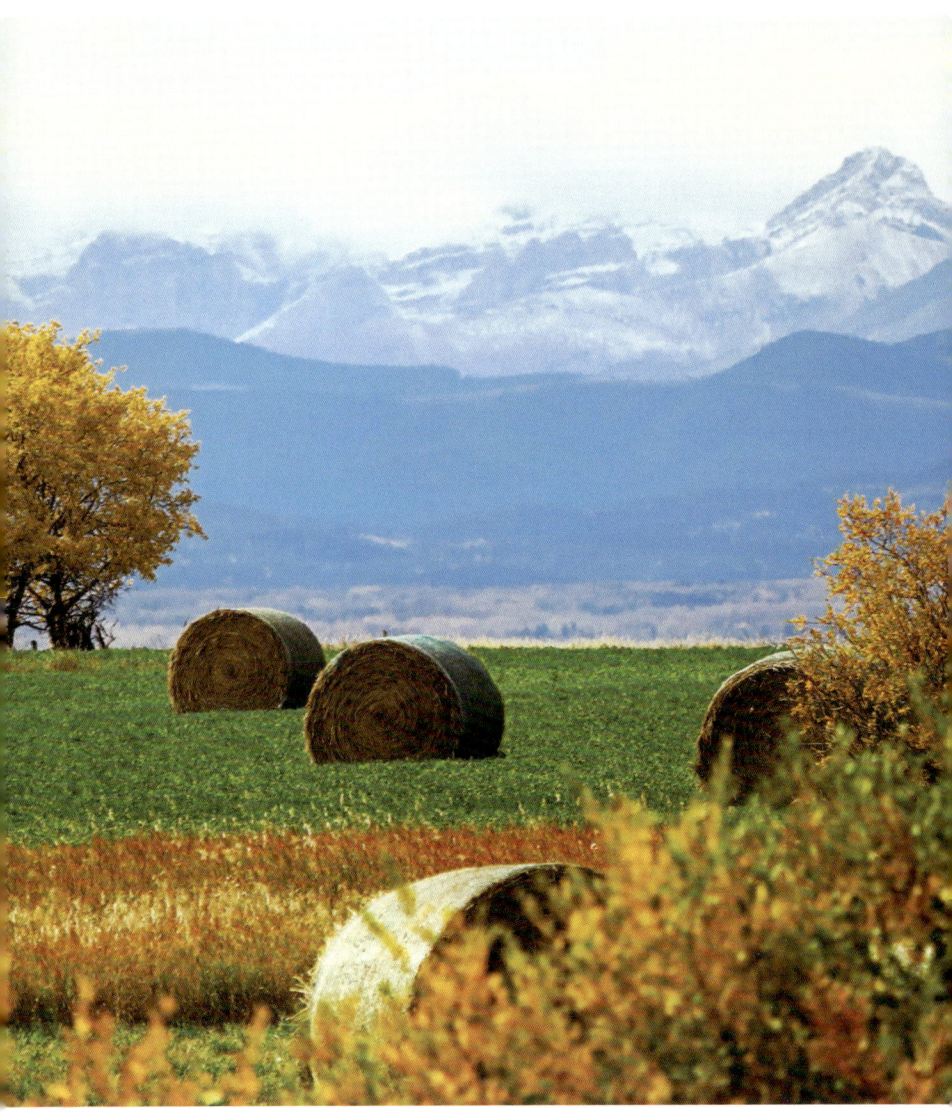

Fall Landscape by Sara Tehranian

Royal Oak Wetlands and Ravines

Walk 10

NW

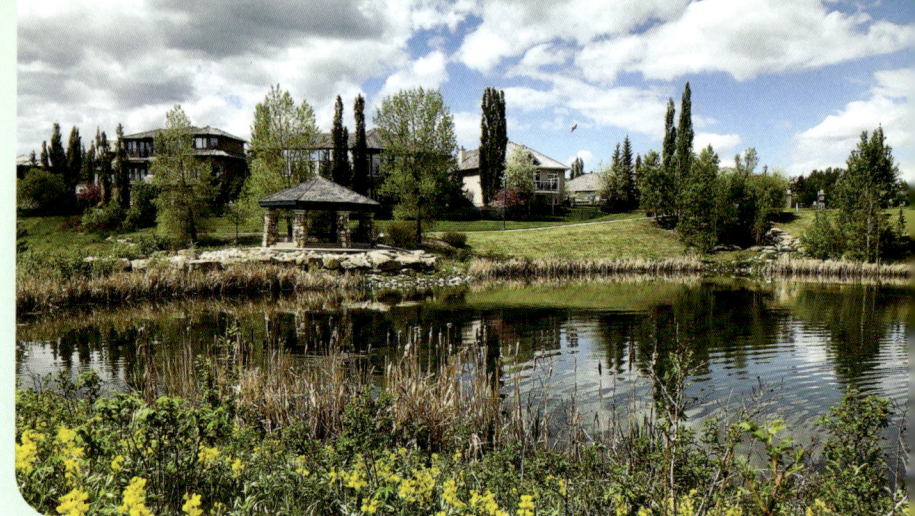

Walk at a Glance:

Wetlands, ravines and Rocky Mountain views are the highlights on this nature intensive suburban walkabout. Tucked into the ravines of northwest Calgary, Royal Oak was established in 1997. A mix of starter family homes and luxury abodes, this family friendly community has nature throughout.

Begin your walk along the paved path through the manicured Royal Oak Pointe Park. A quick zig zag on quiet side streets leads to forested single-track trail in a wild ravine park. Connect to the paved pathway network followed by neighbourhood streets and cut through pathways. A short climb leads to expansive Rocky Mountain views from the green space that parallels Stoney Trail. Continue along the route, on earthy pathways or along the paved path, part of the 150 km

Details

Categories: LRT, Dog, Nature, Neighbourhood & Parks, Vistas, Birds

Start: Royal Oak Point near Royal Oak Way

LRT: Tuscany Station

Facilities: None

Distance & Difficulty

6 km (paved paths, sidewalks and rolling hills)

Highlights, Detours & Destinations

Birdlife is abundant in the wetlands. Check out www.naturecalgary.com to discover Calgary's best and most unique birding hotspots. Maps and bird checklists in English, Spanish, Hindi, French

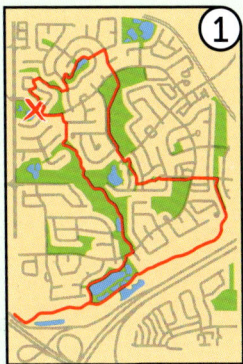

Mattamy Greenway that circumnavigates Calgary, or connect to Walk 11 and cross over Stoney Trail on the pedestrian overpass and explore the community of Arbour Lake. Paved pathways lead to Crowfoot Crossing where you can grab some picnic supplies.

Next up on Walk 10, the Royal Oak wetlands. Listen for the birdlife, especially the distinctive "Conk-la-ree" call of the red-winged blackbirds, as you close in. Keep watch for long necked Great Blue Herons standing incredibly still waiting for their prey to swim by. Circle the ponds before connecting to Elina Ravine followed by the forested single-track trails of Mitra Natural Ravine Park. Climb to the top of the ravine and navigate past homes and along pathways back to your starting point.

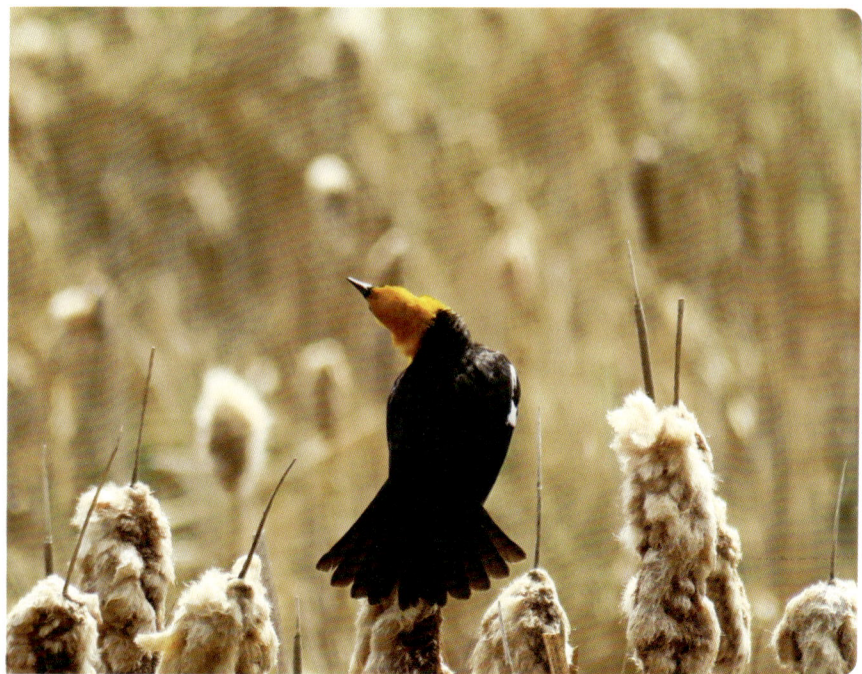

Yellow-headed blackbird by Sara Tehranian

Wetlands at work

Marshes, ponds, swamps, fens and bogs- these are the five types of Alberta wetlands. You'll know what to call a wetland by assessing its source of water, presence of peat and the types of vegetation in and around the water. In Royal Oak the wetlands are ponds, and like giant sponges they soak up rain and snowmelt and slowly release the water in the dry season. A variety of soils and microorganisms help to filter the ponds' water of toxins making it safer for animals and humans to drink. The grasses, shrubs and trees provide food and shelter and when you get up close you may see fish and frogs, muskrats and beavers, paddling ducks and brightly coloured migratory birds.

As you walk past the Royal Oak wetlands, slow the pace and keep an ear out for the boreal chorus frog— Alberta's smallest frog, measuring a mere 2–4 cm. It is more often heard than seen, but if you are lucky enough to catch a glimpse, you'll be able to identify it by looking for the three dark stripes or lines of broken spots on its back and a white upper lip. The male mating call is quite loud, so listen for the sound of a thumbnail being dragged over the teeth of a stiff plastic comb to know the frog is close by. Widely distributed across the province around all bodies of water, the hardy amphibian overwinters by burrowing underground before emerging in the spring. The wood frog overwinters on land under leaf litter and freezes completely solid—frozen frog! How do they survive the freeze-thaw cycle? Their cells flood with glucose to reduce dehydration and damage, an adaptation that keeps them alive at -35! Measuring up to six centimetres and brownish with dark spots, it often has two light-coloured dorsal stripes and sometimes a whitish vertebral stripe. Listen for high-pitched snores and grunts and you'll know the male is floating nearby. Outside of the breeding season this frog spends most of its time on land throughout Alberta and into the far north. In fact, the wood frog is the only amphibian to be found inside the Arctic Circle.

Royal Oak Wetlands and Ravines

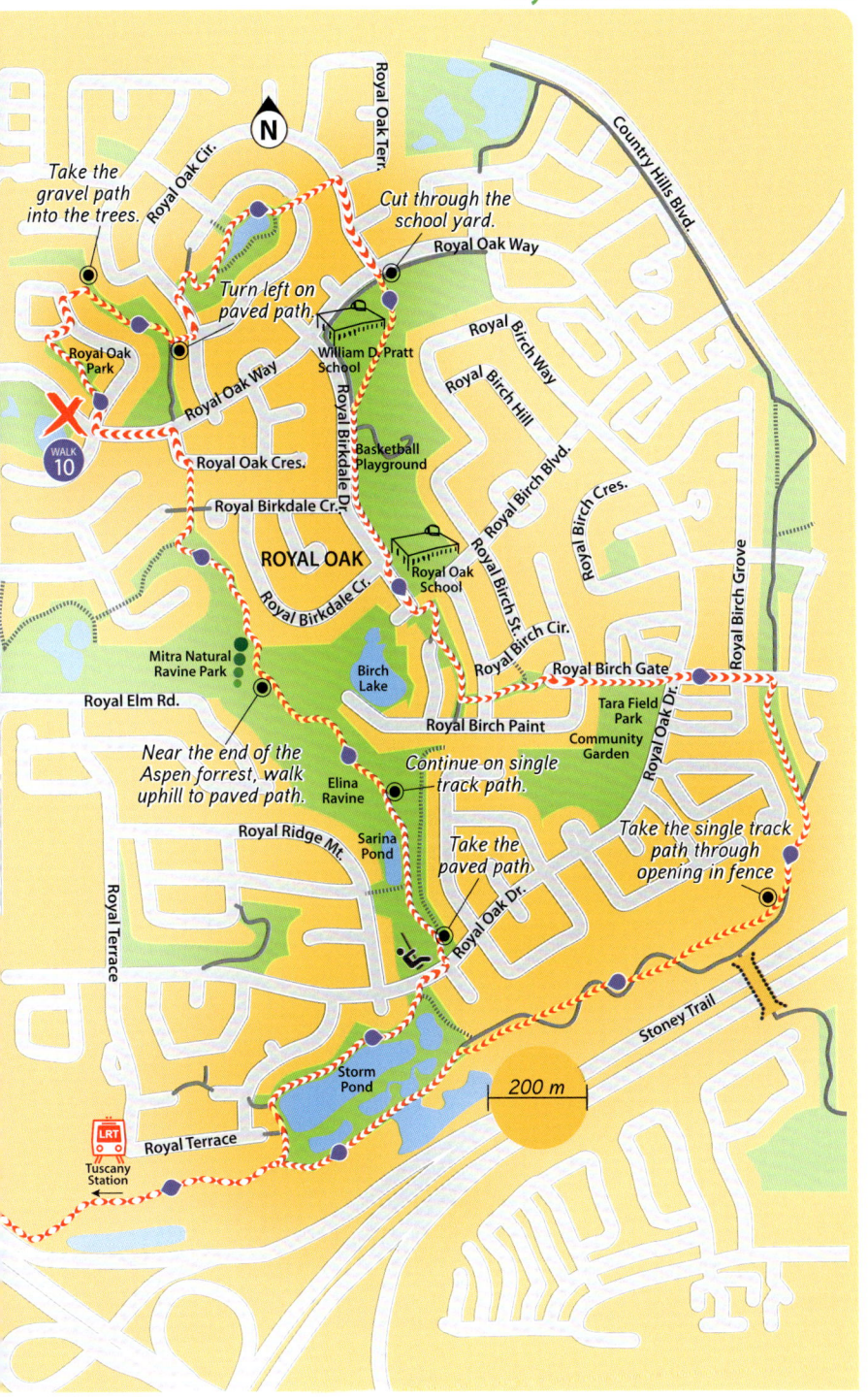

Twelve-Mile Coulee and Arbour Lake, Royal Oak, Scenic Acres

Walks 11 and 12

NW

Walks at a Glance:

Wild walkabouts tucked into suburban neighbourhoods are always a pleasant surprise. Tuscany's Twelve Mile Coulee Park got its name in the early days because it is approximately 12 miles (19 km) from Fort Calgary and was a convenient mileage marker on the stagecoach run from the Fort Calgary main post office to the mission church at Morleyville, a missionary outpost.

The Metis used the term coulée, which means "small valley" or "gully," to describe the type of landscape in the park. It comes from the French verb couler, meaning "to flow," which is appropriate since the spring snowmelt leads to a rise in creek water level.

Details

Categories: LRT, Café, Dog, Nature, Neighbourhood & Parks, Hilly, Vistas, Birds

Start: Walk 11: Crowfoot Crossing, Crowfoot Crescent and Crowfoot Way; Walk 12: Official parking lot off Tuscany Boulevard, just north of Scenic Acres Link.

LRT: Crowfoot or Tuscany Stations

Facilities: Crowfoot Crossing has all services.

Distance & Difficulty

Walk 11: Arbour lake-Royal Oak-Scenic Acres-Twelve Mile Coulee: 8 km (hills, sidewalks, paved paths and single-track trails)

Walk 12: Twelve Mile Coulee-Tuscany: 5.5 km, from Tuscany LRT: 8.5 km (hills, single-track trails and paved paths)

Highlights, Detours & Destinations

Dogs love Twelve-Mile Coulee off leash. Note that the coulee creeks are narrow and small however the current can be strong in the spring and the water levels can be high enough to soak your feet, well into the fall. Saskatoons are abundant in mid-summer. Nearby eats and cafés: Good Earth Café in Crowfoot Crossing, Cadence Café (description in Walk 19), Angel's Drive In and Calgary Farmer's Market (description in Walk 13)

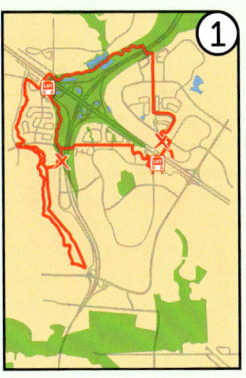

Walk 11 begins in Arbour Lake near the Crowfoot LRT Station. Navigate some busier roads past the Crowfoot Crossing Shopping Centre before connecting to Arbour Lake side streets and the paved pathway that continues over Stoney Trail to the Mattamy Greenway, a 150 km pathway network that circumnavigates Calgary. Soak up big Rocky Mountain views as you descend into the Royal Oak wetlands. Pass by the Tuscany LRT Station and briefly walk Tuscany side streets before leaving the pavement and continuing along single track creekside ravine trails that lead into Twelve Mile Coulee and connect to Walk 12.

Walk 11 climbs out of the coulee and loops back over Stoney Trail, along an off leash cut line while Walk 12 continues the full length of Twelve Mile Coulee where a pups run free, and walkers choose between few trail options. You can walk above the creek, on the slope-side trail, or along the coulee bottom. Adventurous creek-hoppers will enjoy using their creative navigating skills since the trail diverges in many areas and, depending on how much water is in the creek, you may have to backtrack and choose a higher route. This is the kind of exploring that kids and dogs love!

Those who choose to stay high and dry will walk through shrubs of willows, red-osier dogwoods, and American silverberry, as well as stands of trembling aspen, balsam poplar, and white spruce while on the north-facing slopes. The south-facing slopes are drier and host native prairie plants: saskatoon shrubs, rough fescue, Perry oat grass, and spear grasses thrive here. If you're a rockhound, check out the large, bedrock, sandstone outcroppings at the south end of the park. This is Calgary's best and most accessible example of the Porcupine Hills Formation that underlies the entire city.

You can easily adjust your walk length by taking any one of the many trails that climb out of the coulee, all of them unmarked but well used. At the end of the coulee, near Nose Hill Drive, climb to the community of Tuscany and to views of the Rocky Mountains, Canada Olympic Park, and the downtown core. Continue along the paved path at the top of the coulee or pick a trail and descend back into the wilderness. Creek-hop back to your starting point.

Twelve-Mile Coulee and Arbour Lake, Royal Oak, Scenic Acres

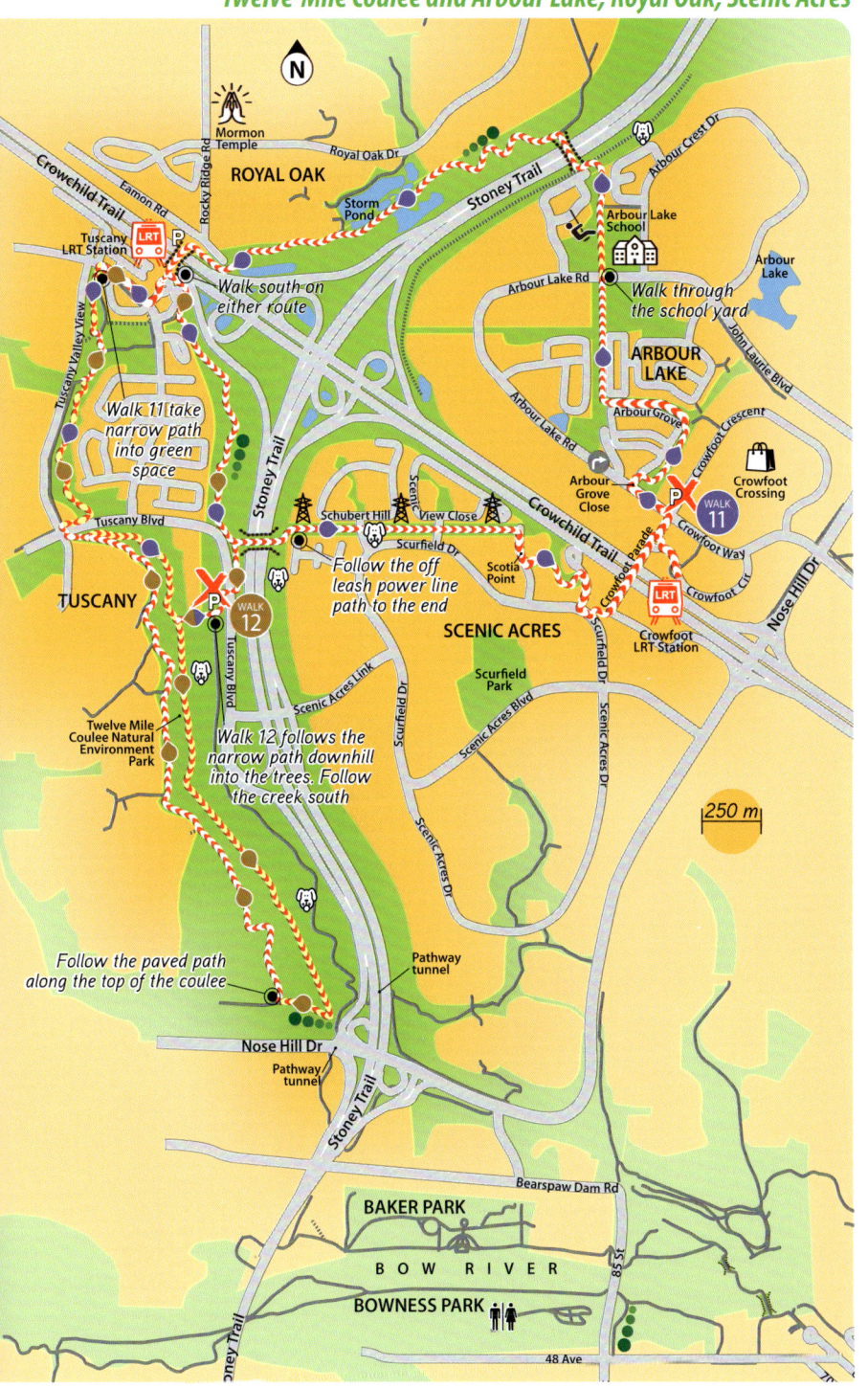

Urban foraging: Saskatoons

Pies, salads, soups, sides and marinades. Hot and cold drinks and even medicine. Nutritious and delicious rewards await all around Calgary, if you know where to look. My favourite foraging is for Saskatoon berries in August. Indigenous people used the berry to make pemmican, which is preserved dried meat, and today, the berry is used to make many delicious foods including pies and jams and marinades. They are abundant on the slopes and ravines throughout Calgary.

- This shrub's name comes from its Cree name "mis-ask-quah-toomina" which was shortened to "Saskatoon" by early settlers.
- This shrub goes by many common names including serviceberry, Indian pear and juneberry.
- After a fire, the Saskatoon shrub may lose its branches, leaves and flowers but the roots will typically survive if the soil is moist. It has been observed there is even more Saskatoon growth after a fire.
- Indigenous usage of the Saskatoon included food, arrow shafts and medicine for liver trouble and intestinal issues.

Plan your saskatoon foraging walk in August at Twelve Mile Coulee, Bowmont Park, Nose Hill Park, Edworthy Park, Sandy Beach, Britannia Slopes, or Fish Creek Park. More info about foraging can be found here: www.northernbushcraft.com

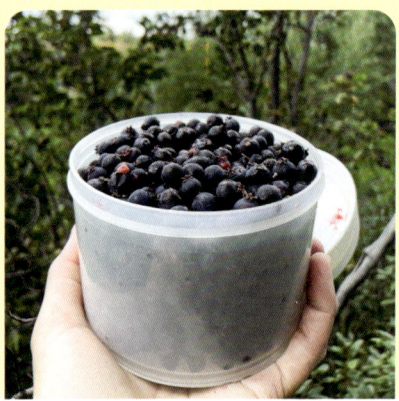
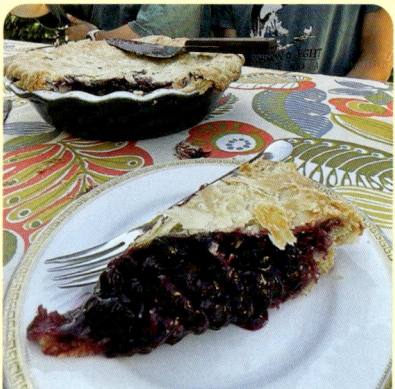

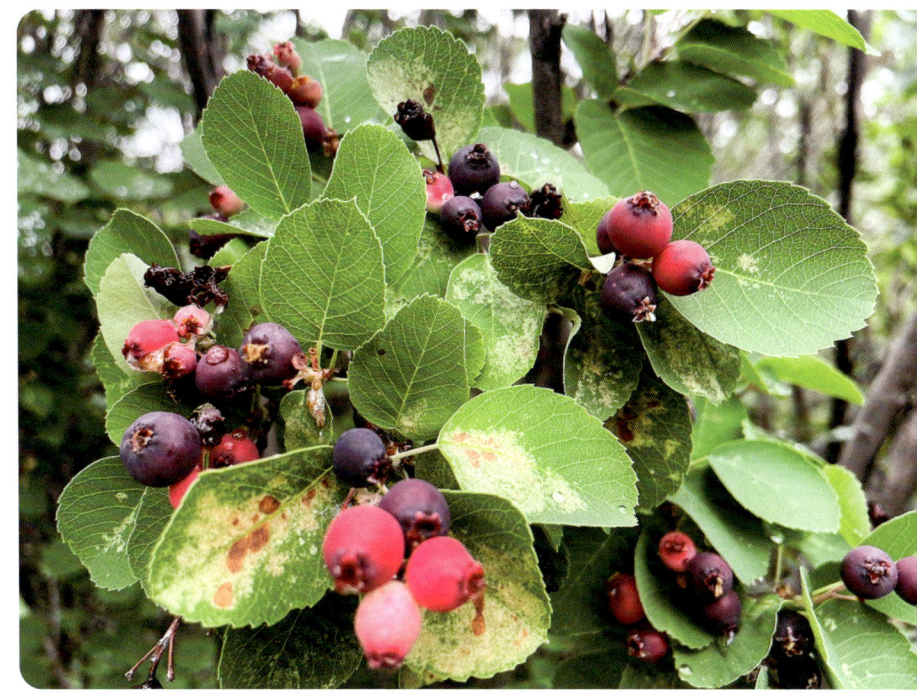

Forager's Saskatoon Pie

It is so rewarding to go for a foraging walk and create this delicious pie. This recipe, adapted from the wonderful Duchess Bake Shop cookbook, is perfection. I often mix with blueberries if I don't have enough saskatoons and the saskatoon flavour still takes centre stage. Serve with vanilla ice cream or whipped cream for the big finish!

Assembly
1 blind baked pie shell
1 ball of pastry for the top of the pie
Whipping cream or ice cream for topping (optional)

Filling
880 g (6 cups)	fresh or frozen saskatoons (or a mix of blueberries and saskatoons)
3 Tbsp	water
3 Tbsp	lemon juice
200 g (1 cup)	sugar
55 g (1/3 cup)	all-purpose flour
¼ tsp	ground nutmeg
1 Tbsp	cornstarch

Procedure
- To make the filling, in a saucepan, combine the saskatoons, water, lemon juice, and sugar. Cook over medium heat until the sugar dissolves and the mixture begins to simmer. Stir in the remaining ingredients and continue to cook until mixture thickens.

- Fill the shell to the rim with saskatoon filling and cover with pastry.

- Bake the pie for 45-50 minutes, until the top is golden brown and the filling is bubbling. Serve the pie warm or let is cool.

Storage
This pie will keep at room temperature for up to three days (if it last that long!)

Bowness Park, Douglas Fir Trail, Greenwood, Farmer's Market, Baker Park

Walks 13 and 14

NW

Bowness Lagoon

Walks at a Glance:

Bowness Park, one of Calgary's most popular outdoor areas for family and friends to congregate, is a hive of activity in the summer picnic season so be prepared for a sensory explosion; bonfires, the smell of burgers, and the infectious energy of friends and families having fun. In the winter, bring your skates (or rent them at the convenient rental hut) and glide along the Bowness Lagoon or skating oval, a frozen outdoor maze. The lagoons are equipped with frequent fire pits so you can warm up your hands. Don't forget to bring a Thermos of hot chocolate!

Walk 13 begins with a mix of paved paths and sidewalks, before crossing the Bow River into Bowmont Natural Environment Park. Your visit to Bowmont Park is brief, but if you like the looks of it you can switch to the Walk 17, the Bowmont Park West route, and continue to

Details

Categories: Café, Dog, Nature, Neighbourhood & Parks, Hilly, Stroller, Historic, Vistas, River, Birds

Start: Walks 13 and 14: Bowness Park, 8900, 48 Avenue NW or Baker Park, 9333 Scenic Bow Road NW

Facilities: Bowness Park: bathrooms, café, restaurant, ice skating on lagoon, ice-skate rentals, fire pits, picnic areas, playgrounds, spray park, wading pool. Baker Park: bathrooms, disk golf course. Calgary Farmer's Market: Open Wednesday-Sunday year round

Distance & Difficulty

Walk 13: Bowness Park, Baker Park, Douglas Fir Trail: 7.5 km (paved paths, optional stairs)

Walk 14: Romeo & Juliet - Greenwood - Farmer's Market - Bowness: 7.5 km (hills, paved paths, sidewalks, and stairs)

Alternate route: rolling single track dirt paths on the Romeo and Juliet trail

Highlights, Detours & Destinations

Plan to attend the 3-day Tour de Bowness (www.tourdebowness.com) bike race and street festival that happens on the August long weekend every year. The holiday Monday is the street festival and the fast-paced criterium bike race through the streets of Bowness. It is a blast to get up close to these high-level cyclists that come from around Alberta. Bowness Park is a hive of activity year-round: Ice skating on the Bowness lagoons or the skate track, crokicurl, and skate rentals and in the summer, there is a wading pool, train for kids, and boat rentals.

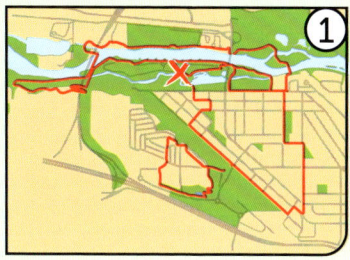

Waterfall Valley. Or stay on route and continue to Baker Park, the little park across the river from Bowness Park. Popular for its disk golf course, it is a great place for listening to gaggling gossiping geese in the fall. Listen for the sounds of cocktail-party chatter and then look up to see Canada geese practicing their V formation. Cross the Bow River on the Stoney Trail pedestrian bridge and enter the Wood's Douglas Fir Tree Sanctuary, one of the few extant stands of the inland variety of Rocky Mountain Douglas fir trees remaining in Alberta. Climb above the Bow River to Valley Ridge before looping back on the paved pathway. If you'd like more wilderness walking, add on the Romeo and Juliet wilderness trail that travels through more Douglas fir forest that is tucked between Bowness and Greenwood. Connect to Walk 14 at a set of stairs that leads to Greenwood Mobile Home Park and the Calgary Farmer's Market, open Wednesday through Sunday. Stop for a coffee, ice cream or a full meal, fill your backpack with local produce, and return to explore the community of Bowness as you navigate side streets, chit-chatting with friendly "Bownesians" (Bow-NEE-zhins), before connecting to the Bow River Pathway the connects back to the park.

Tasty Pit Stops

The Calgary Farmer's Market is the perfect mid-walk pit stop on Wednesday through Sundays. Choose your tasty treat from vendors offering all types of prepared foods as well as ice cream, baked goods, coffee and fresh produce, there is something for everyone. Angel's Drive In is a fun stop for breakfast, lunch, or dinner. Offering a multitude of burgers, milkshakes, fruit shakes, and the classic Breyer's ice-cream cones, this is a perfect stop if you did not have time to make a picnic before leaving home. Or stop by the little café in Bowness Park that operated by the Seasons of Bowness restaurant for a freshly baked cookie and a drink.

Location
Angel's Drive In: 8603, 47 Avenue NW
Calgary Farmer's Market: 25 Greenbriar Drive NW. Open Wednesday- Sunday year-round.
Bowness Park: Café by Seasons of Bowness, Bowness Park. Hours vary based on the weather.

Wood's Douglas Fir Tree Sanctuary

The inland variety of the Rocky Mountain Douglas fir, also known as the Blue Douglas fir, can be found only sporadically throughout Alberta's mountain valleys and foothills. This stand of trees represents one of the last and best collections of this species in Alberta since fires and lumbering have virtually eliminated this variety of Douglas fir trees from the province. The inland variety of the Rocky Mountain Douglas fir is a majestic, imposing tree; the largest species of tree in Alberta, it can measure over 1 metre in diameter and rise to 45 metres tall. With a potential lifespan of up to 400 years, the Rocky Mountain Douglas fir tree is also one of the most enduring tree species in Alberta. Some trees in the sanctuary are several centuries old. Situated close to the river valley and in the transitional zone between parkland and the open prairie, the area of the present-day sanctuary was in previous centuries used by Indigenous peoples to hunt and collect medicines and other natural products. The Rocky Mountain Douglas fir trees in the area possessed a particularly elastic quality and were used by Natives to create bows. This region was known as man-a-cha-pan - loosely translated as "the place where they go for bows" - and provided the Bow River with its name. The continuing preservation of the inland variety of the Rocky Mountain Douglas fir provides a vital reservoir of seeds and gene pools of a species of flora largely decimated in Alberta.

Bowness Park, Douglas Fir Trail, Greenwood, Farmer's Market, Baker Park

BOWNESS PARK, DOUGLAS FIR TRAIL, GREENWOOD, FARMER'S MARKET, BAKER PARK

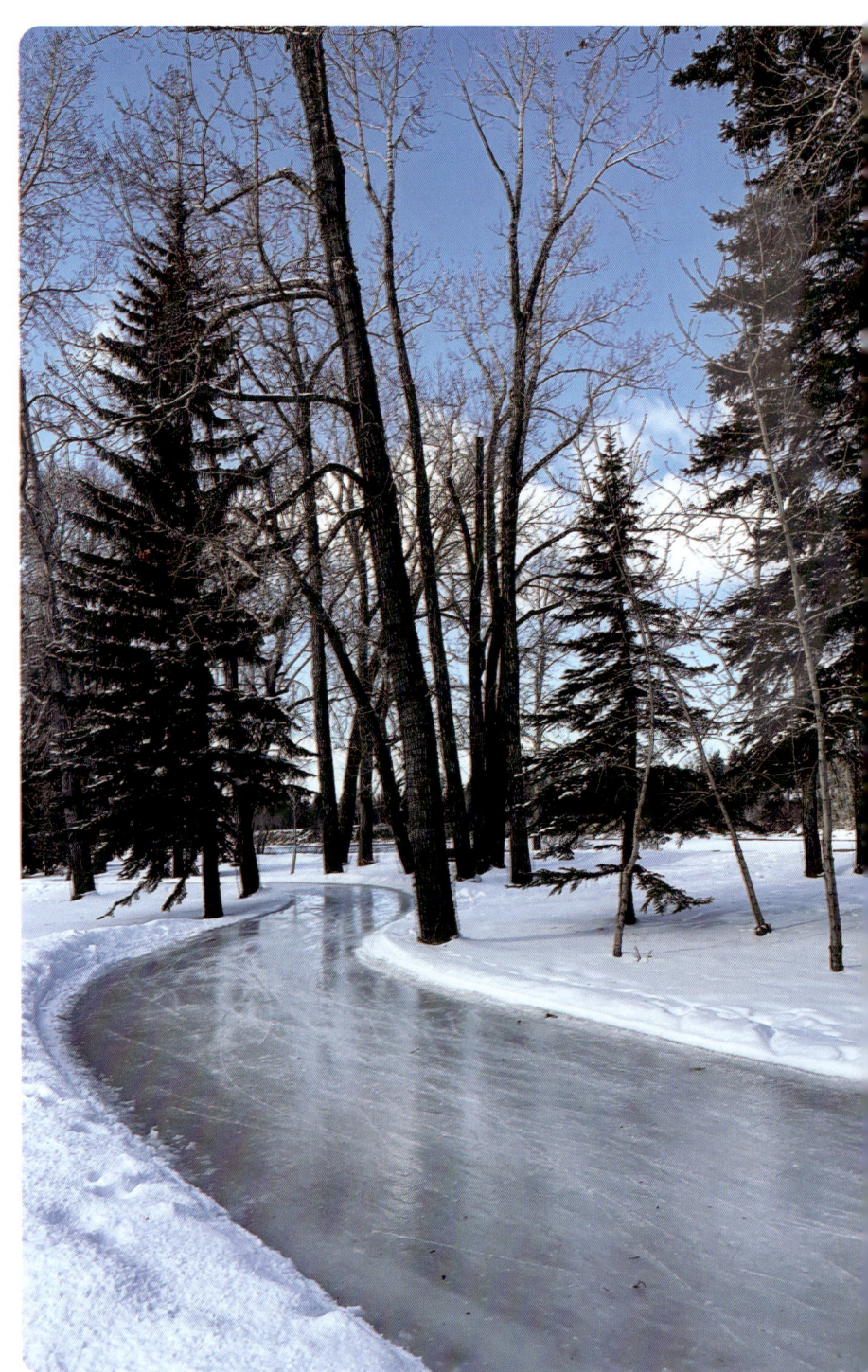

Historic Streetcars to Bowness Park

In a time when automobiles were rare, Bowness Park had a streetcar that took Calgarians from the city to the town of Bowness (Bowness did not become a community in the city of Calgary until 1963). The park became a destination in the early 1920s and 1930s, even before it had many services. Thousands would visit the park on a warm summer weekend. The streetcar that extended to Bowness was the brainchild of landowner John Hextall, an Englishman turned owner of the Bowness Ranche. He donated the two islands that are Bowness Park to the City of Calgary in 1911 in a deal that ensured streetcar service to his new subdivision for the high-end Bowness Estates. The streetcar service was maintained from 1913 to 1950.

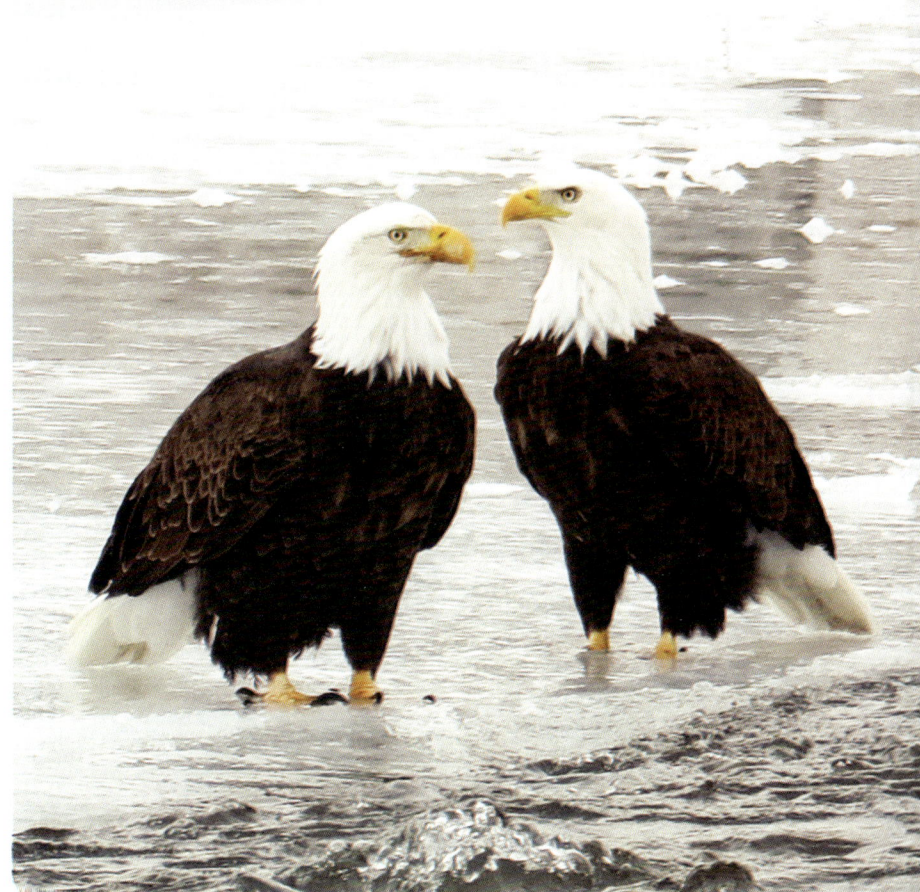

Bald Eagles, Bowness Park by Sara Tehranian

Valley Ridge Ravines and Bearspaw Dam Trail

Walks 15 and 16

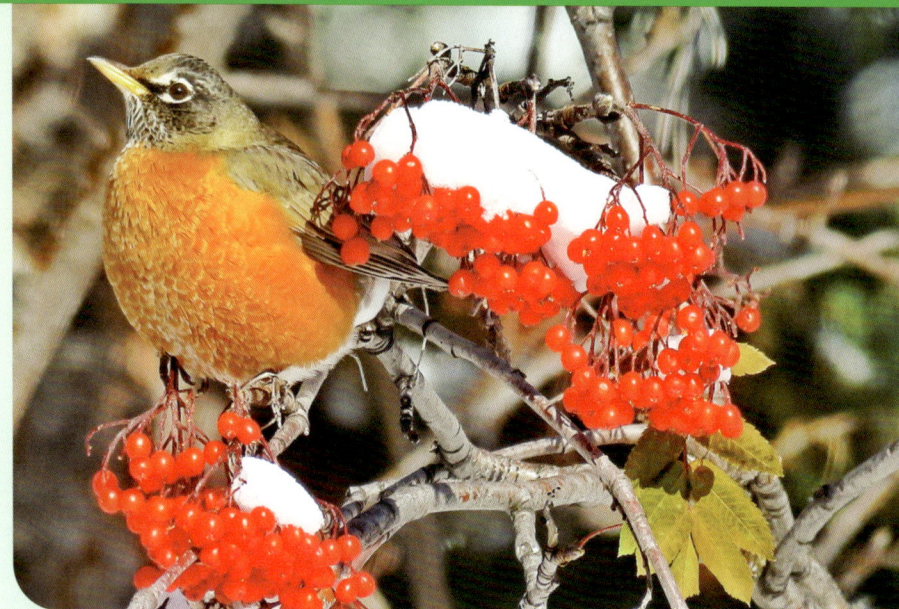

Robin by Sara Tehranian

Walks at a Glance:

Wild and remote yet at the edge of the suburb of Valley Ridge, these rolling wilderness walks follow earthy single-track trails through the forest. Connect the two walks and get the best of all worlds: Bow River views, creek side paths, peaceful climbs to big views and homes, gardens, and flowering fruit trees.

Walk 15 starts above the Bow River where it dips and climbs along a forested path to the Bearspaw Dam, offering intermittent river views and the sense of having left the city behind. You can continue beyond the mapped route along the cut-line trail but be advised that the descent to the river is steep and there are no

Details

Categories: Dog, Nature, Neighbourhood & Parks, Hilly, River, Birds

Start: The end of Valley Woods Landing at Valley Woods Place NW

Distance & Difficulty

Walk 15: Bearspaw Dam Trail: 3.5 km (rolling wilderness path)

Walk 16: Valley Ridge Ravines: 3.5 km (steep hills, single track trails and paved paths)

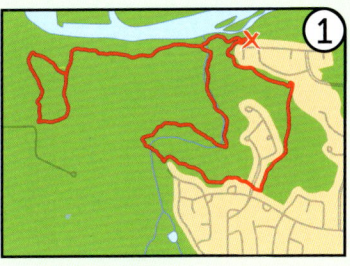

Highlights, Detours & Destinations

The ravine trails on Walk 16 have some steep hill climbs and creek crossings on bridges made of planks. Combine the two routes for hilly hiking training. Drop by the Calgary's Farmer's Market (see Walk 13) on Wednesday- Sunday year-round to grab picnic supplies or relax with a drink or an ice cream post walk.

trespassing signs. Walk 15 circles back and connects to Walk 16 where the trail becomes more challenging with some steep hills. Climb from dense forest to wide open wildflower meadows followed by aspen forest paths. Descend steep slopes before climbing to the paved pathway network that weaves through Valley Ridge. Leave the paved paths and walk behind homes on gravel paths while checking out beautiful gardens and chatting with a local or two, as I always do. A zig and a zag have you crossing neighbourhood streets to more ravine pathways, flowering fruit trees in the springtime and to a forested paved pathway descent back to your starting point.

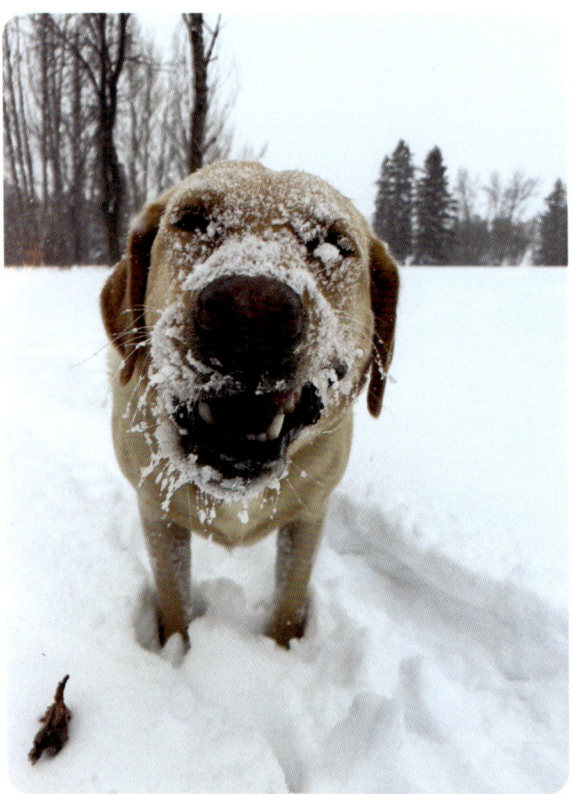

Hilly Hiking Techniques

Practice the "mountaineer" or "rest" step when climbing stairs or hills. Take a step uphill, straighten the stepping leg by letting your heel come back to the ground and then take your next uphill step. If the hill is steep you may want to count one second in between steps. This endurance technique lets you relax your calf muscles and breathe easy, so you have lots of energy for the long haul. The endurance step is a technique used by long-haul hikers. While a slow and consistent pace is the key to endurance, a faster pace will help you build muscle strength and improve your anaerobic threshold. There is a benefit to the muscle burn you feel while hiking uphill. The strong muscles that result from the "burn" help support you on steep slope descents, or when you need a quick burst of energy.

Valley Ridge Ravines and Bearspaw Dam Trail

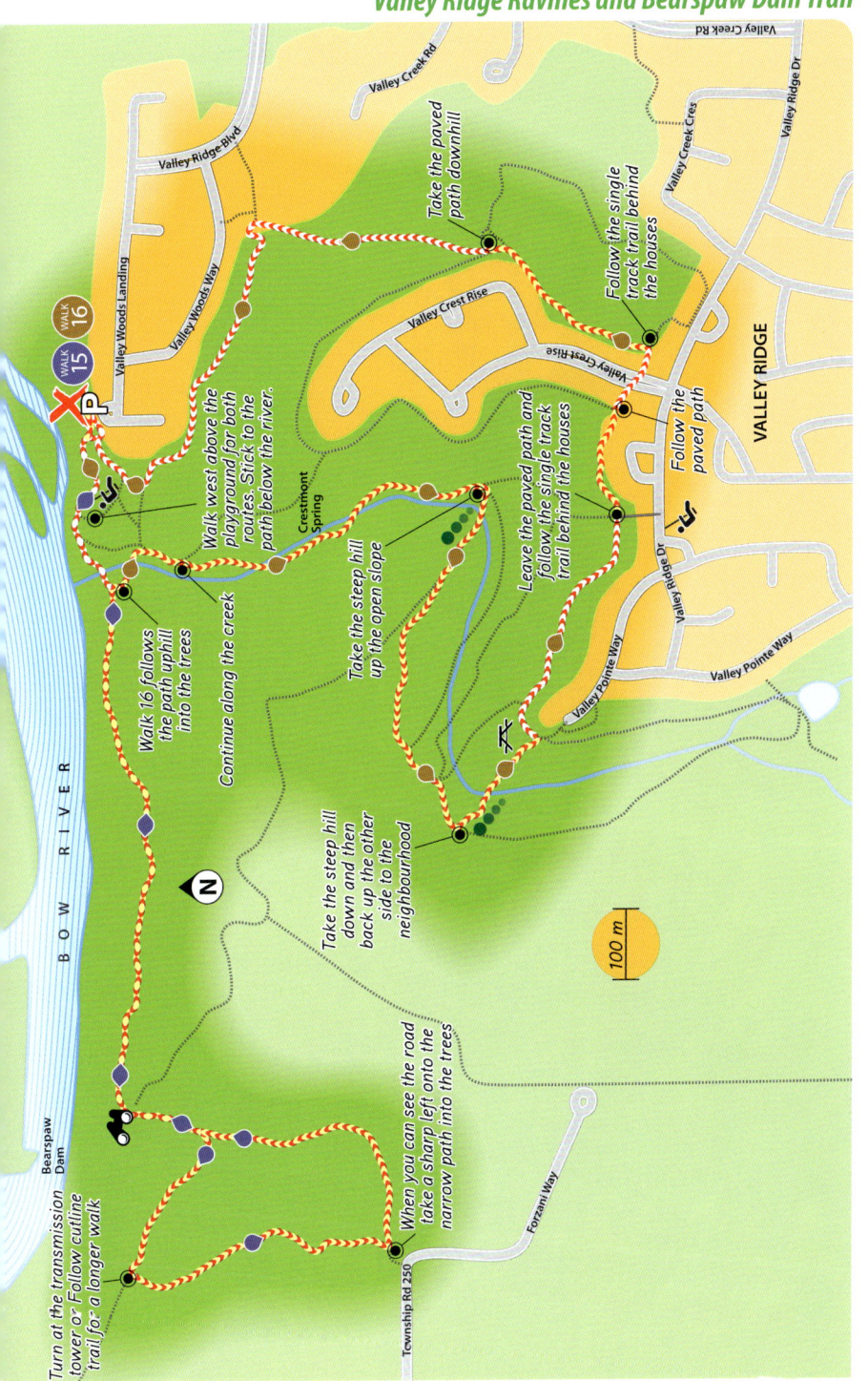

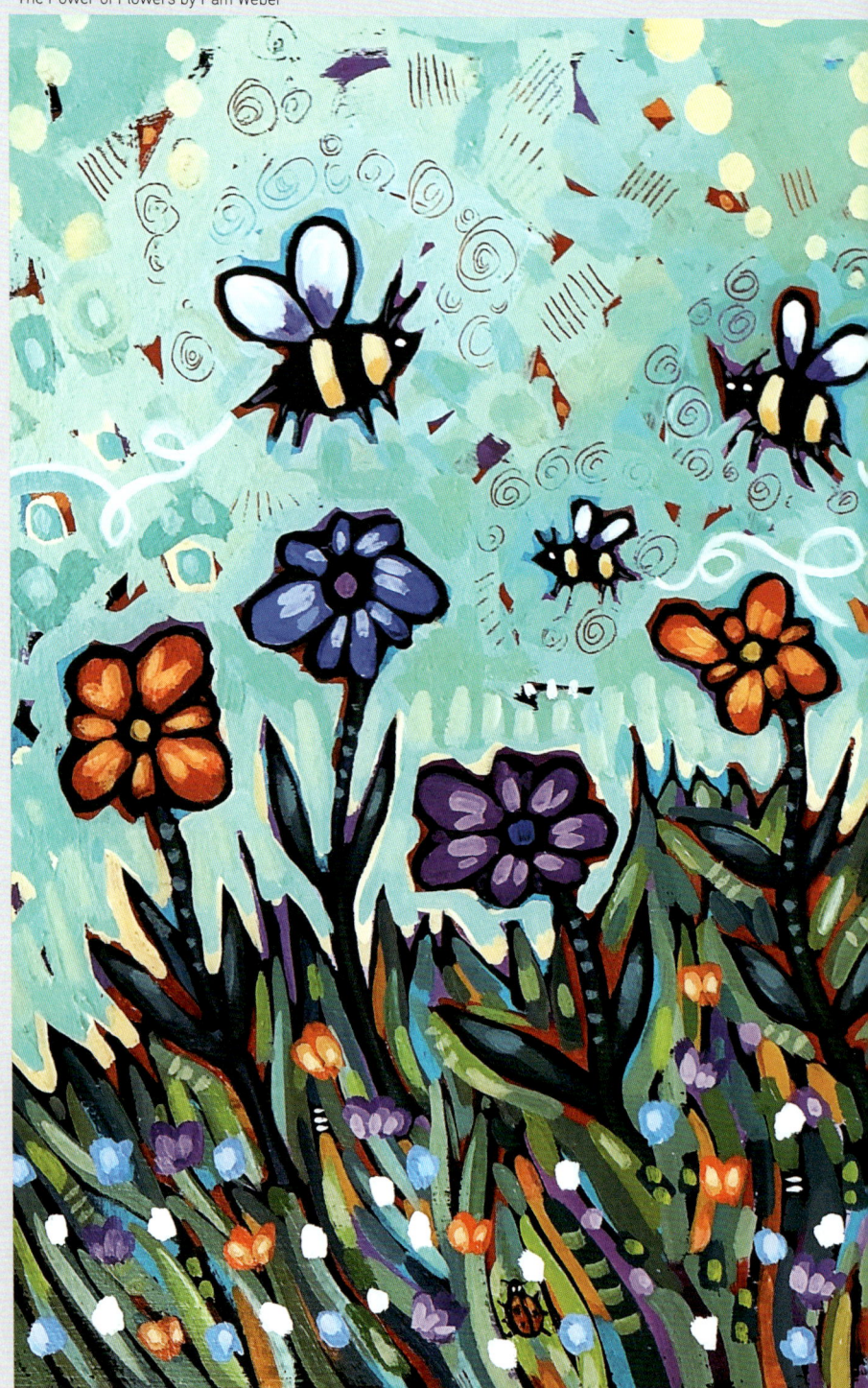

The Power of Flowers by Pam Weber

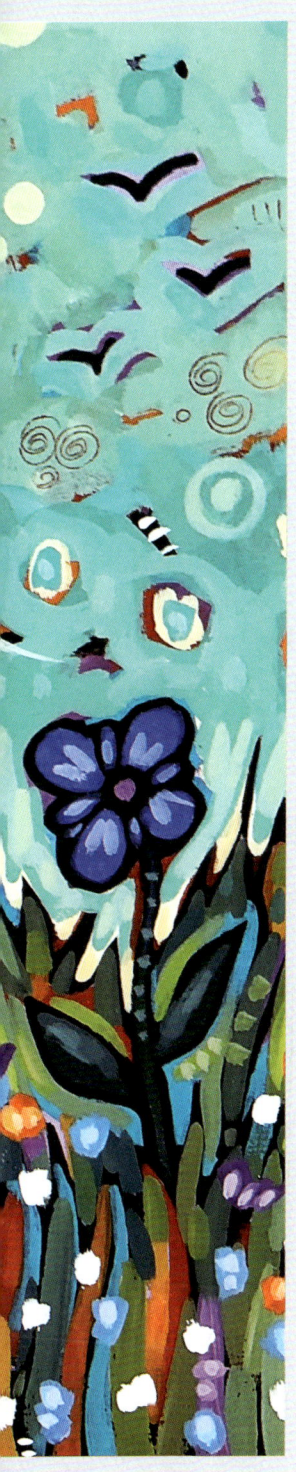

Seven names for Calgary

Calgary was incorporated as a town in 1884, but it was known by many other names before that. The city is situated on the traditional territories of the peoples of the Treaty 7 region in Southern Alberta, which includes the Iyarhe Nakoda Nations (Chiniki, Bearspaw, Wesley), the Tsuut'ina, the Blackfoot Confederacy (Siksika, Piikuni, Kainai). Most of the indigenous names for Calgary refer to where the Elbow River turns abruptly north into the Bow River, making an "elbow-like" curve. The Elbow River gets its name from the distinctive "crook" as it flows towards the Bow River, which gets its name from the reeds that grew along its banks. They were used by local First Nations to make bows.

Wincheesh-pah: This is the Stoney word for "elbow". Stoney means "Stone people" or "people who cook with stones." They were also known as the "Mountain People" who traditionally lived on lands west of Calgary.

Moh-kíns-tsis: The Blackfoot word for "elbow." Another name, Moh-kíns-tsis-aká-piyoyis, meaning "elbow many houses" was also used in 1875. The Blackfoot refers to three tribes; the Siksika, Kainai and the Pekuni. Each tribe was independent, but they all spoke the same language and regarded themselves as allies. They lived in southern Alberta and northern Montana.

Otos-kwunee: The Cree also referred to the region by its rivers, using their word for "elbow". The Cree are the largest group of aboriginal people in Canada today. They migrated to the Prairies during the early 1700s, becoming known as the Plains Cree.

Kootsisáw: The T'suu T'ina word for "elbow." Meaning a "great number of people", land belonging to the Tsuut'ina borders Calgary's western edge. Formerly Sarcee, their traditional territory was far more expansive.

Klincho-tinay-indihay: The Slavey name for Calgary was "horse town." The Slaveys lived in northern Alberta and are a major group of Athapaskan-speaking (or Dene) people.

Fort Brisebois: In 1875, not too long after the Mounties made their march west to Alberta, a fort was built near the meeting of the Bow and Elbow. The officer in charge of the fort, Insp. Ephrem Brisebois, named the post after himself. His superiors were not pleased with this name choice and a year later it was changed.

Fort Calgary: In 1876, the post name changed to Fort Calgary at the suggestion of Lt.-Col. James Farquharson Macleod with the North-West Mounted Police. He named it after the ancestral estate of his cousins on the picturesque Scottish Isle of Mull, which he had recently visited. Calgary dropped "Fort" from its name when it was incorporated a city in 1884.

Bowmont Park West - Waterfall Valley - Bowness

Walks 17 and 18

NW

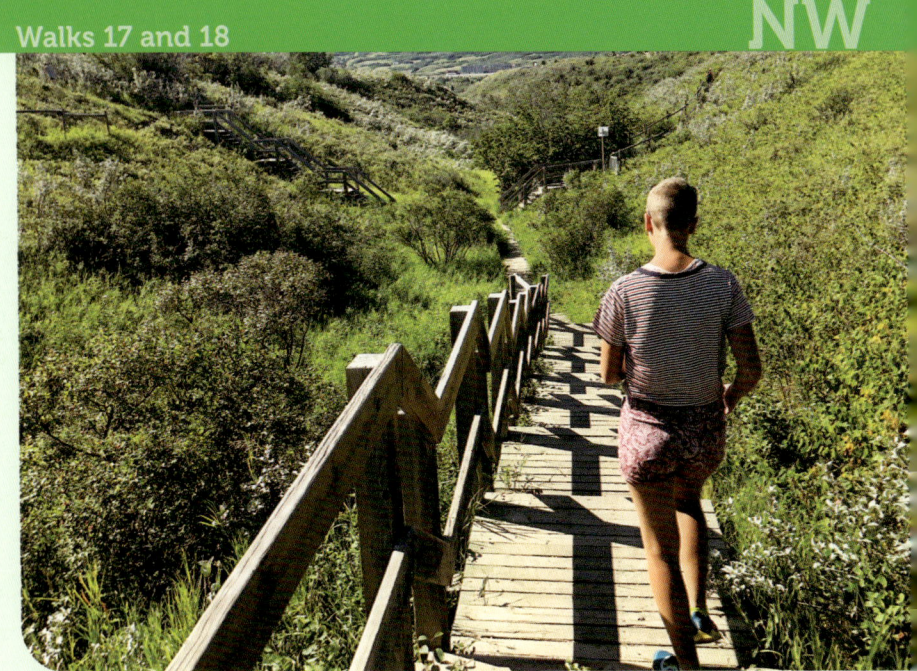

Walks at a Glance:

Waterfall Valley is your halfway point on the Bowmont Park single-track walkabout that skirts the edges of escarpments and descends into ravines. Take the rolling hilly start or warm up slowly on the paved path before climbing to Bow River views.

Choose between the Bowness Loop or the Bowmont Park route. Walk 18, the Bowness neighbourhood walk, crosses the Bow River and continues along the tree-lined Bow Crescent, a three-kilometer side street that hosts a mix of modern and heritage homes sitting on expansive properties along the Bow River. At the end of Bow Crescent, you'll walk past the Little Gallery on the Bow, a series of mini art galleries. Loop back into

Details

Categories: Café, Dog, Nature, Neighbourhood & Parks, Hilly, Vistas, River, Birds

Start: Walks 17 and 18: Park at the official parking area on Scenic Bow Road, just off 85 Street. The parking area is a pull-off on a sharp corner. A Bowmont Park sign hangs on the fence at the park entrance.

Alternate start: Walk 18: Home Road and 52 Street NW. See the map for Walks 19 and 20.

Facilities: None at trailhead. Along the walk is Café Le Matin, 5720 Silver Springs Boulevard and Cadence Café (Walk 19).

Distance & Difficulty

Walk 17: Bowmont Park West and Waterfall Valley: 5.5 km (Many hills, stairs, paved paths)

Walk 18: Bowmont Park – Bowness Loop: 10.5 km (Many hills, stairs, paved paths and sidewalks)

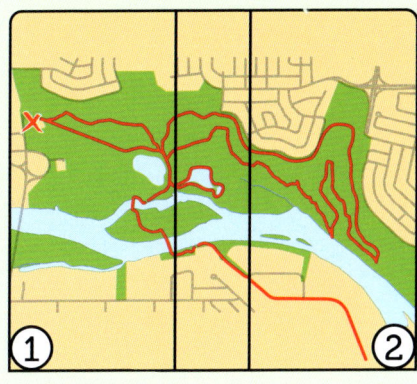

Highlights, Detours & Destinations

Wildflowers blanket the hillside from April through August. Saskatoons ripen in August! Hillside shrubbery and prairie grasses turn golden yellow, burnt orange, and rich red in September. The waterfalls in Waterfall Valley are gorgeous in all seasons. Bring your hiking poles and/or traction devices for your shoes in the winter since single-track trails can be slippery. Nearby eats and cafés: Cadence Café (see Walk 19)

Bowmont Park East and along the Bow River Pathway. Continue west along the paved pathway or dip and climb on the singletrack trails.

Or follow Walk 17, the Bowmont Park route, into Bowmont Natural Environment Park where you'll discover a mix of grasslands, valleys fed with permanent sources of spring water, and shrub-filled offshore islands. Balsam poplar riparian forests still exist here. Once common along riverbanks in the North American prairies, this type of forest is now rare since it depends on flooding for regeneration, and rivers in Alberta flood far less commonly now that they are dammed.

Wildflowers are abundant in the grasslands and appear in April, starting with the purple-headed prairie crocus, followed by the yellow buffalo bean. These blooms are such a welcome sight after many months of the white and brown landscape. Follow the boardwalk trail and descend into Waterfall Valley where a 3-m cascading falls flows over a spongy-looking deposit of tufa. The tufa is composed of mineral deposits that result when

Waterfall Valley

The grasslands in Bowmont Natural Environment Park lie atop 18 m of sediment that was once at the bottom of Glacial Lake Calgary. This lake was formed when the glaciers melted about 12,000 years ago and an ice dam blocked the flow of the runoff. The bedrock below the sediment is called the Porcupine Hills Formation, formed about 65 million years ago. When water seeps through the sediment, it strikes bedrock and then flows sideways, creating the waterfall in Waterfall Valley. The water absorbs calcium carbonate as it travels through the sediment. The mineral is deposited on the algae-covered rocks when the water surfaces, producing tufa. You will see examples of this in Waterfall Valley.

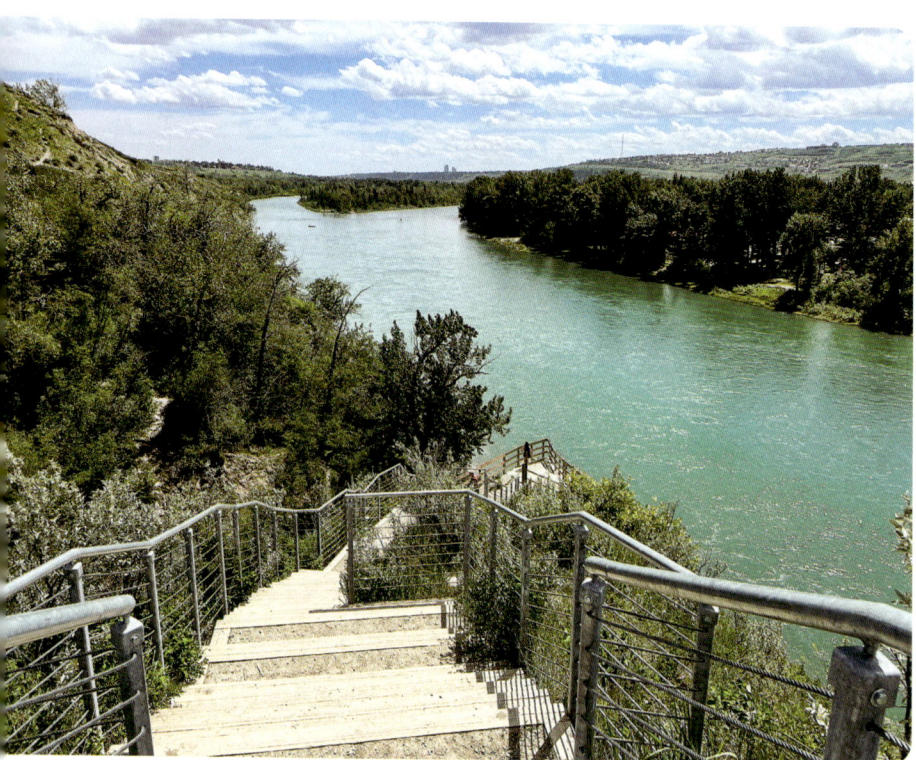

spring water precipitates calcium carbonate over algae-covered rocks. On a very cold winter day when the falls are frozen and the spring water is warmer than the air, you are immersed in a glacial steam bath. Climb back to the escarpment trail and continue east into the poplar stands, dropping closer to the river and then climbing back to the paved Bow River Pathway. This could be the turnaround point, or you could make this a half-day hike by extending your walk along the Bowmont Park East and Dale Hodges Park route.

Continue west along the paved path, enjoying Rocky Mountain views, before descending to the inland ponds. A nice spot for a picnic, the ponds are home to the familiar croak of amphibians. Listen for the boreal chorus frogs and tiger salamanders as you enjoy a snack.

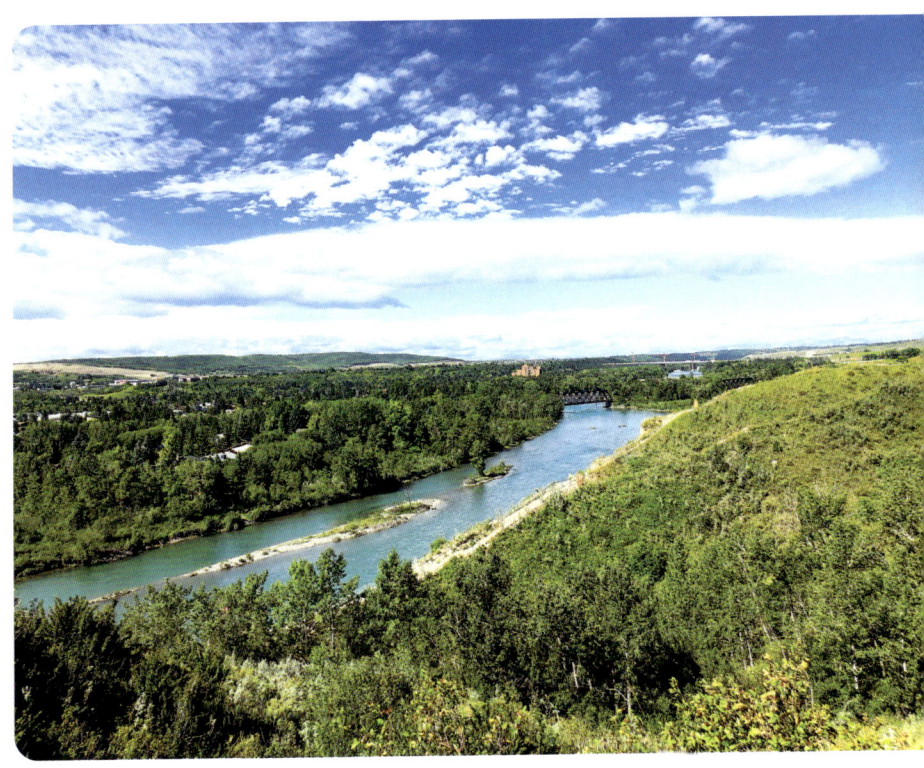

Bowmont Park West - Waterfall Valley - Bowness

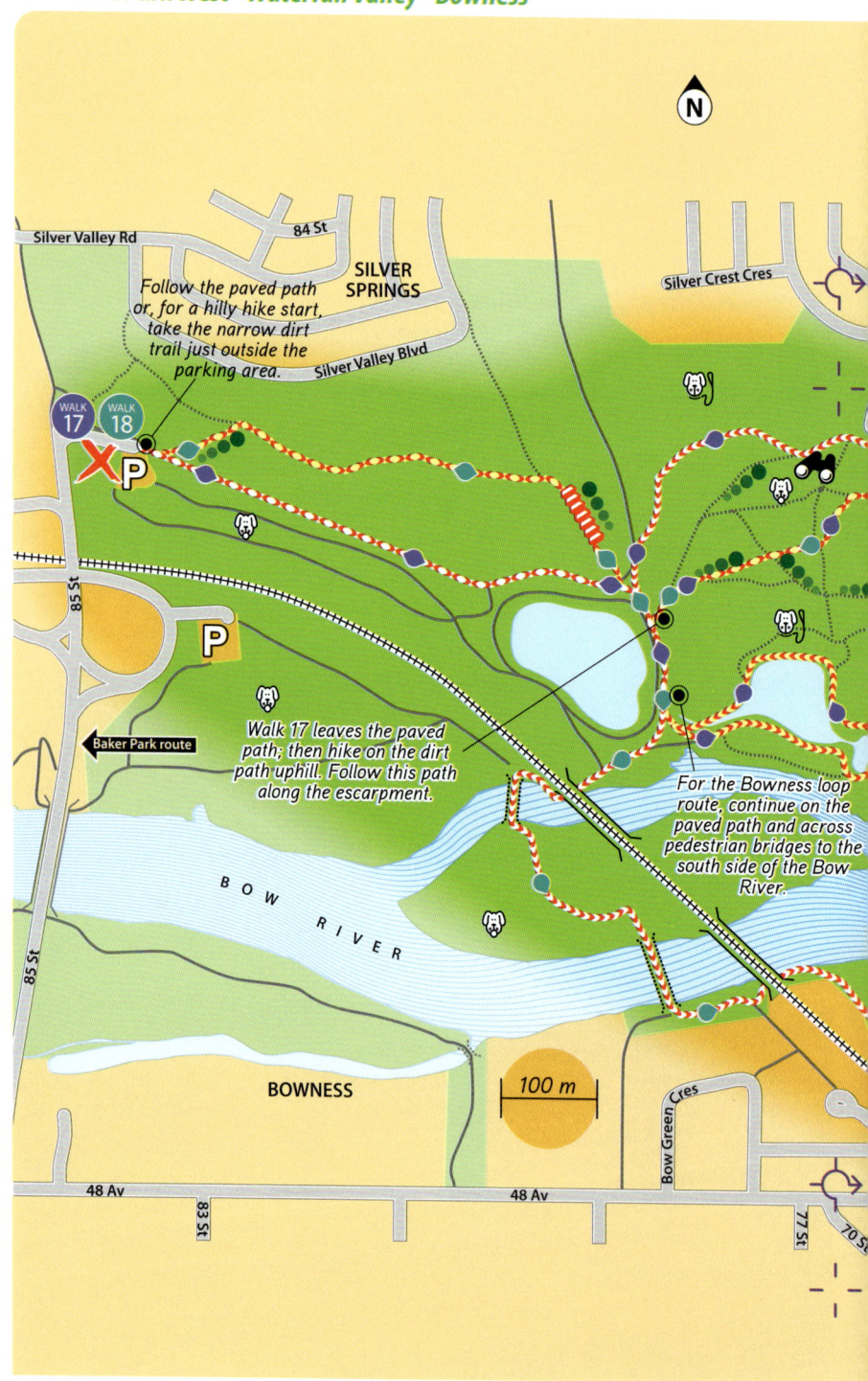

Bowmont Park West - Waterfall Valley - Bowness

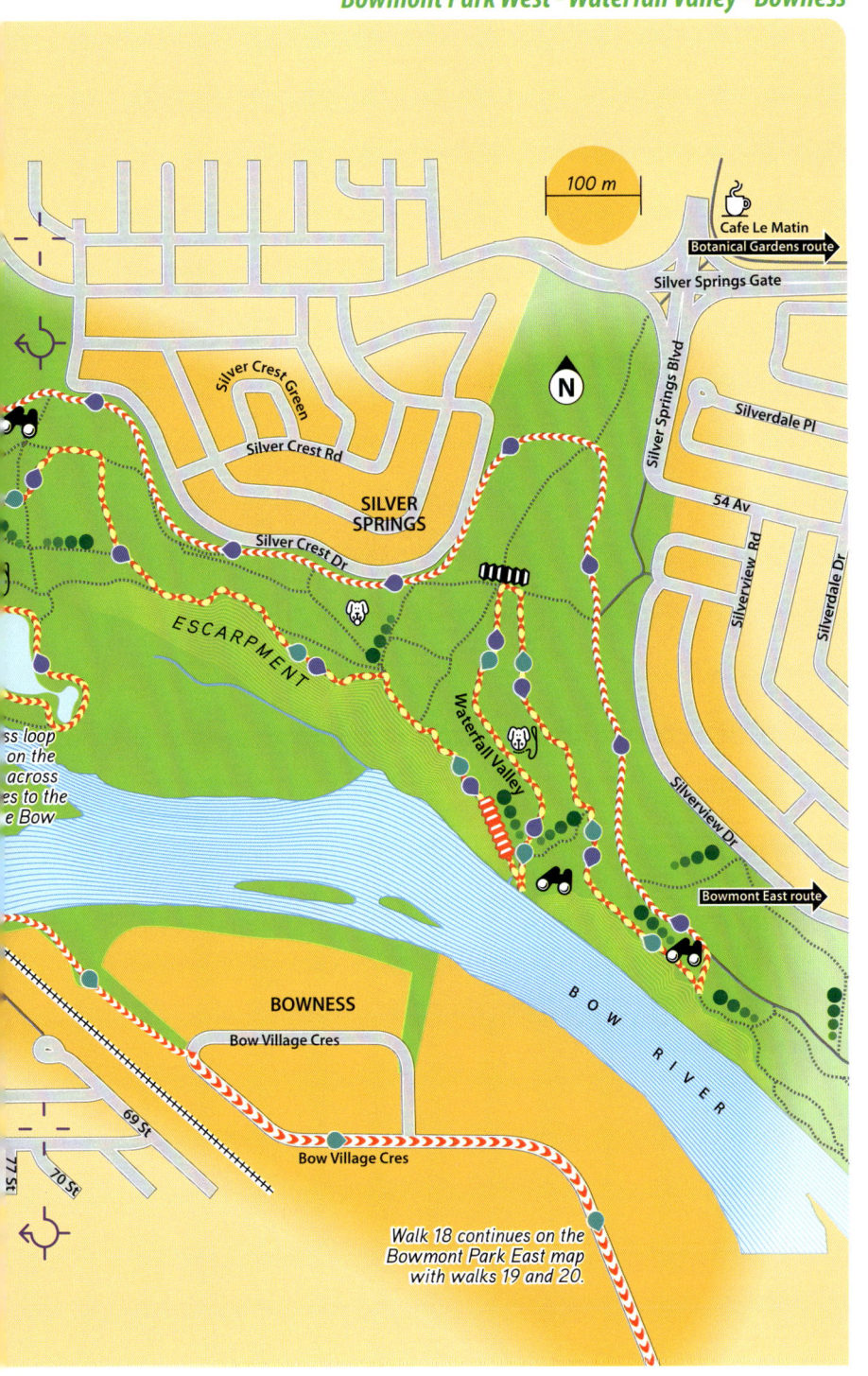

Dale Hodges Park, Bowmont Park East, and Botanical Gardens of Silver Springs
Walks 19 and 20

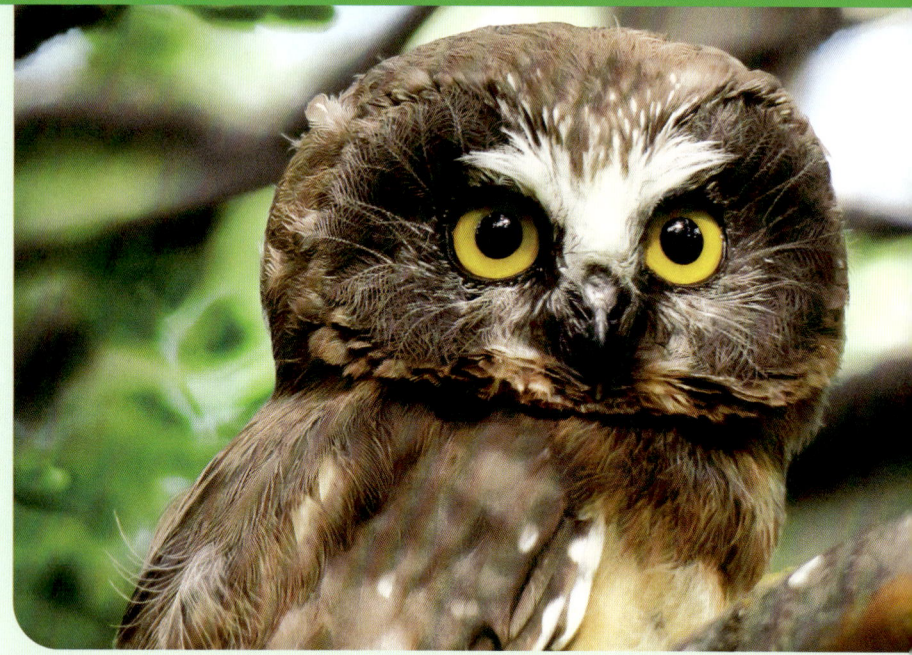

Owl, Dale Hodges Park by Sara Tehranian

Walks at a Glance:

A birders paradise, Dale Hodges Park is tucked in between the community of Silver Springs and the Bow River and borders Bowmont Natural Environment Park, one of my dog's favourite parks to explore with its mix of on and off leash.

Offering a complete nature break, both walks begin on the paved Bow River Pathway and connect to Dale Hodges Park, a former gravel pit that was transformed into wetlands through a unique collaboration between Parks, Water Resources and Public Art.

Walk the trails and boardwalks past polishing marshes, wet meadows and the Nautilus Pond and learn about

Details

Categories: Café, Dog, Nature, Neighbourhood & Parks, Hilly, Vistas, River, Birds

Start: Walks 19 and 20: Park at the official parking area on 52 Street (one-way) just off Home Road

Alternate Start: Walk 20: Official parking lot on Silver Springs Gate NW

Facilities: None at trailhead. Bathrooms in the Botanical Gardens

Distance & Difficulty

Walk 19: Dale Hodges Park and Bowmont Park East: 7.5 km (Paved paths, single track trails and hills)

Walk 20: Bowmont Park to Botanical Gardens: 9 km (Hills, single track trails, paved paths)

Highlights, Detours & Destinations

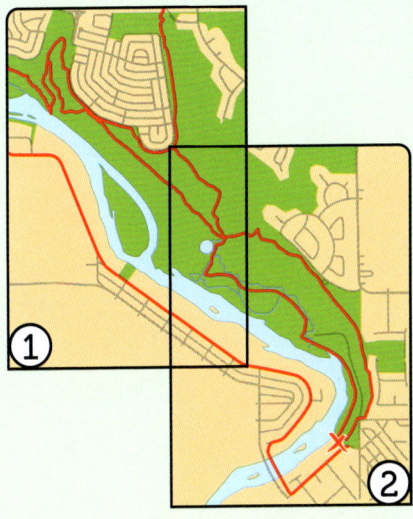

Birders love Dale Hodges Wetlands and dogs love Bowmont Park and the Botanical Gardens. Wildflowers start blooming in Bowmont Park in early April and continue throughout the summer. The Botanical Gardens colour begins in May and continues through October. In late September and early October, the grasses turn autumnal reds and oranges while the aspen groves host yellow leaves - always spectacular against a blue sky. Enjoy the solitude on the trails in the cooler months

the storm water treatment process as it flows to the Bow River. This process is estimated to reduce sediment in storm water by 50%, helping to protect our river system. Calgary is home to over 200 bird species, some migrating and some residents, and many can be seen along the Bow River and in the wetlands. Slow the pace in Dale Hodges Park to see Mallards, Cedar Waxwings, Yellow and Red-Winged blackbirds and maybe the migratory Northern Saw-Whet Owl that might be at eye level in the dense thickets of shrubs. One of the smallest owls in North America, they are about the size of a Robin. Continue past the Nautilus Pond and onto the rollercoaster grassland pathways. Walk 19 continues

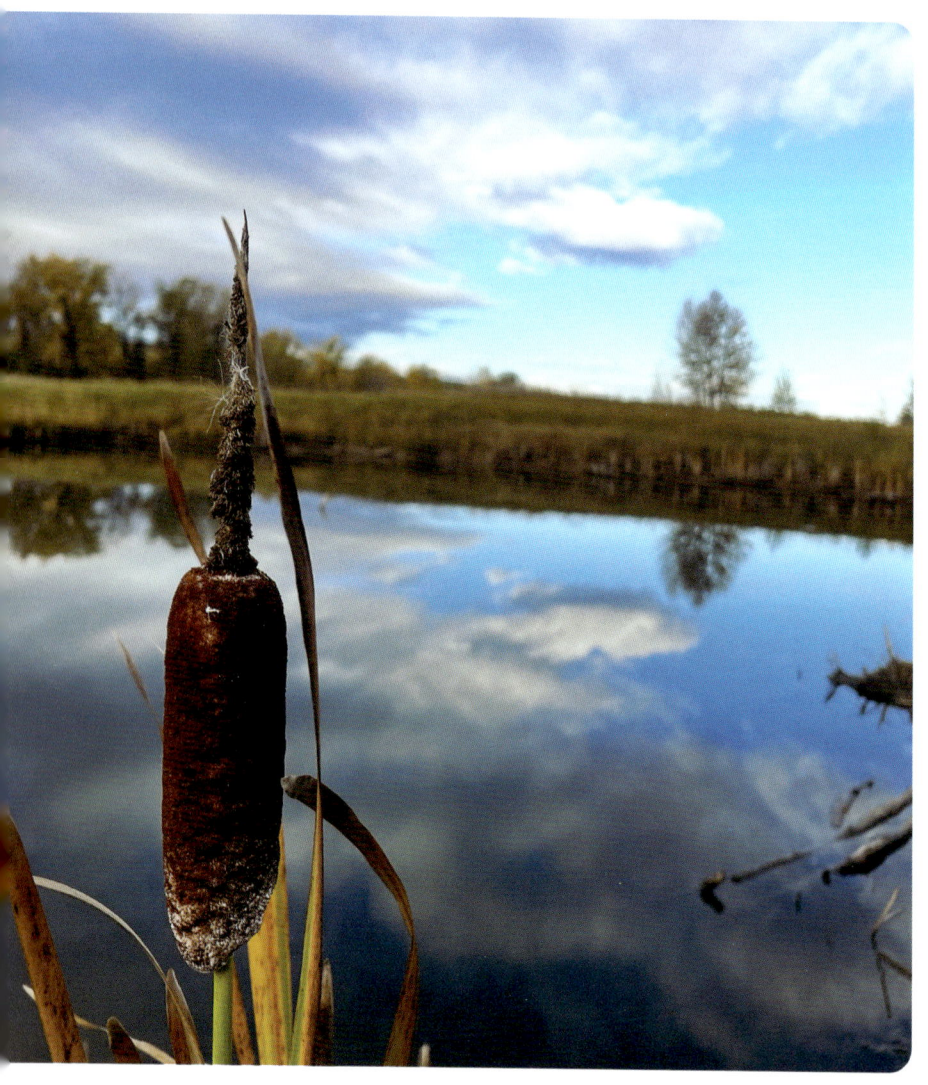

Tasty Pit Stops: Cadence Coffee

Self-described as "a 21st century diner located in the heart of Bowness, where friends meet to enjoy great food, superfine coffee, and fresh baking," Cadence Coffee is a local hot spot. Popular for breakfasts or a cup of coffee and freshly baked muffin, it is a wonderful post-walk destination. It is my favourite post Bowmont Park stop with groups of walkers that join me on guided walks. Cadence is also a great place to grab a picnic lunch before your walk. Made-to-order sandwiches, fresh soups, and lots of salads are available; grab some tasty food and enjoy it during a break at one of the sightseeing lookouts perched on the Bowmont Park escarpments.

Location: 6407 Bowness Road NW

west while Walk 20 heads north to the Botanical Gardens of Silver Springs where a garden oasis awaits.

Bowmont Park's hilly topography is perfect for hikers in training. The high points on the trail offer a bird's eye view of some of the vast and impressive properties along the river in Bowness and ever-present Rocky Mountains on the horizon. Walk 19 continues along the top of the escarpment, past the homes with million-dollar views. Cut inland along narrow pathways, descend the slope, and climb back up again along the switchback trail. Continue through the park to conclude your walk. Now you are all set to visit Bowness for a post-walk drink or meal, or just to check out the shops along Bowness Road.

Black-Capped Chickadee

Calgary's official bird and my favourite flying friend is the chickadee. Year-round residents of Canada, Calgary is home to three species, the black-capped, boreal and mountain chickadee. One of the friendliest backyard birds, they stay close while people are around, especially when those people are offering up seeds from the palm of their hands. Their tell-tale sound is chicka-dee-dee-dee-dee but they also have ones that sound like they might be saying cheeseburger, Hey baby and I did-it. Chickadees are social birds often flocking together with other species during the winter including nuthatches and woodpeckers. They learn the alarm calls of other birds and use it to their advantage to hide from incoming predators. Chickadees are excellent insect and spider control, particularly during nesting. In the short time it takes to get chicks out of the nest (about 3 weeks), chickadees will need between 5000-9000 insects to feed their brood! Caterpillars, aphids and spiders make up much of this diet, but they aren't overly picky.

They eat berries, seeds, nuts, frozen insects and spiders in the winter and switch to fresh insects, spiders and other animal material in the summer. Seeds are stored underneath tree bark; in tall hollow stems and clusters of pine needles and any other nooks and crannies they can find. In the fall and winter, the brain of chickadees gets bigger! The part of the brain responsible for spatial memory (the hippocampus) grows so they can remember where they cached the thousands of seeds they collect, and studies show that they can find them a month after they have cached them.

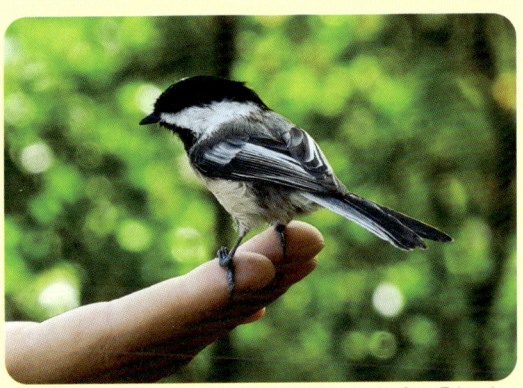

Chickadee by Sara Tehranian

Dale Hodges Park, Bowmont Park East, and Botanical Gardens of Silver Springs

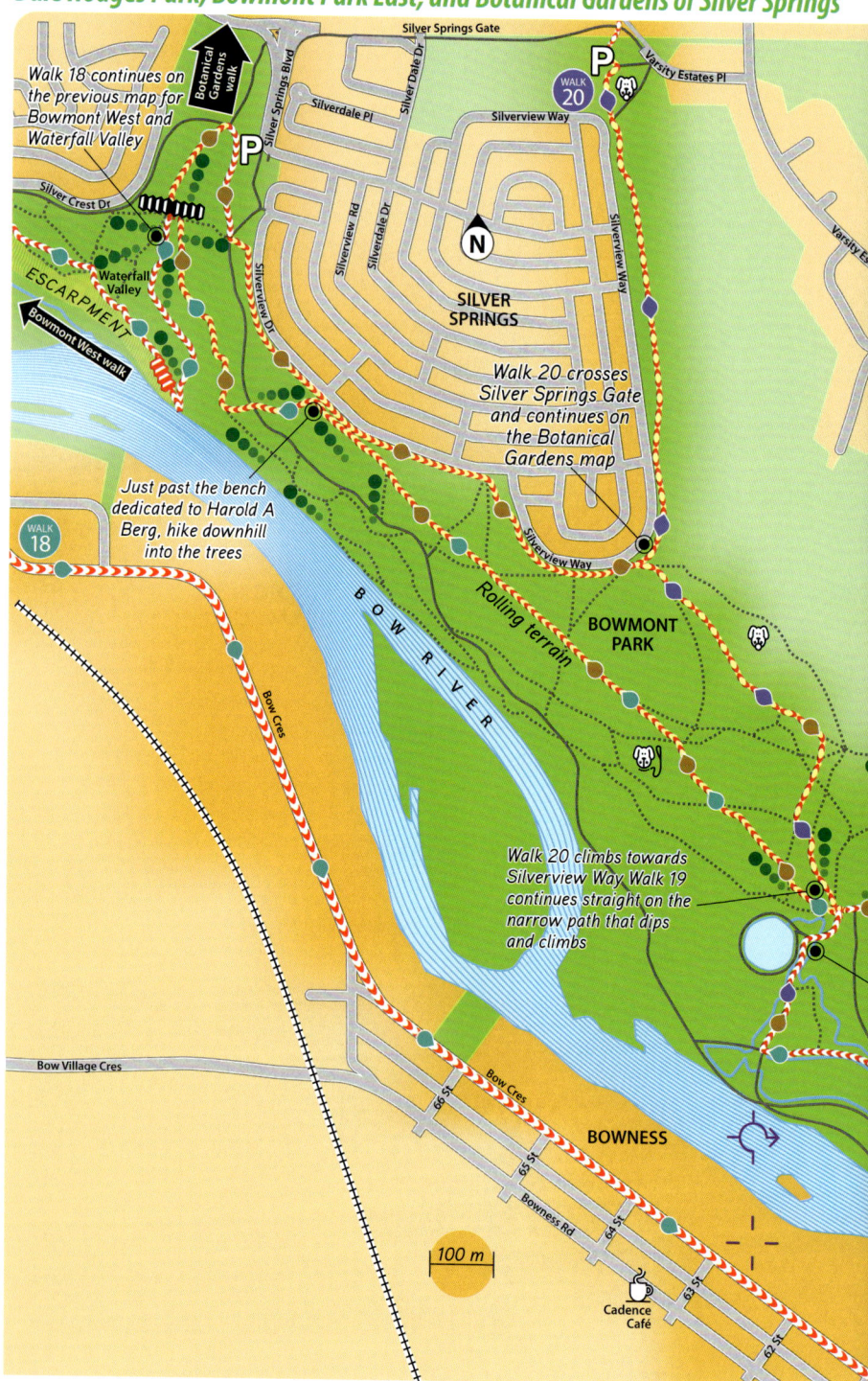

Dale Hodges Park, Bowmont Park East, and Botanical Gardens of Silver Springs

Botanical Gardens of Silver Springs

Walk 21

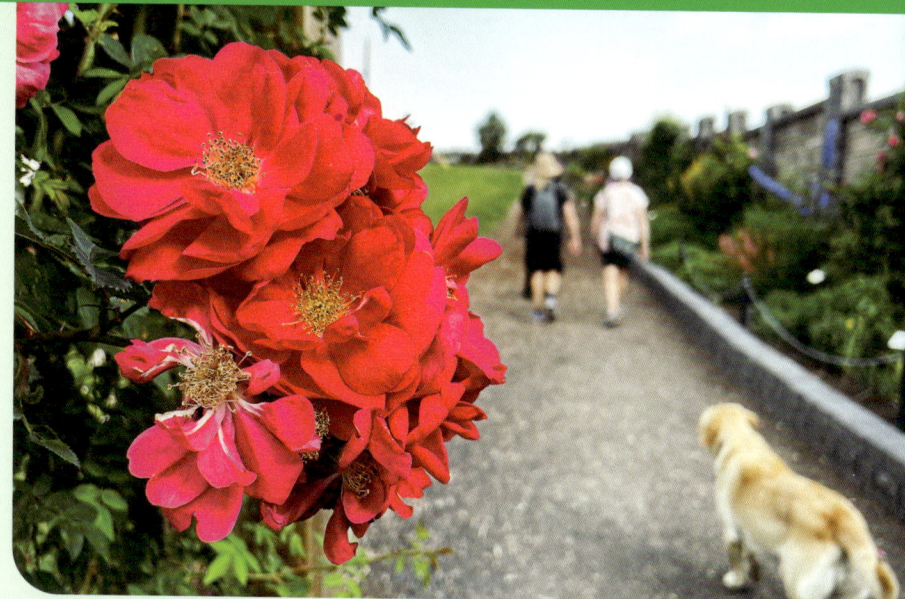

Walk at a Glance:

Thousands of volunteer hours have created a garden oasis in the community of Silver Springs. Dogs are welcome and the entire area is off leash. In 2006 the garden opened and since then has grown to over a kilometre of individual gardens connected by walking paths, nestled amongst three birthplace forests. Gardens range from traditional gardens displaying plants that grow well in Calgary to more focused gardens that demonstrate various aspects of gardening.

Specialty gardens include a theme garden as a tribute to Shakespeare and his writing, a low H_2O Garden featuring plants that require little water and Canada's largest Labyrinth that is a swirl of flowering wild thyme in the Springtime. Circle inward amongst the masses

Details

Categories: Dog, Nature, Stroller, Birds

Start: 37 Silver Springs Drive NW. Parking area is beside the baseball diamond in Sarcee Park on the south end of the Gardens

Facilities: Bathrooms and picnic tables

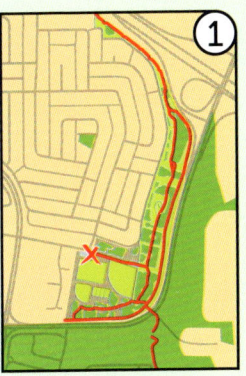

Distance & Difficulty

2.8 km (mostly flat, gravel paths)

Highlights, Detours & Destinations

Year-round: Dogs love the gardens as they are off leash

Spring: One of the most spectacular sights in the Gardens and Birthplace Forest is the Labyrinth in spring when the wild thyme is in bloom. Other blooming plants in the spring are the fruit trees, peonies and lilacs

Summer: July-August is peak blooming period for many plants. The roses are exceptional with over 100 individual species

Fall: Asters and Chrysanthemums and gorgeous Stonecrop (Sedum)

Winter: The gardens are decorated for Christmas

of delicate, star like flowers offering up spicy and therapeutic scents. Over a hundred species of roses bloom in the summer in the rose garden and a rock and crevice alpine garden hosts the hardy plants that survive harsh climates and short summers. And be sure to walk there in August when the cheery sunflowers are in their towering golden glory.

The gardens are the perfect place for a stroll year-round but are especially vibrant in the summer through fall. And if you are in the mood for a longer walk, or perhaps a picnic overlooking the Bow River, then connect follow Walk 20 into Bowmont Park and add some Bow River and Rockies views to your colourful gardens trek.

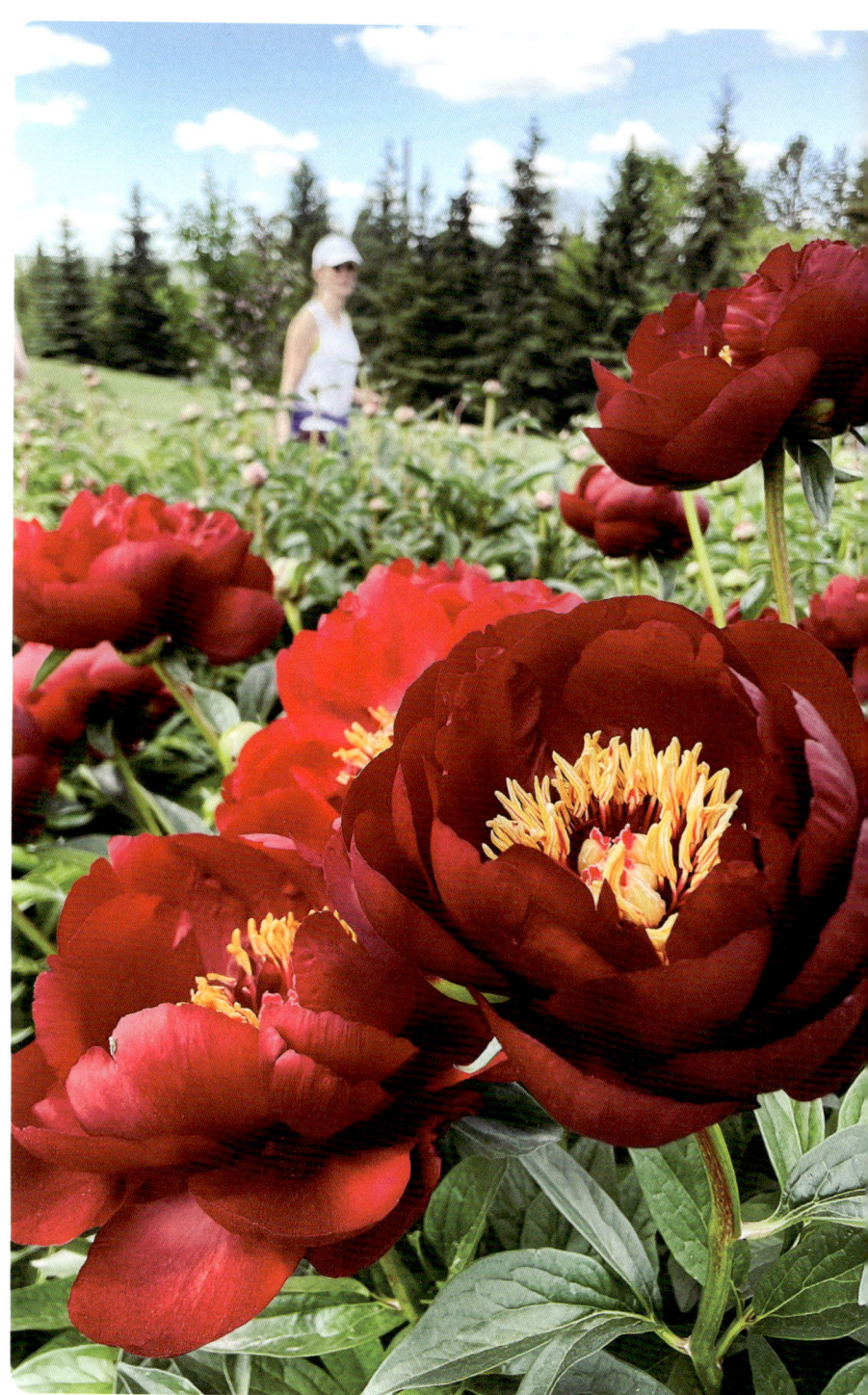

Botanical Gardens of Silver Springs

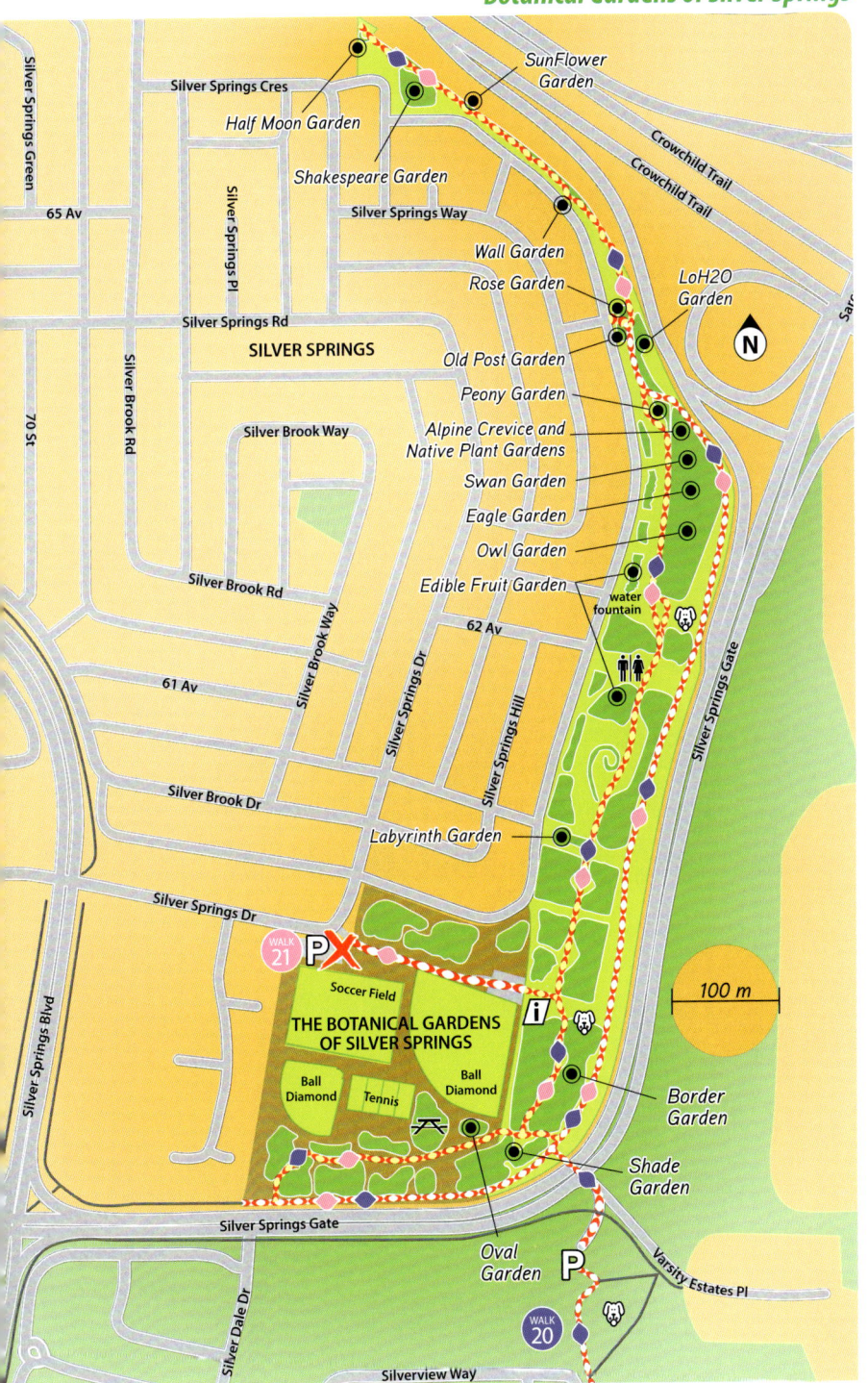

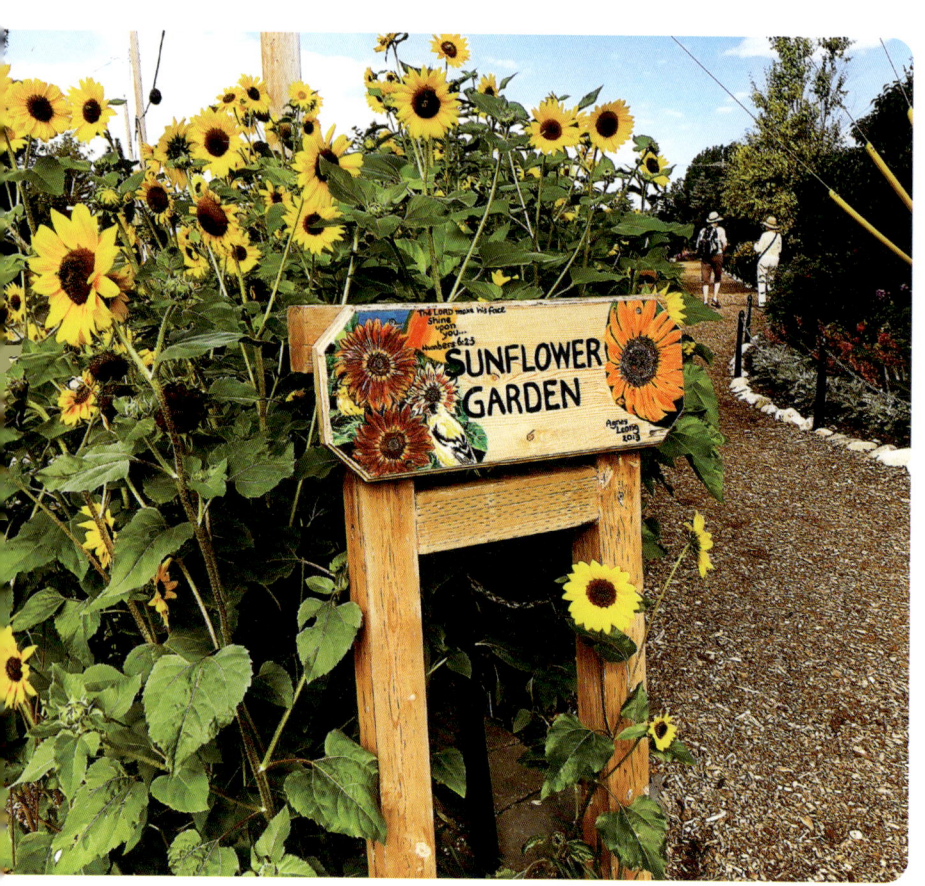

Chinook Gardening

Snowstorms in the summer and patio days in the winter: this is normal in Calgary. In the winter, when warm moist air from the West Coast hits the mountains, winds called Chinooks descend on Calgary. Chinook means "snow eater," but it could also mean "snowplow" in Calgary since we depend on it to clear snow-filled side streets. Calgarians love to brag to relatives and friends in eastern Canada or even in Edmonton about the huge temperature changes we experience during some Chinooks. "It went from -20°C to +20°C in one day," we report to snow-weary Canadian friends. While rapid changes in temperature make for great variety —and Calgarians do welcome those warm, dry, Chinook winds during the winter— Chinook thaws make gardening under the arch a challenge. For example, warm January temperatures melt the snow and expose plants to the inevitable return of frigid days. Chinook-exposed plants may be tricked into beginning what are normally springtime processes, such as the growth of new root hairs, leaves, and flower buds, which then makes them vulnerable to injury from cold and frost. All of this said, Calgary gardeners are hardy and enjoy a good challenge. Despite the havoc a Chinook can wreak, Calgary gardens are beautiful from June into September.

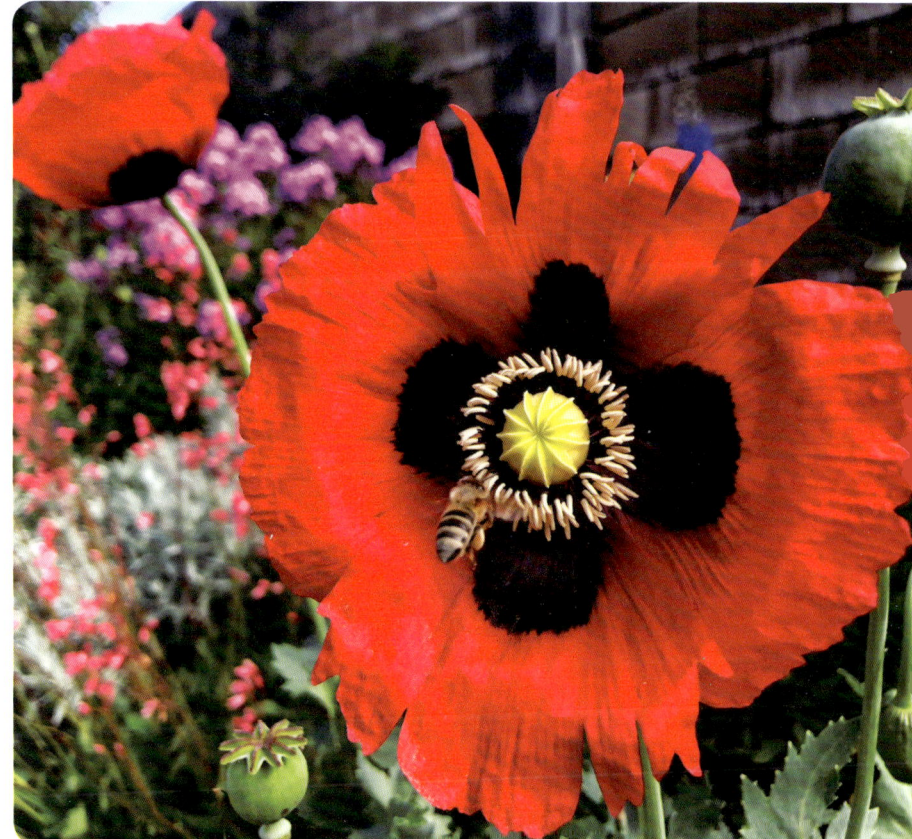

Varsity, Dalhousie and Edgemont Ravines

Walks 22-27

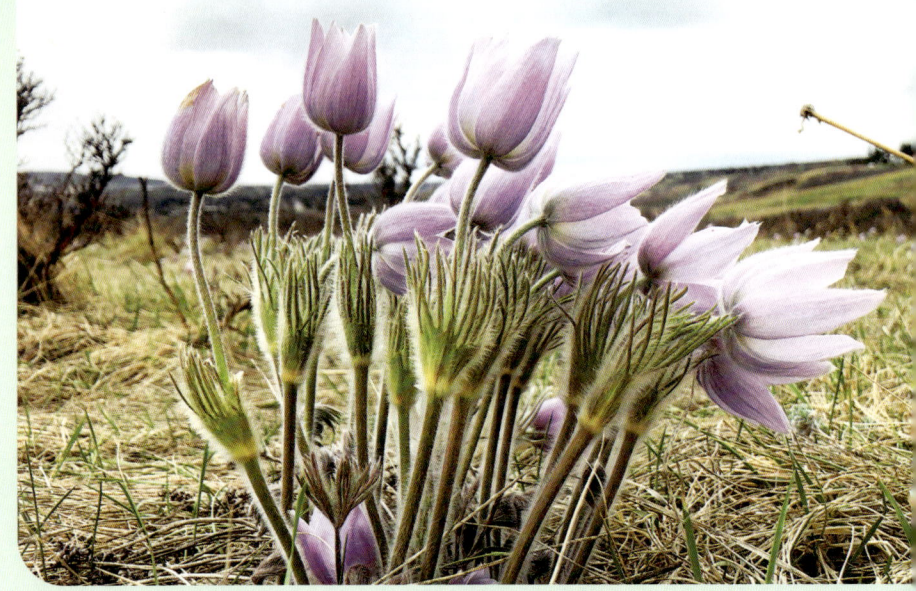

Walks at a Glance:

Sloping and vast, the manicured Varsity, Dalhousie and Edgemont Ravines are part of the connector pathway network that climbs from the Bow River Valley to Calgary's northern communities. These walks are interconnected and travel through a mix of manicured ravine parks and onto wilder exposed slopes that are covered with wildflowers from April through August and host impressive windswept snowdrifts throughout the winter. And with a high point of 1245 m, Edgemont offers expansive views of Calgary.

Walks 22 -24 follow paved paths through the ravines and into the neighbourhoods of Varsity and Dalhousie. Pups love the off leash in Varsity Ravines and kids love the sloping hills that are perfect for tobogganing in the

Details

Categories: LRT, Café, Dog, Nature, Neighbourhood & Parks, Hilly, Stroller, Vistas, Birds

Start: Walks 22 and 24: Euphoria Café, 8 Varsity Estates Circle NW

Walks 23 and 25: Official parking lot at Edgemont Hill and Edgemont Drive NW

Walk 26: Friends Café, 104, 45 Edenwold Drive NW

Walk 27: Edgemont Community Association, 33 Edgevalley Circle NW

LRT: Dalhousie Station

Facilities: Café at the start of Walks 22, 24 and 26

Distance & Difficulty

Walk 22: Varsity Ravines and neighbourhood: 4 km (paved paths and sidewalks)

Walk 23: Dalhousie Ravines and neighbourhood: 4 km (Paved paths and sidewalks)

Walk 24: Varsity - Dalhousie Ravines: 8 km (Paved paths and sidewalks)

Walk 25: Edgemont Hills and Ravines: 10 km (Hills, single track trails, paved paths, and sidewalks)

Walk 26: Edgemont Hills Loop: 5 km (Hills, single track trails, sidewalks)

Walk 27: Edgemont Ravines Loop: 5 km (Hills, paved paths and sidewalks)

Highlights, Detours & Destinations

Year-Round: Dogs love these walks for all the of leash in Varsity Ravines and the Edgemont slopes

Spring-Fall: Enjoy wildflowers on the Edgemont slopes and a nature hit with many birds at the wetlands in Edgemont Park Ravines

Winter: Bring your sleds for some tobogganing fun in Varsity Ravine Park

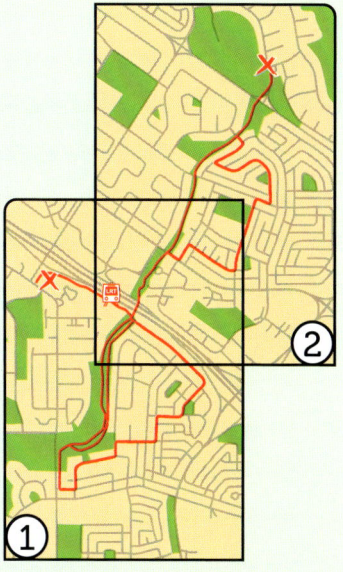

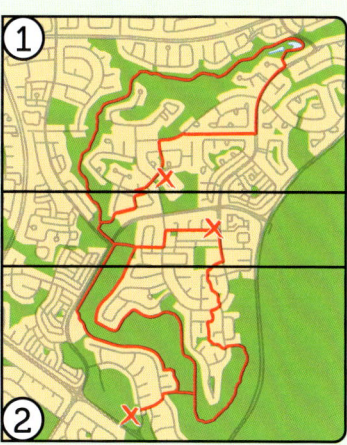

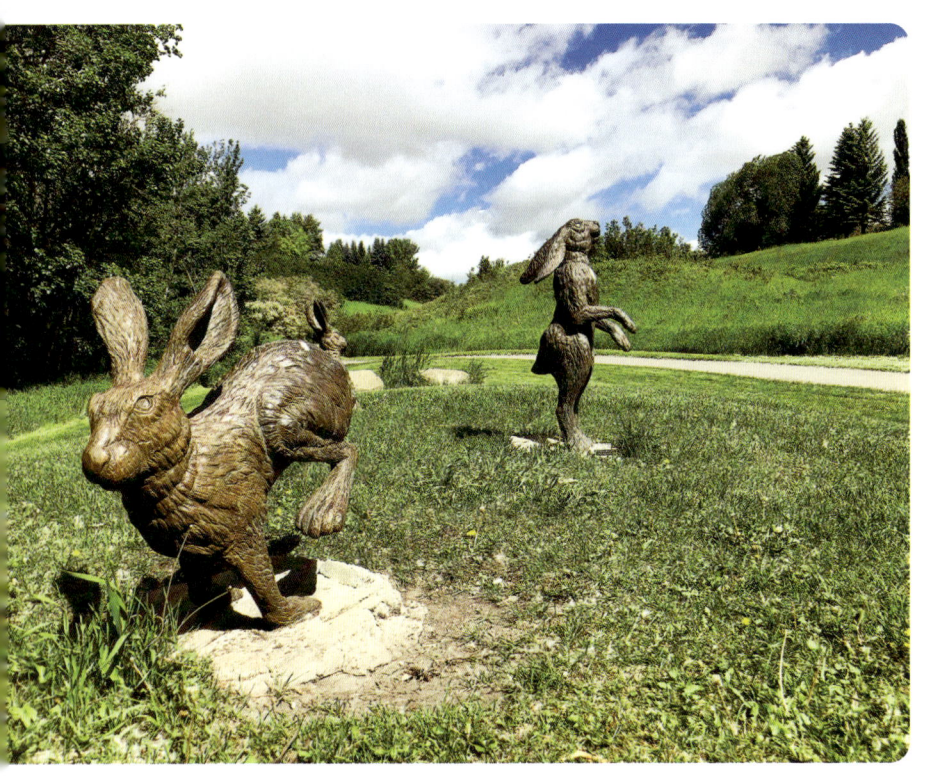

Geological Calgary

Three distinctive levels make up the Calgary we know today. The upper level beneath Paskapoo Slopes and Nose Hill is the oldest surface. It consists of sandstones that are part of the Paskapoo Formation. Dalhousie, Brentwood, Altadore, and Wildwood are on the middle level that formed by glacial erosion and was covered by lake deposits. The deepest level is the Bow River valley that contains the downtown and the communities of Sunnyside, Bowness, and Bridgeland. The deepest level formed during the final rush of glacial meltwaters that eroded downwards.

During the last glacial period, about 22,000 years ago, ice sheets from the mountains in the west and from the Canadian Shield in the east met in the Calgary area. These glaciers pushed back and forth against each other, receding and advancing several times, carving the Bow Valley and leaving blankets of chaotic glacial sediment and giant erratic boulders in their wake. As the glaciers melted away, around 17,000 years ago, the vast eastern glacier from the Canadian Shield blocked the Bow River and Elbow River valleys. The water that melted from the retreating ice was dammed by the glacier to form "Glacial Lake Calgary," between Calgary and Cochrane. Lake levels varied as the ice sheet melted and re-advanced, depositing lake bottom silts and clays where the communities of Brentwood, Varsity, and Silver Springs, as well as the Foothills and Children's hospitals, are now. The highest shoreline of Glacial Lake Calgary is about where John Laurie Boulevard is today. By about 16,500 years ago, the glacial dam had melted to the point where Glacial Lake Calgary could drain away. The massive outflow of water helped the Bow River valley cut down to its current position. Calgary's geological past is the foundation for the variety of urban walkabouts in my book.

snowy months. Be sure to check out the Monsters Inc. door tucked into the Crowchild trail retaining wall in Varsity.

Walks 25 and 26 explore the southern part of Edgemont, with a mix of sidewalk strolling and wide-open green-space climbs. Dogs run free on the off-leash slopes while their people enjoy summer wildflowers and big views. Walk 25 crosses Edgemont Boulevard and connects to Walk 27 in Edgemont Ravines where both walks follow the paved pathway through the manicured multi-use park with art installations and playgrounds. The ravine trail offers a relatively flat trek through a pleasant green space.

Turn the corner at the T-junction and the park becomes less manicured, more natural, with some steeper hills. Thick willow shrubs consume the north-facing hillside, creating a sheltered home for mule deer. Listen for the wetlands of Edgemont Park Ravine. Before reaching the ponds, the bird chatter is loud and clear. Cattails line the sides of the water and attract red-winged blackbirds, which have a distinctive sing-song call.

Circle the wetland and climb the slope to continue the walk along quiet neighbourhood streets, or make it a linear route, an out and back walk. Turn on your heels and follow your breadcrumbs back to your starting point.

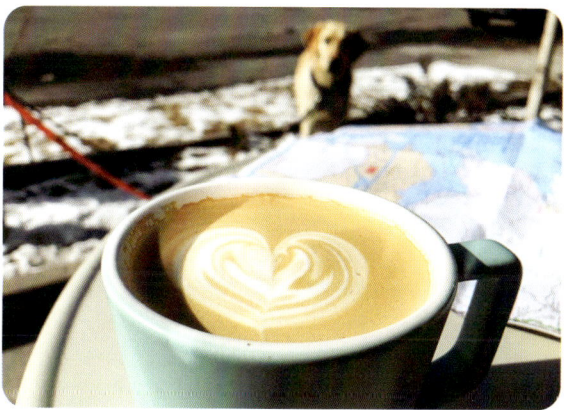

Varsity and Dalhousie Ravines

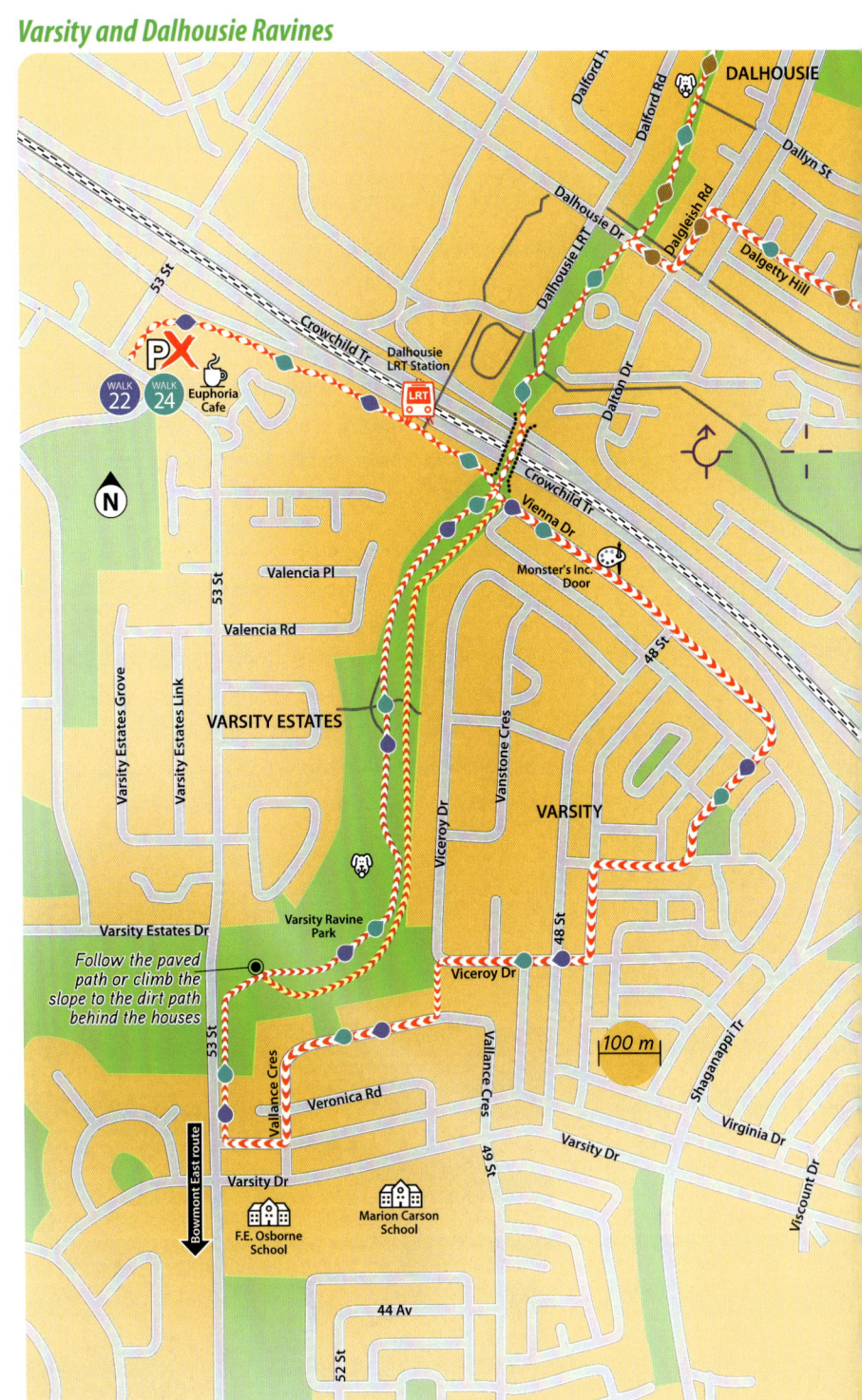

Varsity and Dalhousie Ravines

Edgemont Hills and Ravines

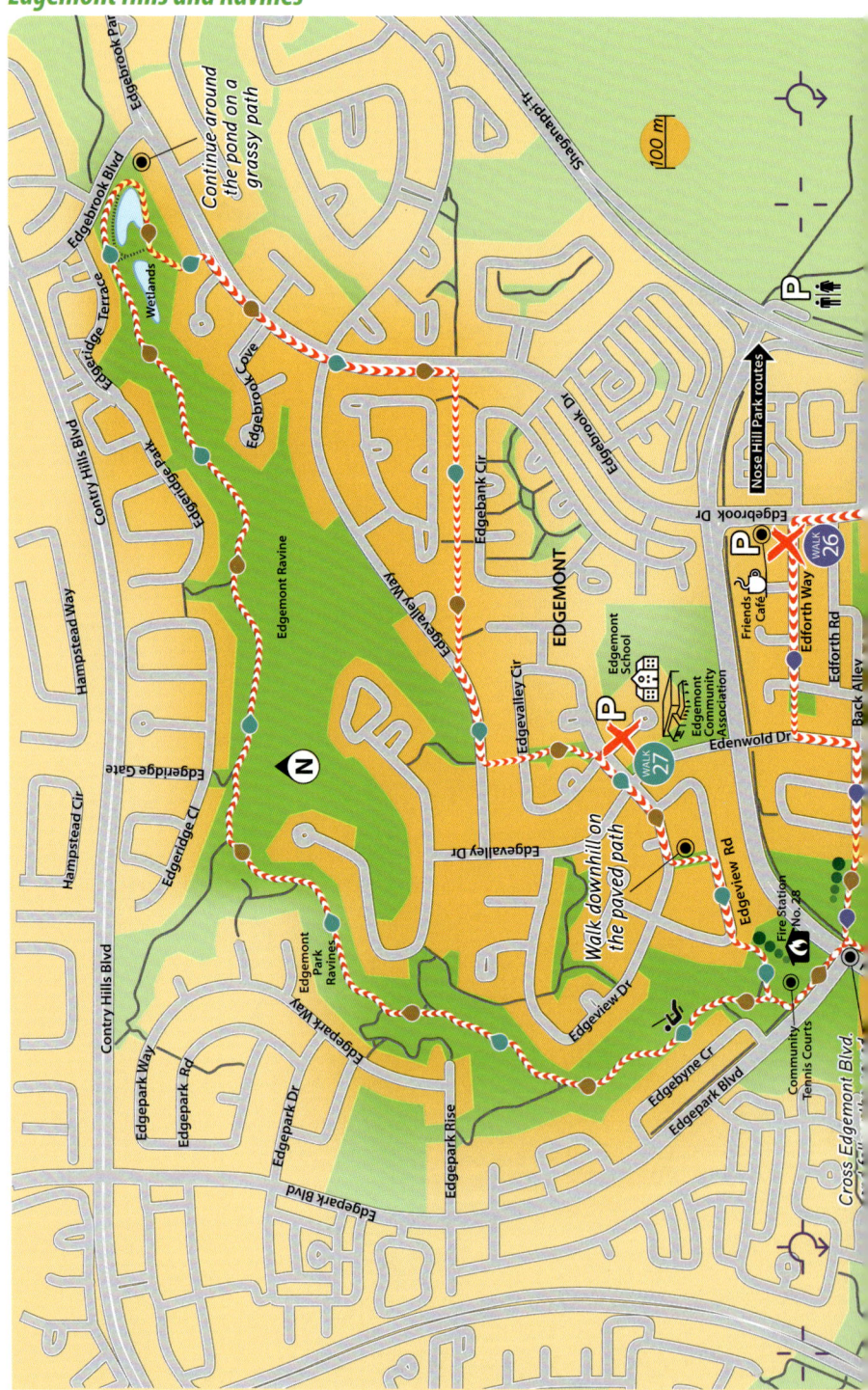

Edgemont Hills and Ravines

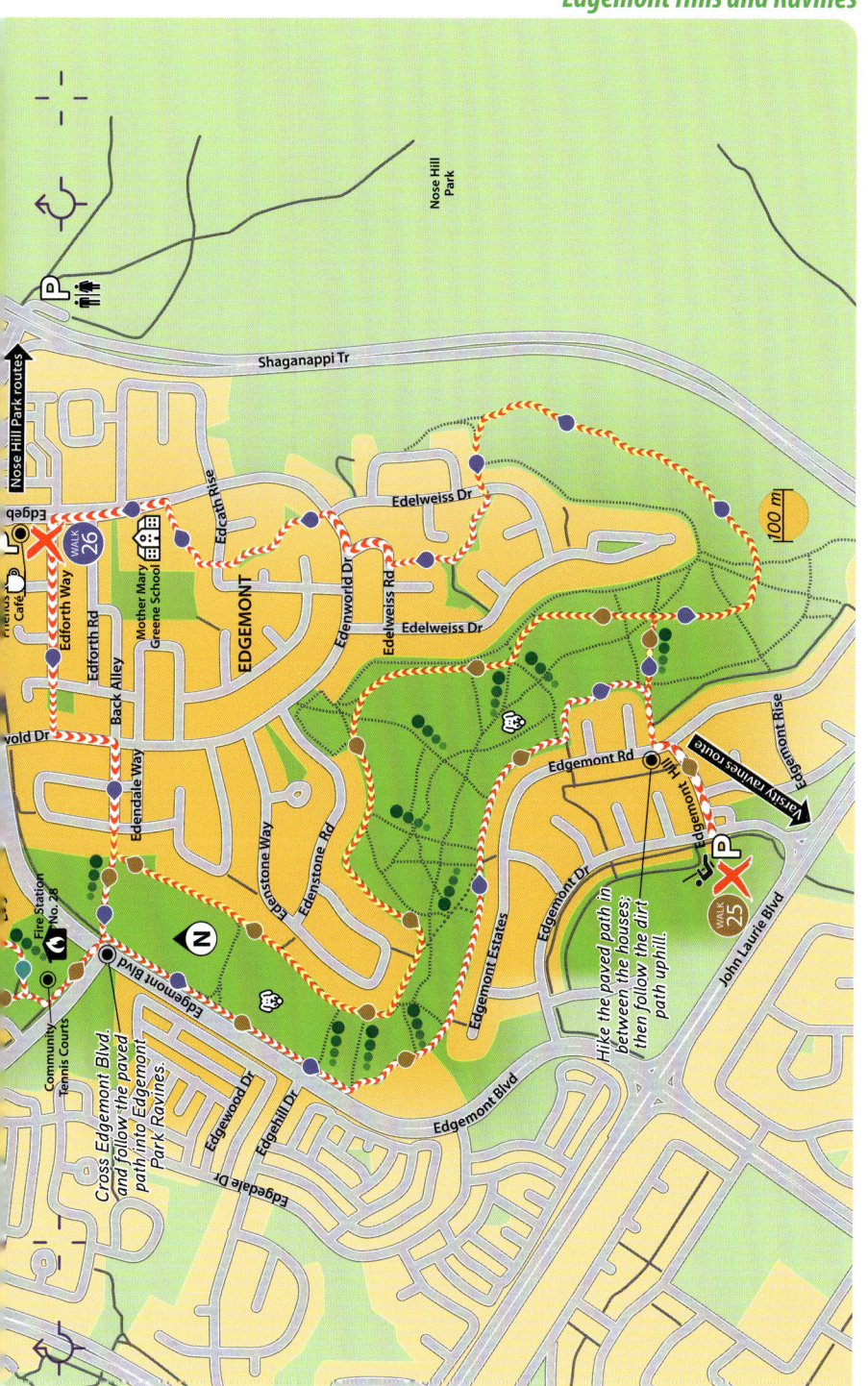

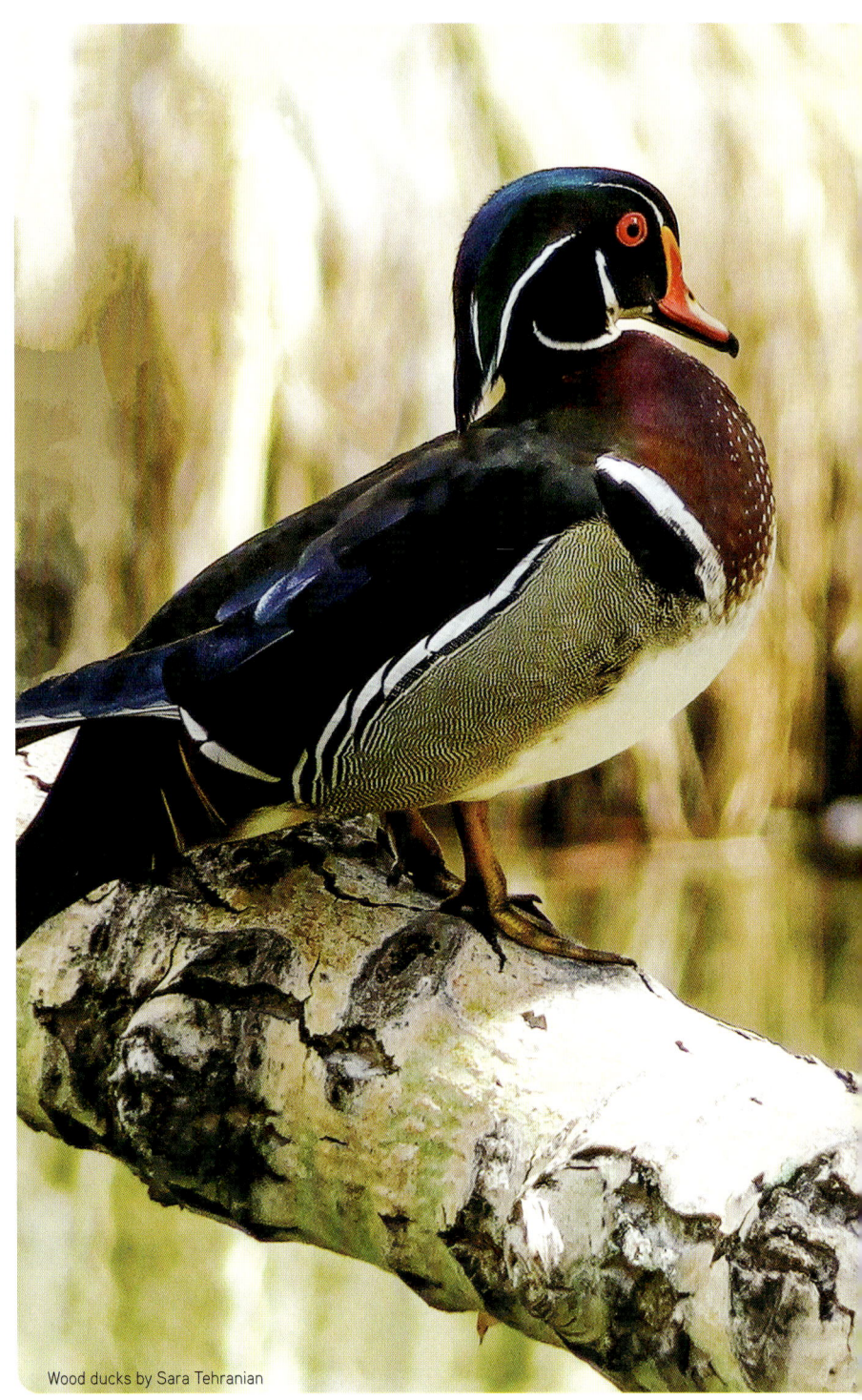
Wood ducks by Sara Tehranian

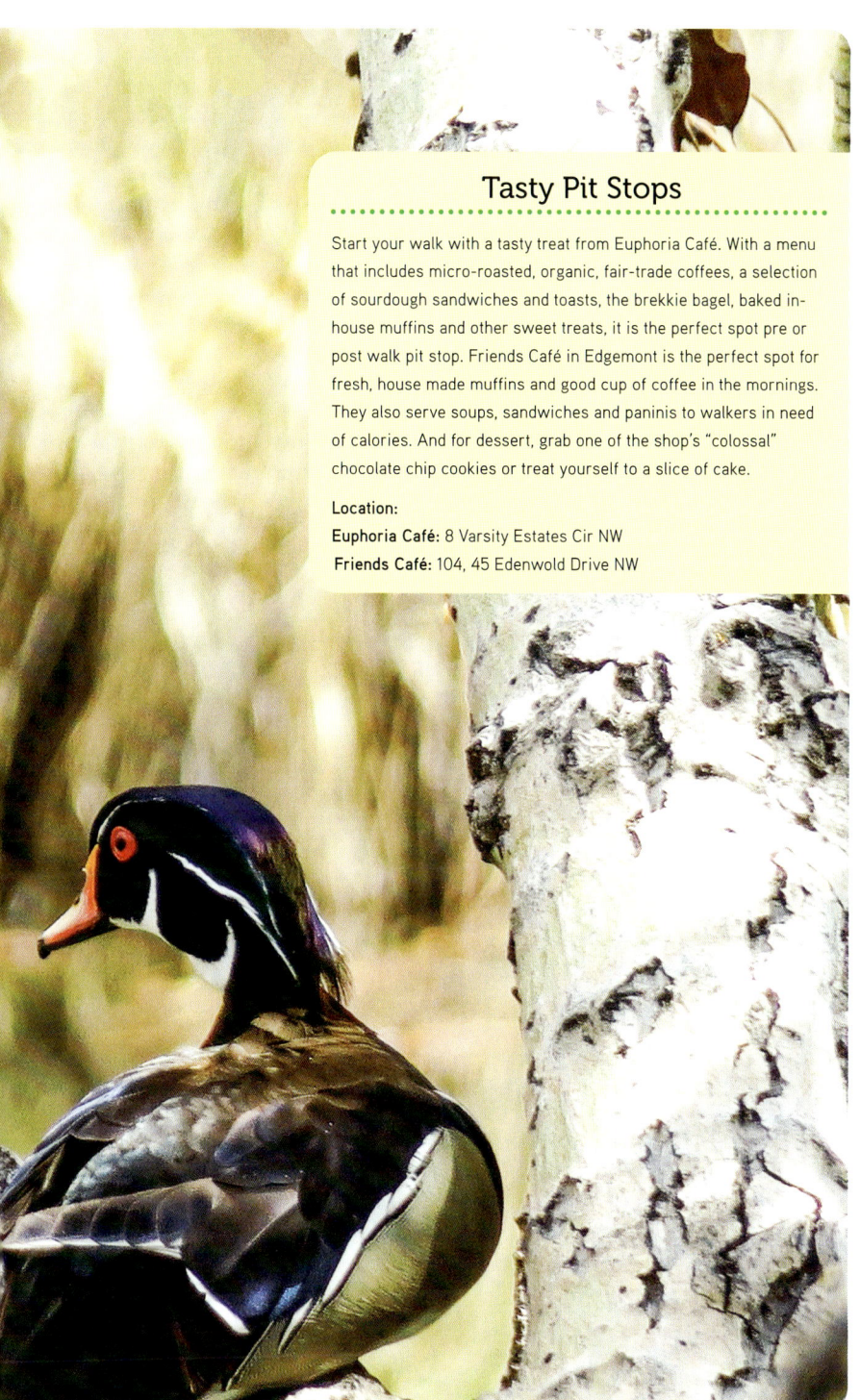

Tasty Pit Stops

Start your walk with a tasty treat from Euphoria Café. With a menu that includes micro-roasted, organic, fair-trade coffees, a selection of sourdough sandwiches and toasts, the brekkie bagel, baked in-house muffins and other sweet treats, it is the perfect spot pre or post walk pit stop. Friends Café in Edgemont is the perfect spot for fresh, house made muffins and good cup of coffee in the mornings. They also serve soups, sandwiches and paninis to walkers in need of calories. And for dessert, grab one of the shop's "colossal" chocolate chip cookies or treat yourself to a slice of cake.

Location:
Euphoria Café: 8 Varsity Estates Cir NW
Friends Café: 104, 45 Edenwold Drive NW

Nose Hill Park

Walks 28-30

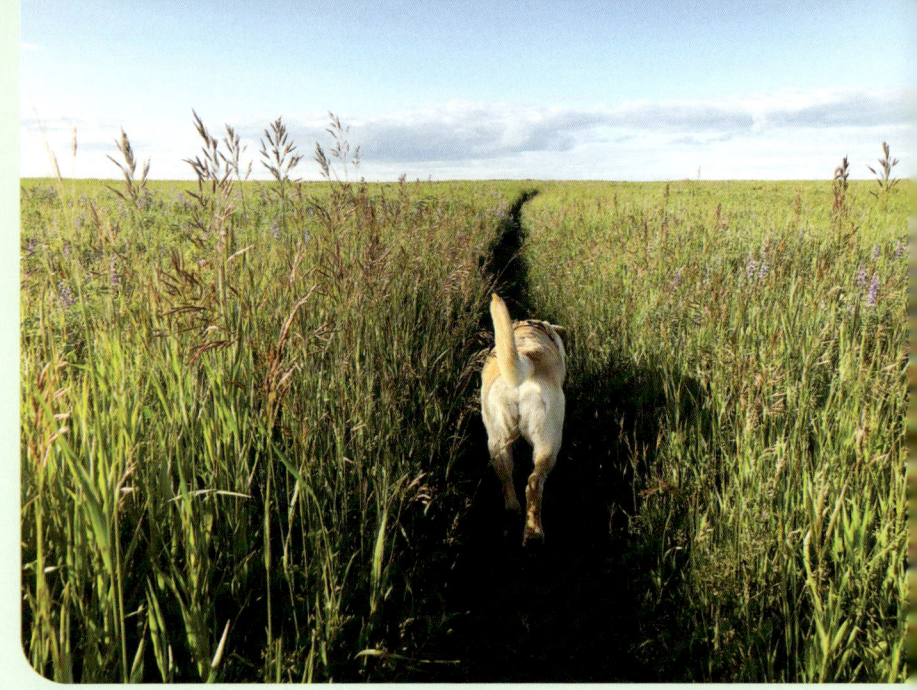

Walks at a Glance:

At 11 square km, Nose Hill Park is one of the largest municipal parks in Canada. It is also Calgary's highest point so be prepared for spectacular views. Once on top of the plateau, look around and you will see that Broadcast Hill (the hill where Canada Olympic Park is built) is also flat and at the same elevation as Nose Hill. Hills south of the city near Priddis are the same.

Details

Categories: Café, Dog, Nature, Hilly, Vistas, Birds

Start: Walks 28 and 29: Parking lot at Brisbois Drive and John Laurie Drive or John Laurie Drive and 14 Street or 64 Avenue and 14 Street; Walk 30: Parking lot at 14 Street and Berkley Drive NW or Shaganappi Trail and Edgemont Boulevard NW

Facilities: Year-round bathroom at Edgemont Drive and Shaganappi trail parking lot. Seasonal bathrooms at other parking lots. Get coffee, treats or lunch at Friends Café near Edgemont Parking lot (see description in Walk 27)

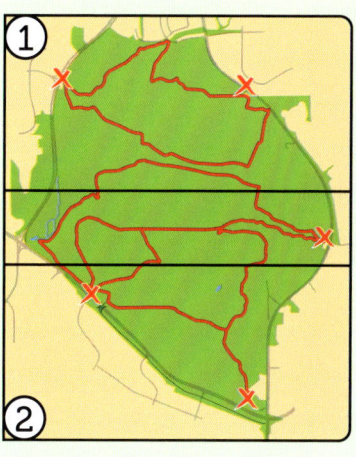

Distance & Difficulty

Walk 28: Many Owls Valley and Medicine Wheel: 7 km (stairs, hills, paved and gravel paths)

Walk 29: Mountain Views and Many Owls Valley: 9.5 km (hills, paved and gravel paths)

Walk 30: Porcupine Valley and Aspen Grove: 7.5 km (stairs, hills, paved and gravel paths)

Highlights, Detours & Destinations

Year-Round: Dogs love all the off leash on Nose Hill, but be mindful of the wildlife, like coyotes, porcupines and deer. If you are new to the hill, be aware that navigating can be a challenge. Pay attention to the landmarks and very cautious when walking in poor visibility (snowstorms, fog, or darkness). The power lines at the far north end of the hill extend from the Berkley Gate parking lot to the Edgemont parking lot. If you can see the airport, you are on the 14 Street side of the hill. In the southeast corner there is an antenna visible that is close to the 14 Street and Calgary Winter Club parking lots

Spring- Fall: Purple-headed prairie crocuses emerge on the 14 Street side of the hill in early April. Over 200 types of wildflowers blanket the hill through the summer. Birders can watch for the 170 plus species of birds that visit Nose Hill. Winter: Soak up the glorious snow drifted landscape

These plateaus are the remnants of a 60-million-year-old, swampy, forested landscape into which the Bow and Elbow rivers, and the glaciers that followed their valleys, have incised by 175 m. That is something to think about while you catch your breath.

The three walks in the book interconnect. Walk 28 begins in the southern part and climbs to the plateau where stunning downtown Calgary views from the Siksikaitsitapi Medicine Wheel are your reward. Walk 29 travels from east to west through meadows to mountain views while walk 30 explores the hilly north end, dipping

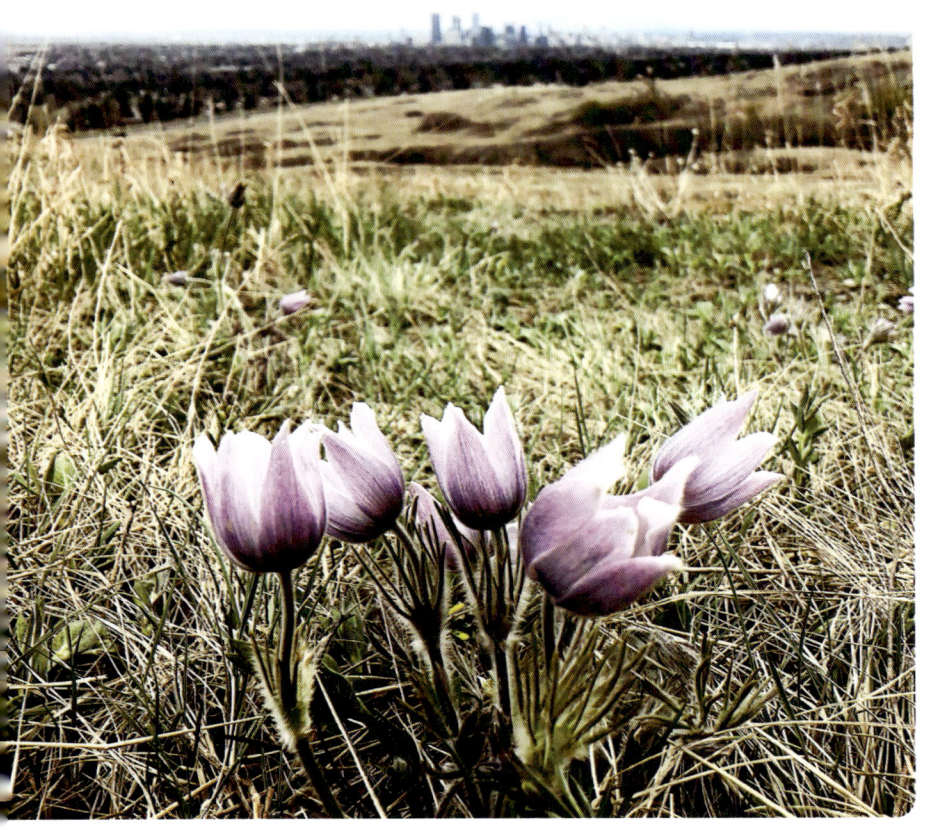

Grass Facts

Hardy grasses dominate the prairies and make up a large part of Nose Hill. These flowering plants are pollinated by the wind. They have no colourful flowers because they do not need to attract insects for pollination. Grasses benefit from grazing by large mammals like cattle and deer. Grazing removes the dead plants (the dry grass we see above ground) and allows the sun to reach new growth in the spring. Seeds eaten by grazing animals are dispersed, ready to go, with their own supply of fertilizer.

and climbing into shady aspen filled coulees and enjoying panoramic plateau views. Once you have the lay of the land you can create your own route or connect all three walks and make a day of it!

From April through October over 200 flowering plants colour the hill's landscape. Amongst the prairie grasses that dominate Nose Hill you'll also find mushrooms, mosses, and many animals. In the fall, shrubs and grasses become a kaleidoscope of rich red, burnt orange, and golden yellow. Learn more about all plants on Nose Hill from the Alberta Native Plant Council, @albertaplants on Instagram or www.anpc.ab.ca. Wildlife is abundant on the hill, and I often see coyotes, groups of mule deer and the occasional waddling porcupine at dusk. Dogs love the extensive off leash areas and birders should be excited to hear that over 170 bird species have been seen on Nose Hill - bring your binoculars.

All the walks offer superb views. And depending on where you are on the hill, you'll see the Front Range of the Rocky Mountains and the foothills, the prairies stretching out to the east, the compact downtown core rising prominently in the south and flights arriving and departing from the airport. Enjoy the solitude of this wilderness wonder in the heart of the city.

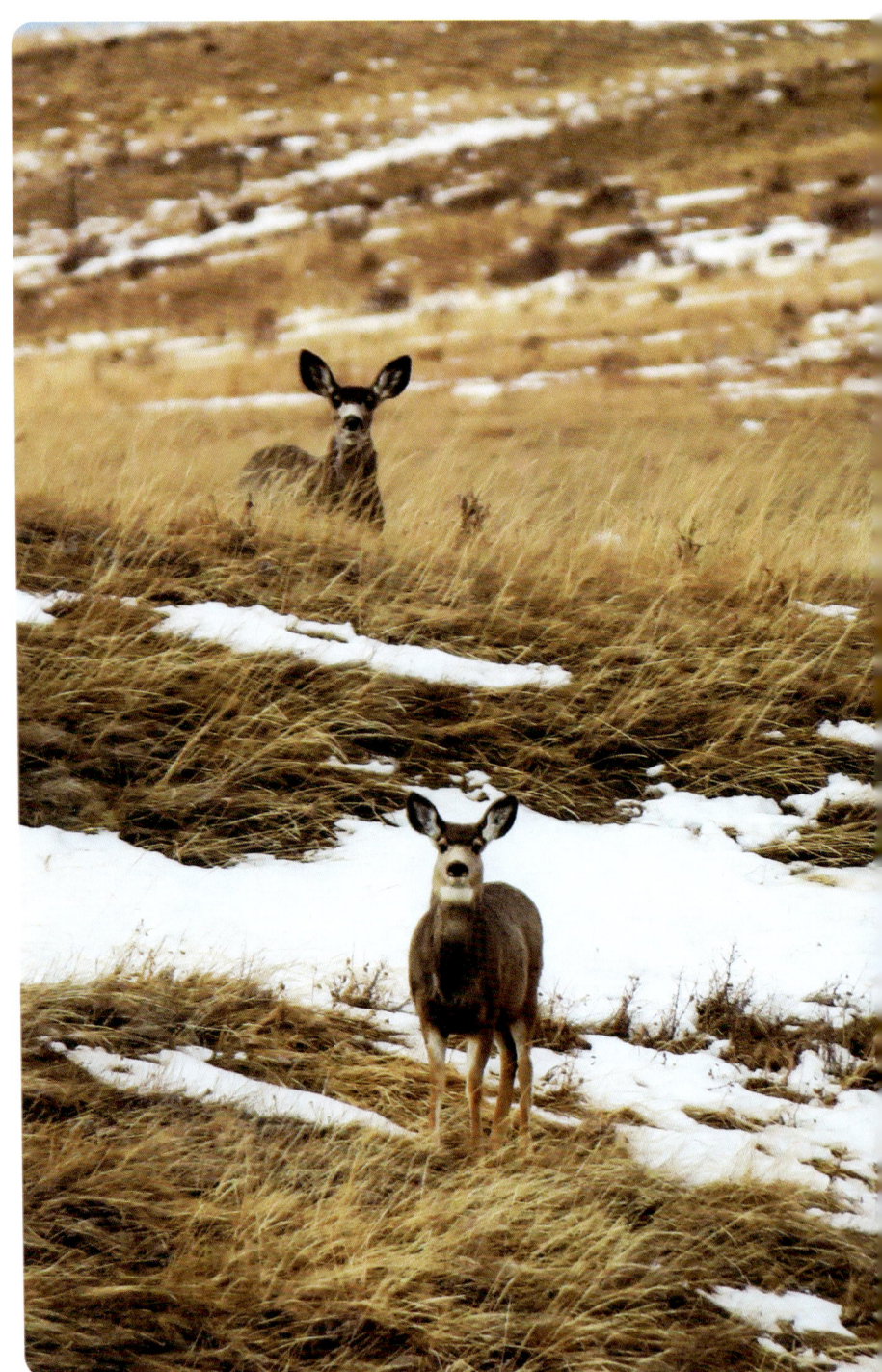

Mule Deer on Nose Hill by Sara Tehranian

Itchy Buffalo and Erratics

When the glaciers carved their way across Nose Hill, they left behind many large boulders known as glacial erratics, which bear no compositional resemblance to local rocks. One hundred years ago, buffalo roamed Nose Hill. In the spring, the buffalo would rub against these stones as they began to molt, trying to remove irritating hairs. You can see the evidence in the form of deep, smooth depressions and shiny spots that remain on the stones today.

Siksikaitsitapi Medicine Wheel

As you circle around the east side of Nose Hill, be sure to stop, reflect, and enjoy spectacular views from the Siksikaitsitapi Medicine Wheel. Built in 2015 by members of the Blood Nation, this modern landmark is a tribute to the historical and spiritual connection between people and the land, and it marks Nose Hill as part of the traditional Blackfoot territory. This new circle was arranged beside a half-buried circle of stones that was left behind by Indigenous scouts thousands of years ago. Medicine Wheels are ancient symbols used by various Indigenous peoples across North America for thousands of years. They represent the interconnectivity of all life, the various cycles of nature, and the spiritual belief system of the Indigenous peoples who created them. The Nose Hill Siksikaitsitapi Medicine Wheel is a tribute to these traditions, embodying the principles of harmony, balance, and respect for the environment. An important cultural site, everyone is welcome in the circle to reflect, meditate, or pray. It is suggested that you enter from the east side and leave to the west.

Nose Hill Park

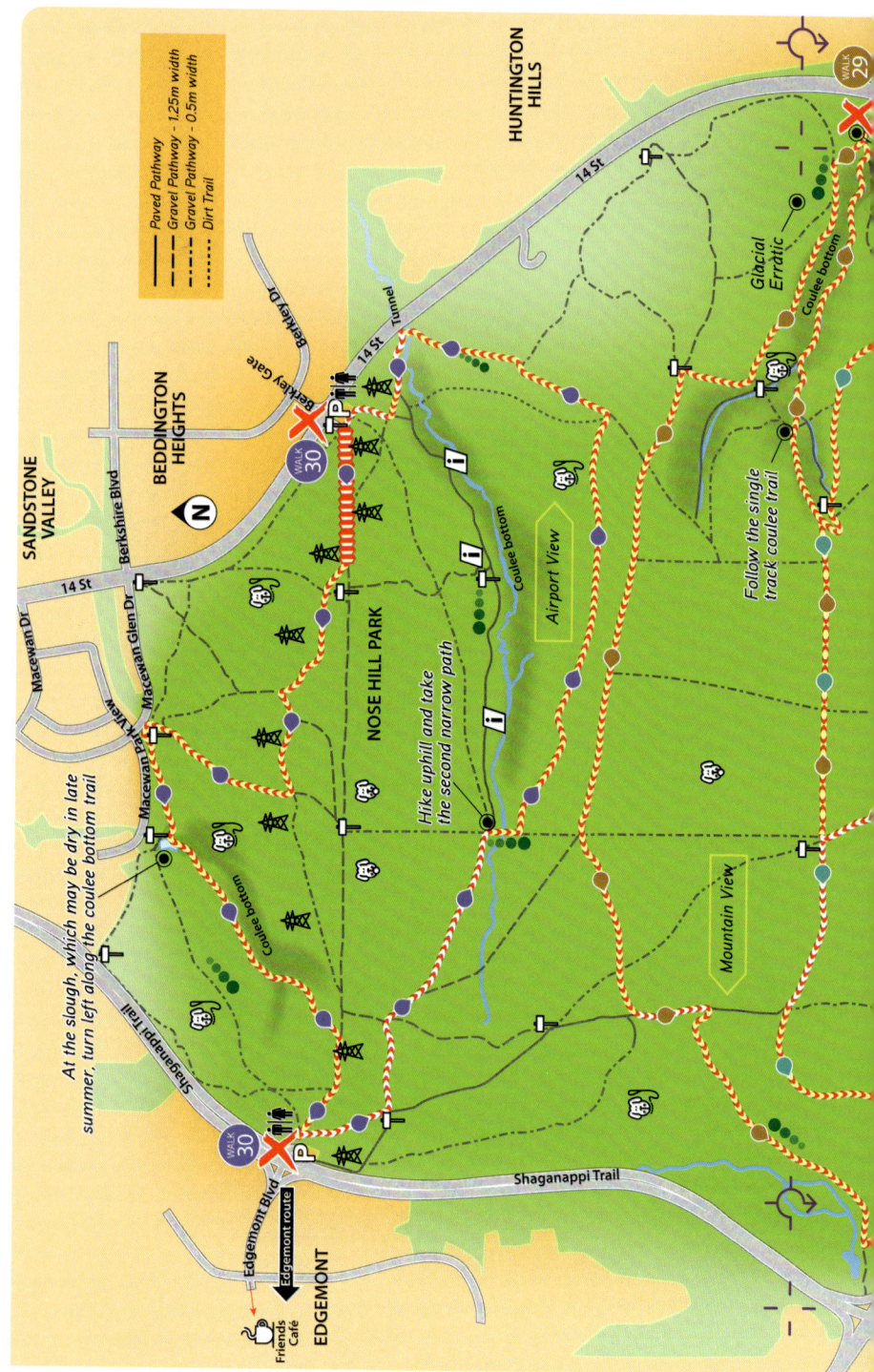

Nose Hill Park

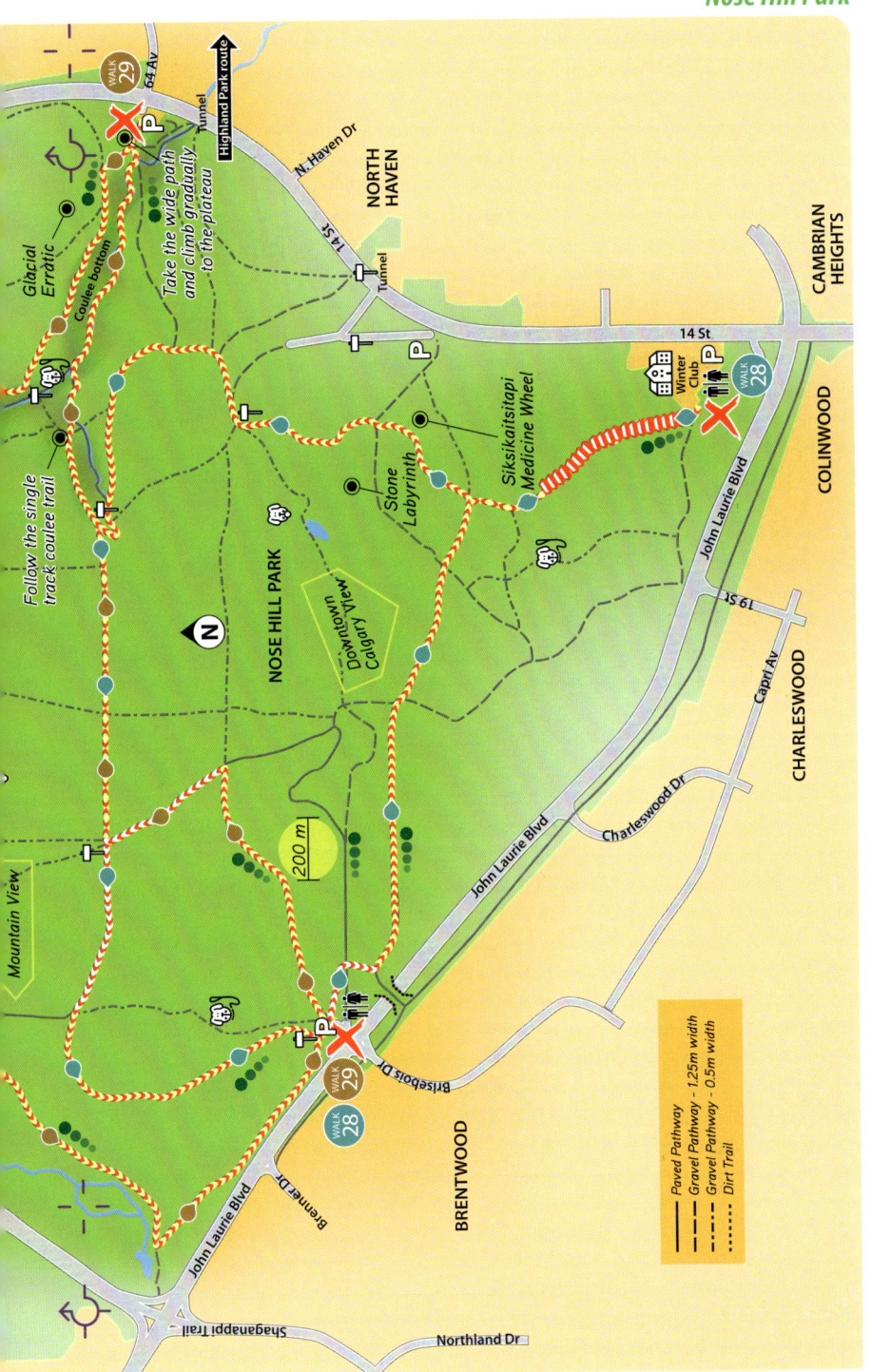

Huntington Hills, Nose Creek, Thorncliffe, Highland Park, Queens Park

Walks 31 and 32

NE

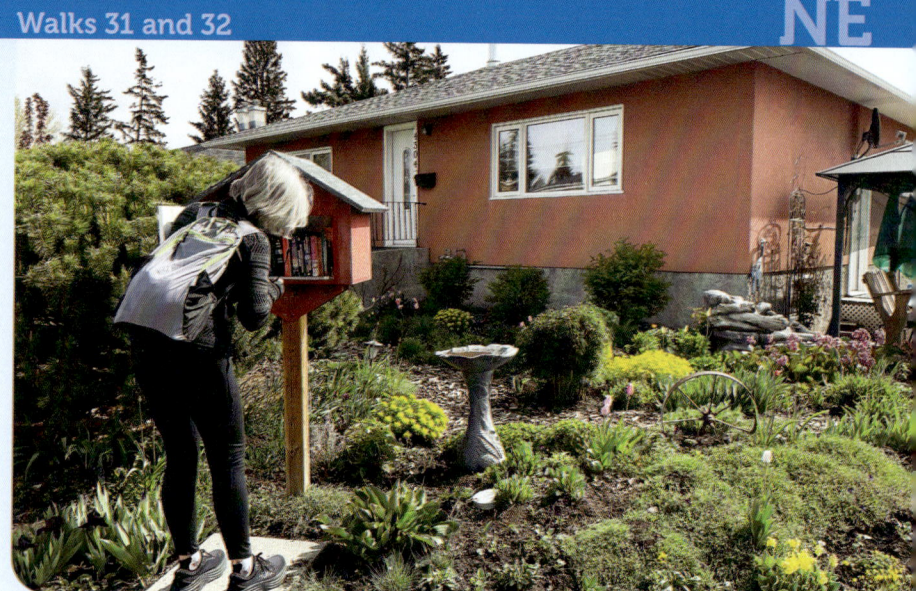

Walks at a Glance:

This I know is true: going for a walk makes me feel good, great in fact. In his book Happy City: Transforming Our Lives Through Urban Design, Charles Montgomery points out that the effects of walking on mental health are clear: "Walking works like a drug, bringing happiness to all who choose to take that first step". Starting out from two popular parks, both Walks 31 and 32 connect communities in interesting ways, with tunnels and cut through paths past schools, community centres and into green spaces and parks.

Details

Categories: Café, Dog, Nature, Neighbourhood & Parks, Hilly, Stroller, Vistas

Start: Walk 31: Nose Hill Parking lot, 14 Street and 64 Avenue NW; Walk 32: Confederation Park, 30 Avenue and 7 Street NW or Laycock Park, 5979, 6 Street NE

Facilities: Year-round bathroom, Confederation Park. Cafés, bakeries and a brewery along both walks

Distance & Difficulty

Walk 31: Nose Hill- Huntington Hills- Nose Creek – Thorncliffe: 8.5 km (sidewalks, paved pathways and single-track trails)

Walk 32: Cambrian Heights- Highland Park- Queens Park: 7.5 km (paved pathways and sidewalks)

Highlights, Detours & Destinations

Many cafés and diners nearby. Walk 31: Haven House Café; Walk 32: The Bullet Coffee House, Ola Luna Bakery Café, Deerhead Café Diner, Congress Coffee, Turca Breakfast House. See the sidebar for details.

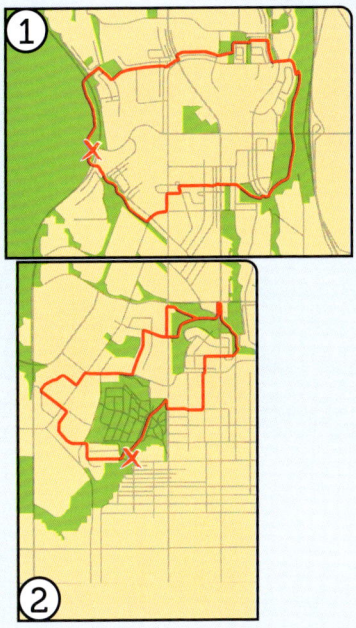

Walk 31 travels from Nose Hill to Nose Creek and into Laycock Park, a multi-use park with baseball diamonds, basketball courts and an accessible playground along the Nose Creek Pathway. It is named in honour of the Laycock family who pioneered agriculture in the Calgary area when Alberta was still part of the Northwest Territories. Climbing out of the Nose Creek Valley, Walk 31 continues through Greenview and Thorncliffe to Egert's Park. An alternate return route follows the pathway to North Haven and past a popular local café before connecting via tunnel to Nose Hill Park.

A neighbourhood hill climb is the start of Walk 32, which begins in Confederation Park. Big views of Calgary's downtown skyline are the reward in Cambrian Heights.

The walk continues along side streets, past homes and gardens, a bakery café and connects to an old golf course turned unofficial off leash park in Highland Park. Tasty detours and live music (see sidebar) tempt the walker to go east before retracing their steps to Queen's Park.

Connecting communities on foot is the best way to get to know a city and the sense of freedom and happiness that walking provides to everyone is simple and cheap. Let's walk!

Tasty Pit Stops

Coffee plus walking equals happiness! Walk 31 has an alternate route that leads you past Haven House Cafe, a cozy spot serving up lattes, coffee, tea, fresh baked goods, meat buns, sandwiches and snacks. They've also got an artisan market. Walk 32 passes by the Ola Luna bakery café that offers up scrumptious pastries, cake and other decadent desserts. A couple of outdoor tables make this a sit and stay option in the warmer months or a grab and go pastry and coffee when the weather is cool. Take a detour and walk east to the Deerhead Café, a cash only little hole in the wall diner with seating for perhaps a dozen or two. It's old school, unpretentious, plain and simple with a blue-collar working person's vibe. They're open for breakfast, brunch, and lunch to 3 p.m. Congress Coffee is a community-driven independent coffee house in the NE community of Tuxedo/Highland Park/Greenview. Capturing the heart of the café scene of the 1990s, Congress is a return to the basics – dark, rich coffee, great conversation, community-focused initiatives, and lots of live music. The Bullet Coffee House has coffee and baked goods to go, and picnic tables just outside. Turca Breakfast House serves up Turkish Cuisine that includes dishes such as gözleme (savory pastries), menemen (scrambled eggs with tomatoes and peppers) or simit (a sesame-crusted bread ring).

Location
Haven House Cafe: 1107 48 Avenue NW
The Bullet Coffee House: 728 Northmount Drive NW
Ola Luna Bakery Café: 1047 40 Avenue NW
Congress Coffee: 215, 36 Avenue NE
Deerhead Café (cash only): 3704 Edmonton Trail NE
Turca Breakfast House: 2604 4 Street NW

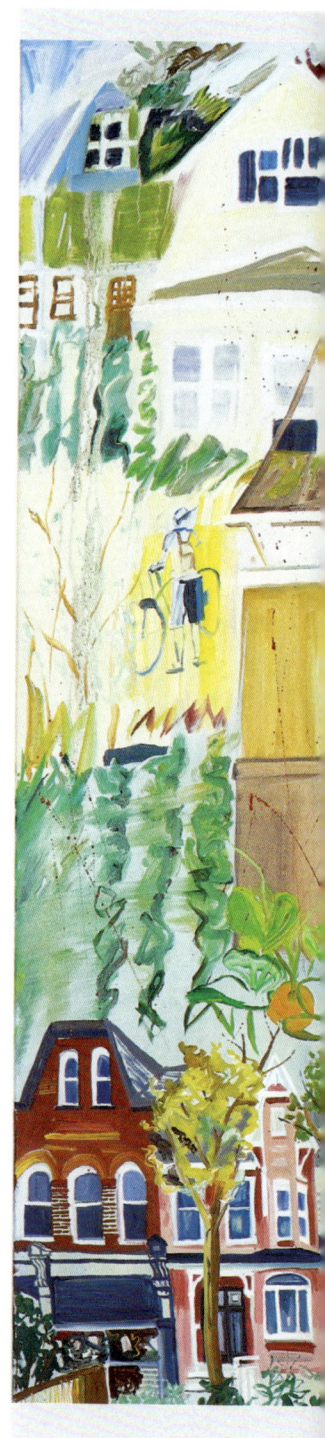

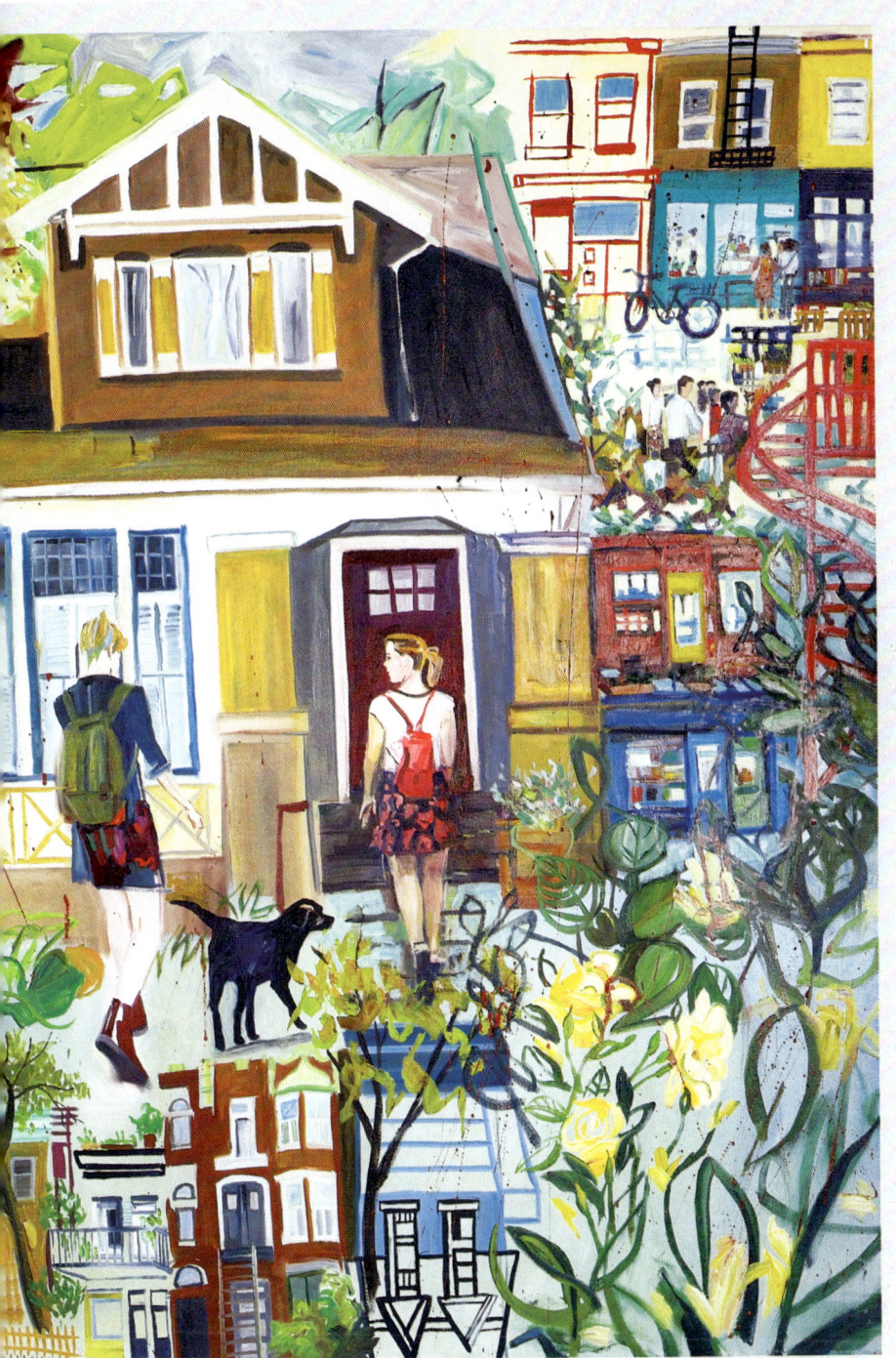

Within Walking Distance, Urban Garden Series by Jill Thomson

HUNTINGTON HILLS, NOSE CREEK,
THORNCLIFFE, HIGHLAND PARK, QUEENS PARK

Huntington Hills, Nose Creek, Thorncliffe, Highland Park, Queens Park

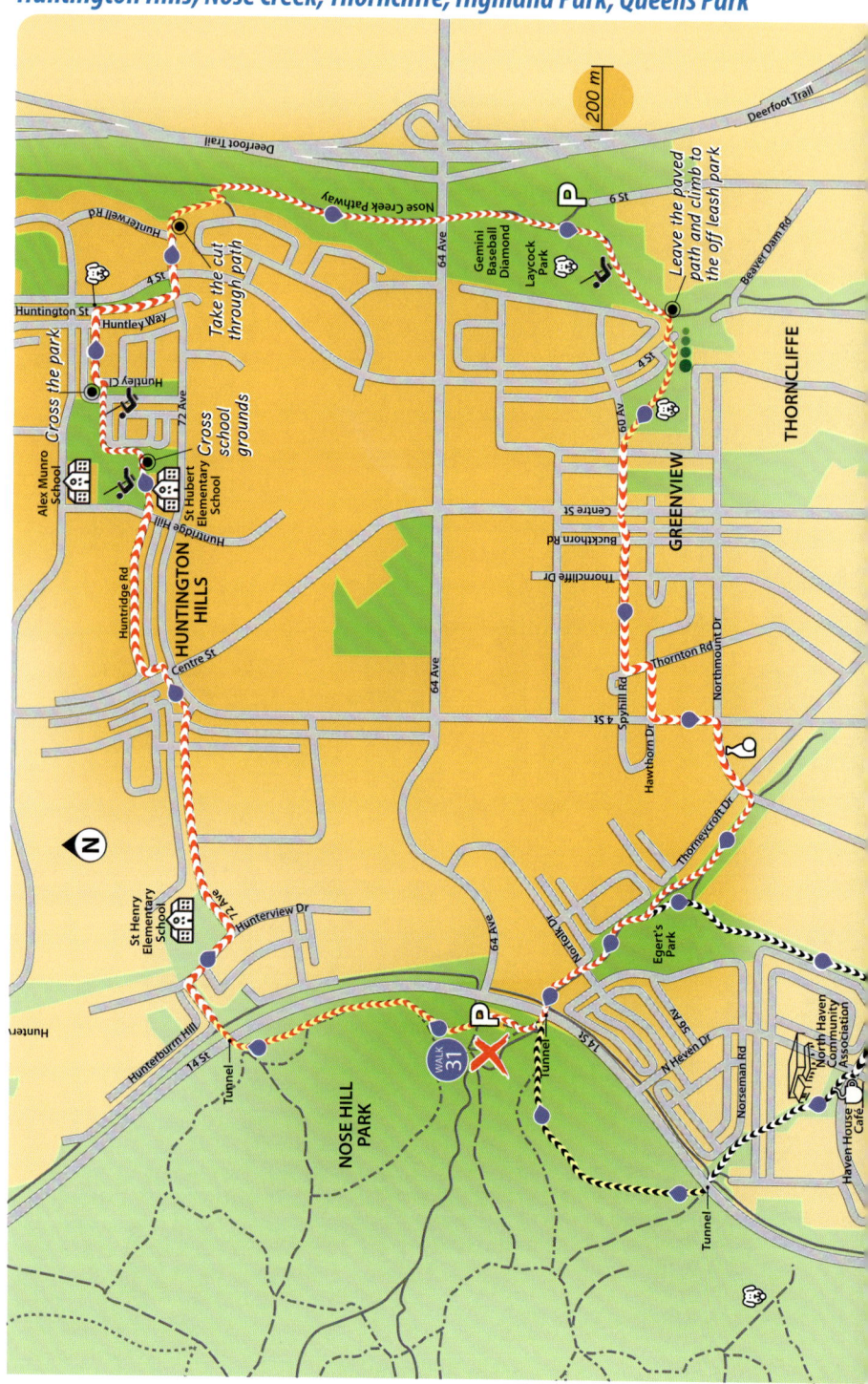

Huntington Hills, Nose Creek, Thorncliffe, Highland Park, Queens Park

West Nose Creek / Confluence Park

Walk 33   NE

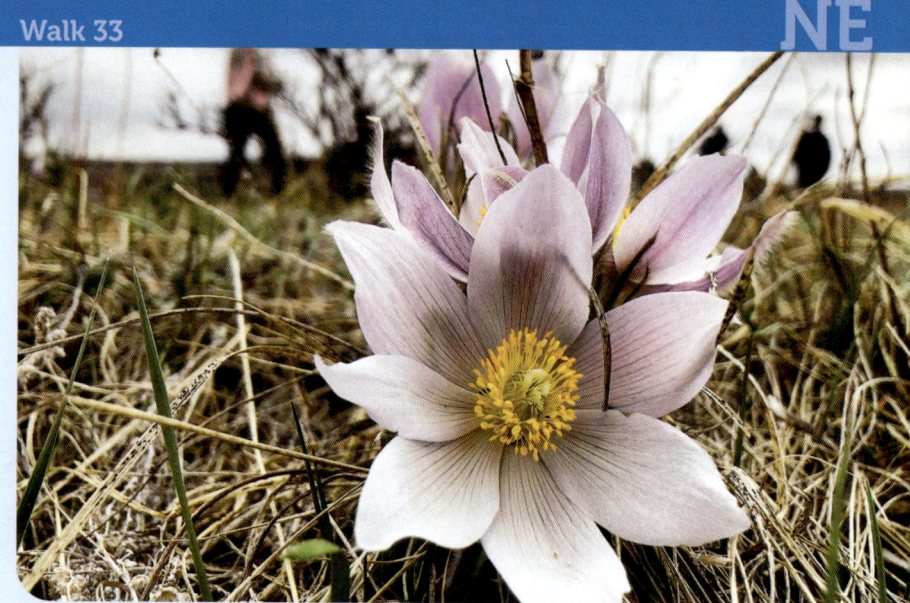

Walk at a Glance:

A burbling creek has cut a valley worthy of the river that it once was, offering you views of sandstone escarpments. The route follows paved and gravel paths just below busy city streets, but make no mistake, this is a wilderness walk. Meander along the valley floor, through rough fescue grassland, alongside and across Nose Creek.

The valley was forged by runoff from the last glaciation and, therefore, is considerably younger than the Bow and Elbow River valleys. Split Rock, a 2-m-high glacial erratic, is a significant feature along the route. Once part of Mount Edith Cavell in Jasper National Park, the boulder had a long ride on glaciers to arrive in Calgary.

Details

Categories: Dog, Nature, Hilly, Stroller, Vistas, River, Birds

Start: Official parking lot at the corner of Beddington Trail and Beddington Boulevard NE

Facilities: None

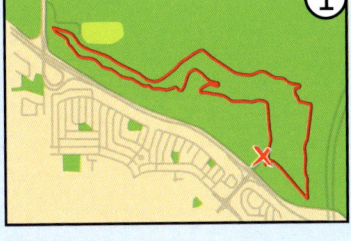

Distance & Difficulty

5 km (some hills, paved and gravel pathways)

Highlights, Detours & Destinations

There is a small off leash park at the start of this walk. Dogs and kids love to run in the unofficial trail network to the north of West Nose Creek

West Nose Creek Park is home to a riparian zone, a narrow green space along the edge of a body of water. The diverse group of plants and animals found in this habitat are different from those a few metres away on either side. You'll walk past willows along the riverbanks and shrubs along the north-facing slope. Keep an eye out for beavers. The park is one of the best locations in Calgary to view beaver dams and lodges. Birders will be pleased to learn that a variety of waterfowl, and several species of swallows and raptors call West Nose Creek Park home.

West Nose Creek / Confluence Park

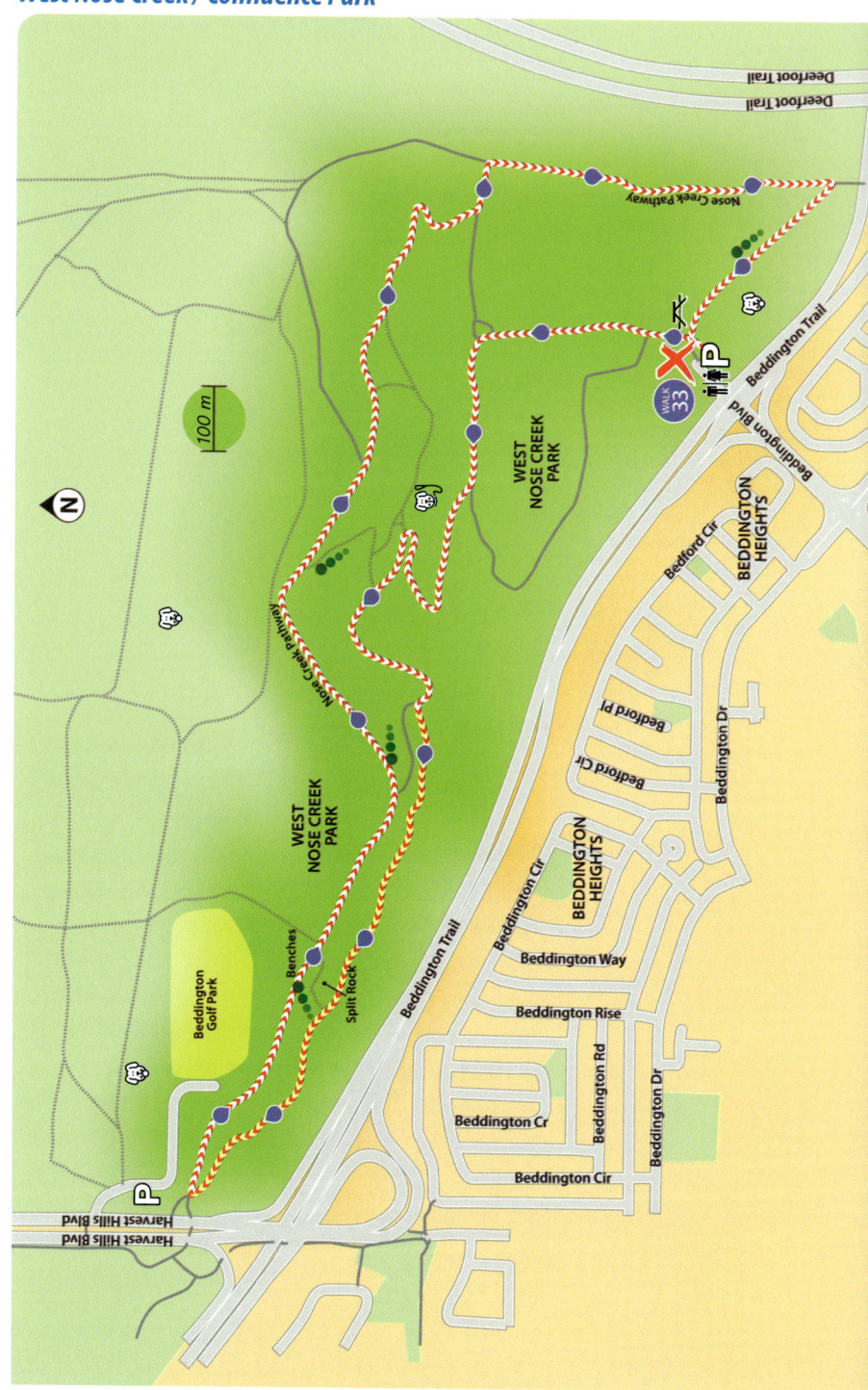

Interpretive signs along the route offer historical tidbits. One to note is that a stone quarry operated near the west end of the park for many years, and stone from the quarry was used to build many of the historic buildings in Calgary: the first and second courthouses, the McDougall Block in the downtown core, and Victoria and King Edward schools, to name a few.

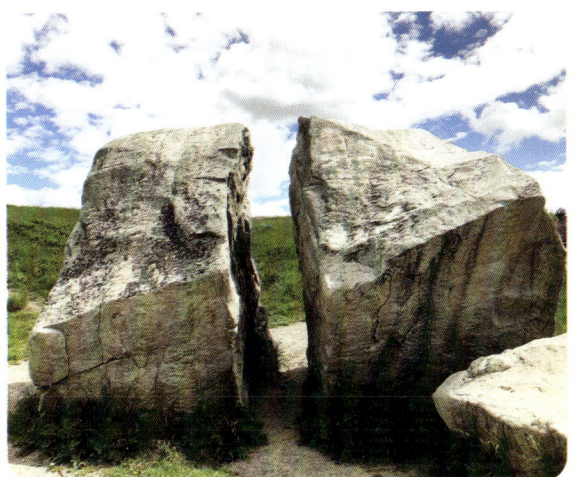

West Nose Creek Park

Add a Bounce to Your Step to Feel Happy

Feeling glum? Add a bounce to your step on your next walk. If you walk like a happy person, light on your feet, shoulders back, head up, and arms relaxed and swinging by your side, then you will feel happier. We know that going for a walk, even a short walk, can make us feel better. Research shows that the mood benefits of regular, modest exercise, including walking, are a result of improved brain function, perhaps due to increased blood flow to the brain. A study published in the Journal of Behaviour Therapy and Experimental Psychiatry suggests your gait may also affect your frame of mind. The study adds to the growing body of research regarding the power of body language on the mind. Previous studies have shown that you can reduce stress and feel happier simply by smiling. Want to feel more confident and assertive? Practice some "power poses" like leaning over a desk with hands planted in front you. If you walk like a depressed person, slumped shoulders, head positioned forward, and only swinging your arms slightly, you are more inclined to focus on the negative. Depression can be a self-perpetuating cycle: because you feel bad, you remember bad things, and because you remember bad things, you feel bad. So, think like an actor and get into character. Project to the world how you want feel, even if you do not feel that way inside. Walk like a happy person, and you will feel happier.

Winston Heights - Renfrew - Tuxedo Park - Nose Creek - Vista Heights

Walk 34 NE

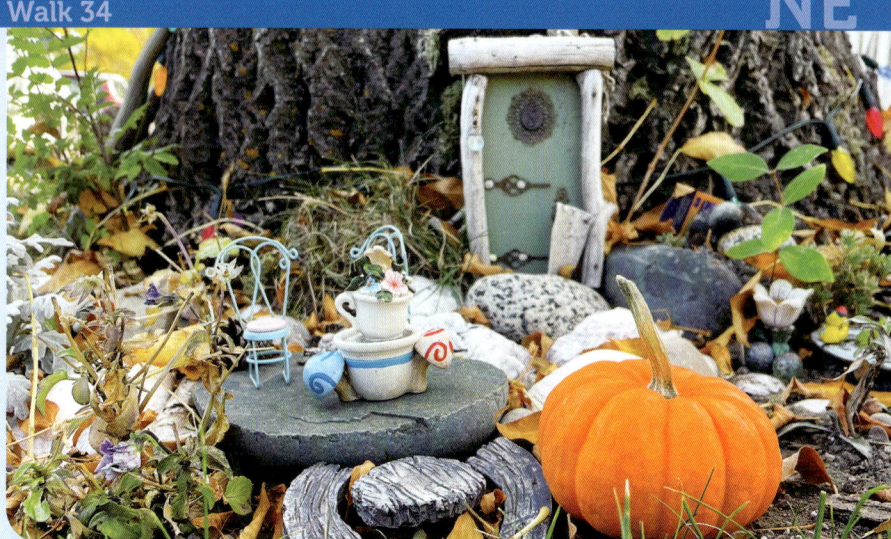

Walk at a Glance:

Larger than life: that is my first impression when I look west from Airways Park in Vista Heights. From this northeast viewpoint, the Rocky Mountains tower above Calgary's compact core. Walking the paved path along the escarpment, you hear the roar of a jet engine flying just above your head. Is the plane landing on the pathway? It's an exciting walk already!

The Calgary International Airport is just north, and the flights arriving and departing are steady. This is not surprising since Calgary is a hotbed of economic activity, a destination for work and recreation. Continue down the winding trail, cross over Calgary's busiest highway and continue south along the Nose Creek Pathway, a pleasant strip of nature that runs parallel to Deerfoot Trail.

Details

Categories: Café, Dog, Nature, Neighbourhood & Parks, Hilly, Stroller, Vistas, River, Birds

Start: Winston Heights / Mountview Community Association, 520 27 Avenue NW or Vista Heights, Vista Street near Valleyview Road NE

Facilities: None

Distance & Difficulty

Winston Heights start: 9.5 km (hilly, paved and gravel paths)

Vista Heights start: 7.5 km (hilly, paved and gravel paths)

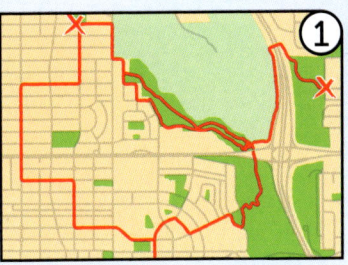

Deerfoot Trail, Calgary's fastest freeway, was aptly named after the runner, Api-kai-ees, a Siksika long distance runner who became a local hero in Calgary's early days. He was recruited by a syndicate of local gamblers around the time Calgary was incorporated as a town in 1884. The syndicate started calling him Deerfoot. Described as a "human thunderbolt" he more than lived up to the name as he defeated racers from as far away as Europe.

Climb the switchback path to the community of Renfrew. Developed in the 1940s, Renfrew is now an inner-city neighbourhood that is attractive for its sense of community and convenient location. During the Second World War, Renfrew was home to the Royal Canadian

Winston Heights - Renfrew - Tuxedo Park - Nose Creek - Vista Heights

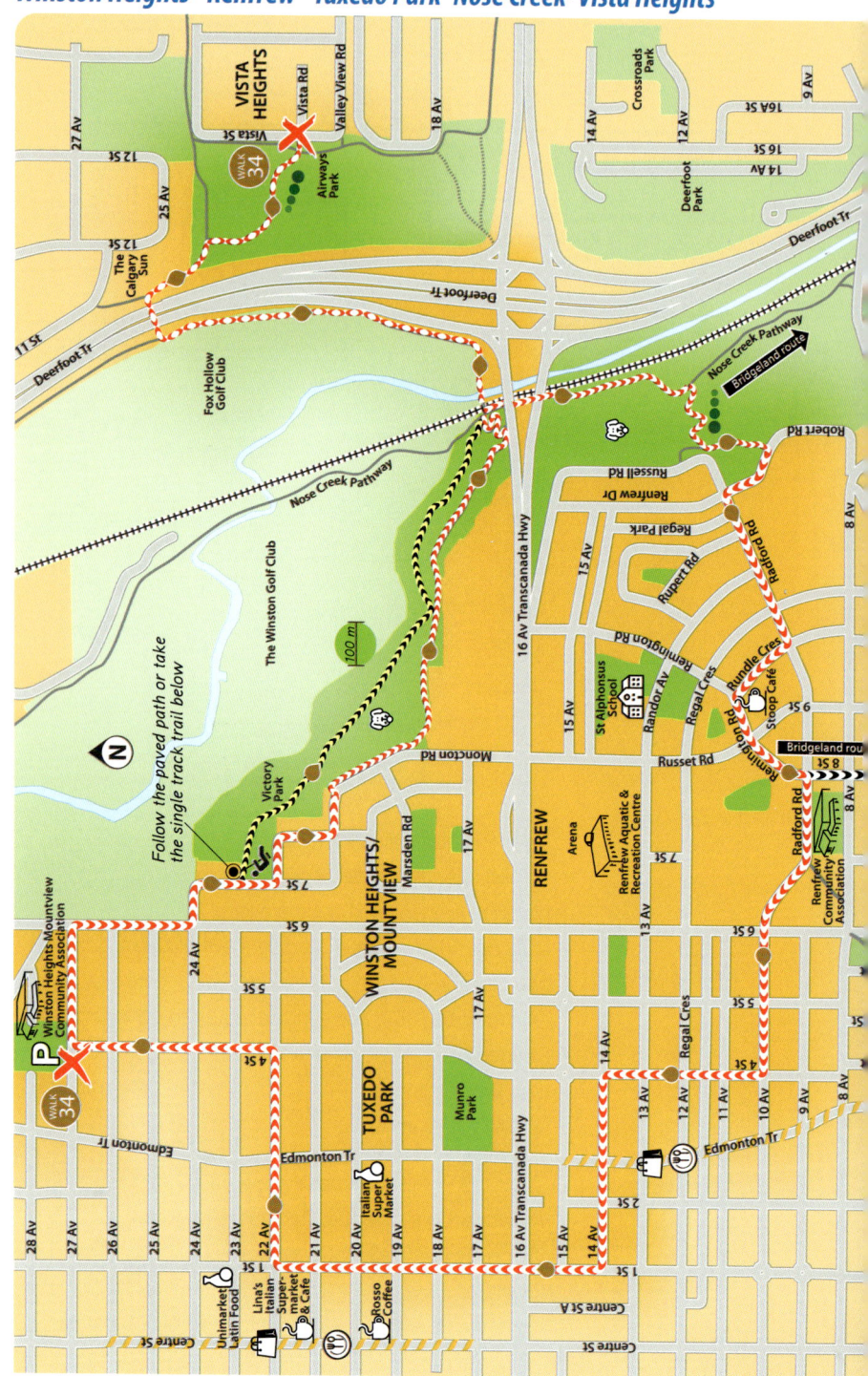

Air Force training base and the Calgary Airport. You'll notice that the community's original homes stand out for their conservative size as new builds rise up and out, expanding to fill lots. The tree canopy spreads across many streets, creating an urban forest. Cross Edmonton Trail, a street with all services and some interesting shops. Meander farther along Renfrew's side streets before crossing the Trans Canada into Tuxedo Park.

Walk east through neighbourhoods in transition. Proximity to Calgary's core means that real estate in Winston Heights / Mountview is increasing in value, and new homes reach high and wide alongside the 1950s bungalows and small wartime houses. You are now back at the Nose Creek Valley escarpment, where you can choose the off-leash single-track path or the paved path along the top of the slope. Descend into the Nose Creek valley and enjoy the slow pace of the creek before the sensory explosion of Deerfoot hits and you climb back into the roar of Calgary's success.

Tasty Pit Stops

Plan a stop at the Stoop Café in Renfrew. This local hotspot that is tucked into the neighbourhood is known for their breakfast sandwiches. They have many other types as well like spicy Capicollo paninis, fig jam and cheese, to roast beef. Rosso Coffee in Tuxedo Park has excellent coffees, baked goods and a nice sitting area make this a top-notch choice. Or drop by Lina's Market Café which features pastas, pizzas, pastries, tiramisu, specialty coffees, and gelato. Enjoy a sit-down breakfast inside or on the patio, a lunch or dinner in the café or pick up a homemade pizza, some veggies, fruit, bread and cheese and a mini tiramisu and have a picnic en route. Prepared lasagna, pasta sauces, and tiramisu are all made on site. Or grab some bread, meat, and cheese and have a picnic. Rows of quality Italian ingredients provide all you need for dinner planning. Continue your walk, well fed and happy.

Location:
Lina's: 2202 Centre Street N
Rosso: 2102 Centre Avenue N
Stoop Café: 1027 Russet Road NE

Bridgeland - Bow River - Nose Creek

Walk 35 NE

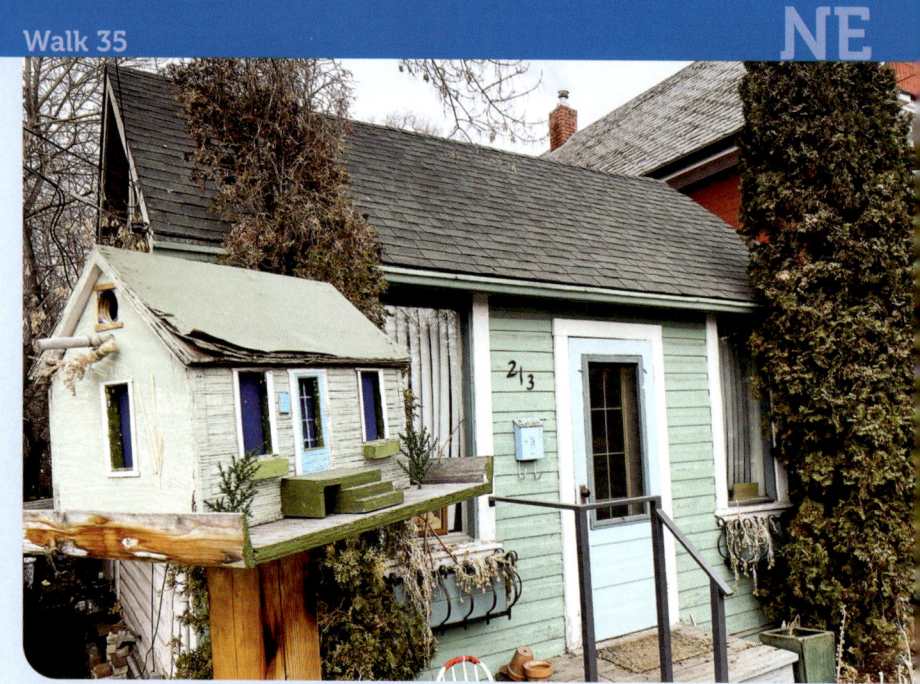

Walks at a Glance:

Bridgeland has a character that comes partly from its immigrant history and partly from rejuvenation. Germans and Russians who moved to Canada in the 1880s and decided to make their start in Calgary were the first people to settle in Bridgeland (then Riverside), where land was cheap. The area became known as Germantown, then, at the beginning of the twentieth century, Little Italy –a name that still resonates– when the immigrant population in the area included many Italians, as well as Ukrainians.

Details

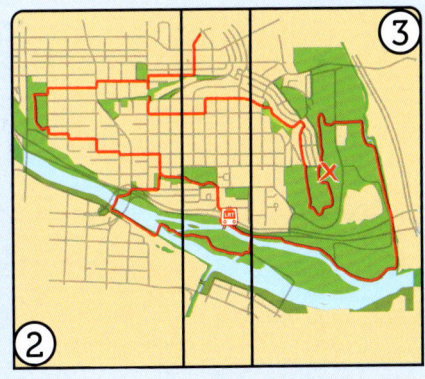

Categories: LRT, Café, Dog, Nature, Neighbourhood & Parks, People watch & shop, Hilly, Stroller, Historic, Vistas, River, Birds

Start: Tom Campbell's Hill, Child Avenue and Hill Road NE

LRT: Bridgeland or Zoo Stations

Facilities: None

Distance & Difficulty

9.5 km (hills, stairs, sidewalks, and paved pathways)

Highlights, Detours & Destinations

Keep watch for a possible moose sighting while passing the Calgary Zoo. Dogs love all the off leashing in Tom Campbell's Hill. Extend your off-leash time by walking north along Nose Creek Pathway from Tom Campbell's Hill. Pups can run free from the Renfrew off leash to the Winston Heights off leash

Today, the community is a mix of homes that date back to the early 1900s, modern abode and condo towers. This inner-city neighbourhood that was historically inexpensive, a working-class community, is now settled by people who love the central location. Because the neighbourhood is conveniently situated along the LRT line as well as the Bow River Pathway, its residents take advantage of public transit and self-propelled travel.

Our route follows the Bow River Pathway east, past the Canadian Wilds enclosure at the Calgary Zoo, which is visible from the main pathway. As you pass by, keep an eye out for the moose and grizzly bears that live in

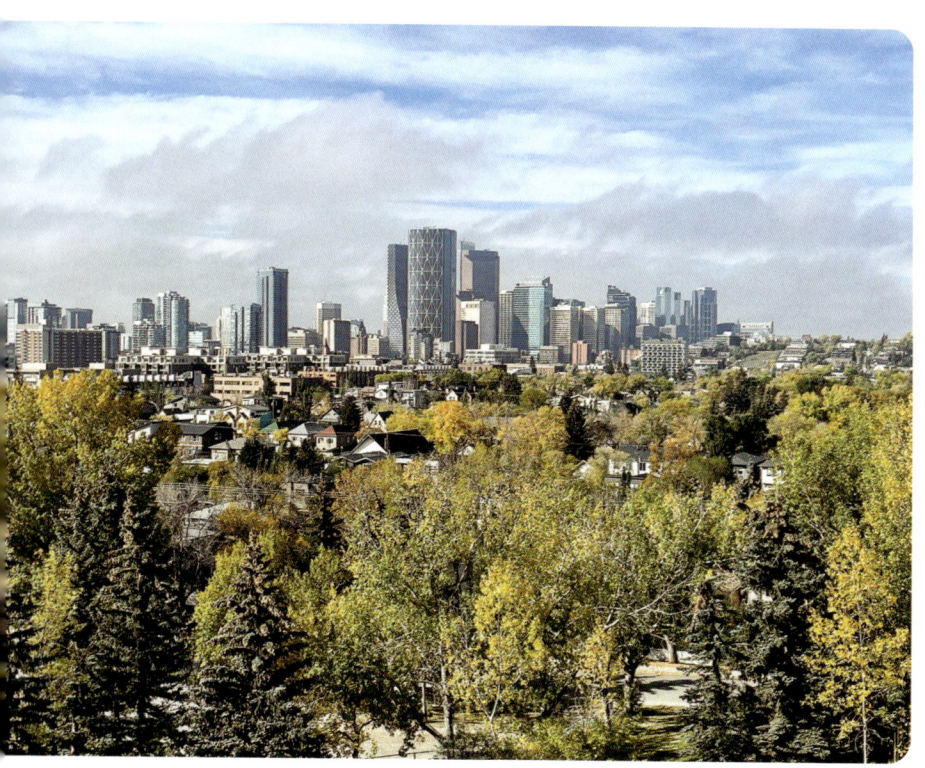

Biophilic Bridgeland: The Urban Forest

From the escarpment trail above Bridgeland, it is hard to see the streets and houses for all the trees. Researchers call this a "biophilic community" or "green streets," where nature is integrated into the community from the ground up. Urban forests that canopy streets and include pocket-sized green spaces are the norm in Calgary's older neighbourhoods thanks to William Pearce and William Reader, two of Calgary's early parks superintendents. William Pearce envisioned a city of trees, and he devoted a lot of time and effort to develop the early boulevard plantings and parks that make the inner-city neighbourhoods great places to walk. You can thank him for the boulevard of trees along Memorial Drive. William Reader was also responsible for planting hundreds of trees, despite tough economic times in the early 1900s, a lack of water, harsh winters, and dehydrating Chinook winds. Studies have shown that green streets lead to positive health outcomes; residents are healthier, more productive, and more generous. Nature is good for us, and a canopy of green is the one reason that walking in these areas is so pleasing, so enjoyable. Biophilic Bridgeland, from sidewalk to treetop, is a natural urban oasis.

the enclosure. The pathway turns north and becomes the quieter Nose Creek Pathway. At Telus Spark (the science centre), walk up to the top of Tom Campbell's Hill, an off-leash natural park. The hill's name originates from a large sign that stood for many years advertising Tom Campbell's Hats. Soak up the views and pat a few pooches before continuing into the neighbourhood. A pathway along the edge of the escarpment offers a bird's eye view of the leafy streets of Bridgeland. Look for the landmark, copper-domed, Ukrainian Catholic Church. The church marks the set of stairs that you'll climb to the next viewpoint.

As condo towers rise up and Bridgeland and surrounding communities become more compact, independent shops and restaurants enjoy success along First Avenue and Edmonton Trail. Density brings variety, followed by life on the streets. Bridgeland is bustling, a place to see and be seen. Grab an ice cream, a freshly roasted coffee or a picnic supper and soak up the sights in this wonderful inner-city neighbourhood.

Tasty Pit Stops

Bridgeland has many spots to replenish lost calories. From Spring through Fall check out the Farmer's Market at the Bridgeland Riverside Community Association on Murdoch Park. It runs Thursdays from 3:30-7:30 pm. Relax with an ice cream at Made by Marcus, Village Ice Cream, or the best soft serve ice cream and coffee at Lukes. Drop by Bike and Brew, Bono Ethiopian Coffee Roasters, Baya Rica Café or Phil and Sebastian for your coffee hit or visit the Bridgeland Distillery for cocktails and spirits. Fuel up on ramen at Shiki Menya or sushi at IKUSA Izakaya and the Tokyo Market. Or drop into the Bridgeland Market for all your picnic needs, fresh breads and other baking, cheeses, meats, dips, fruit and veggies, they have everything you need. Grab a seat in the common area on First Avenue or at Murdoch Park and watch the world go by.

Bridgeland - Bow River - Nose Creek

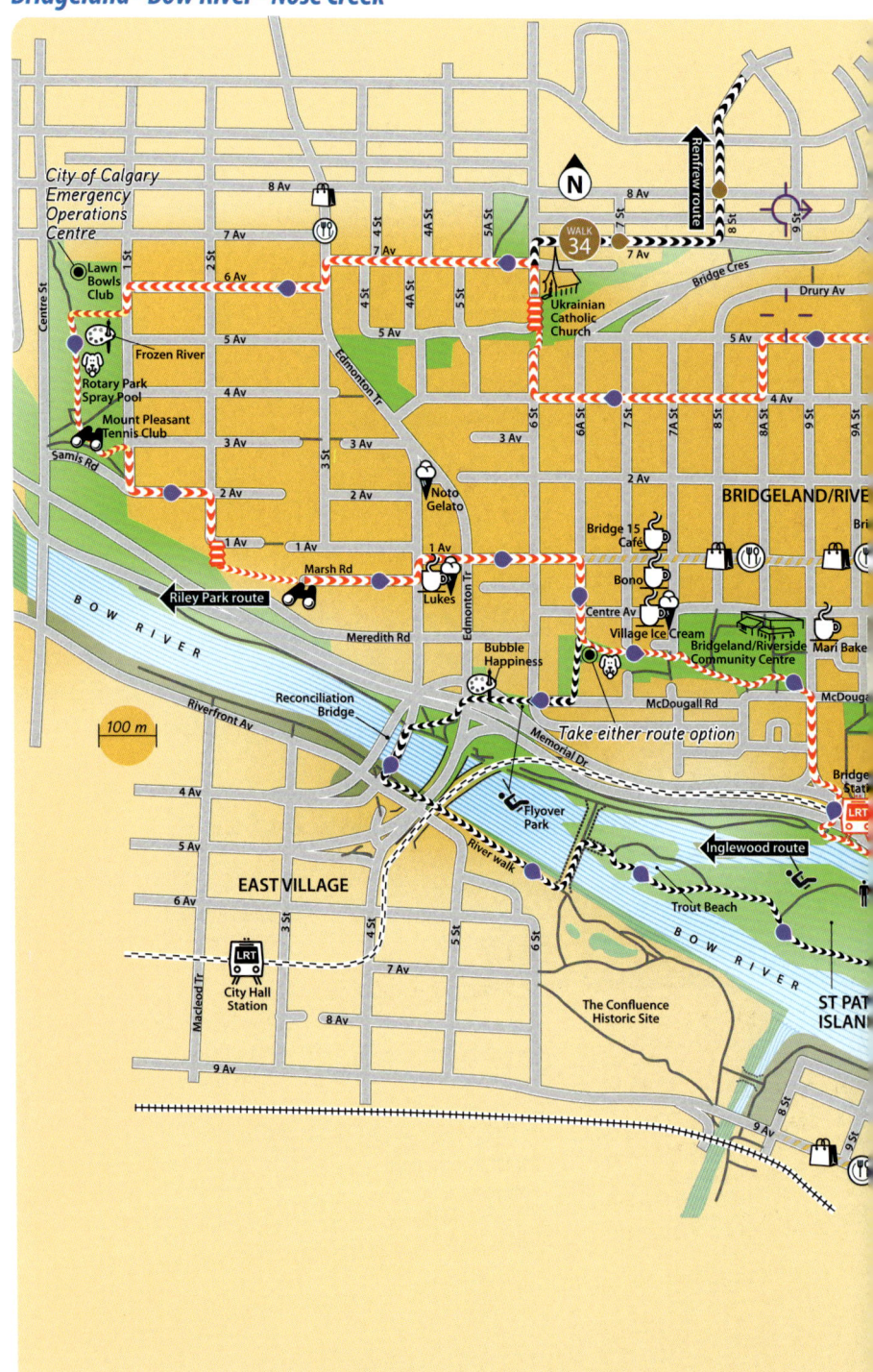

Bridgeland - Bow River - Nose Creek

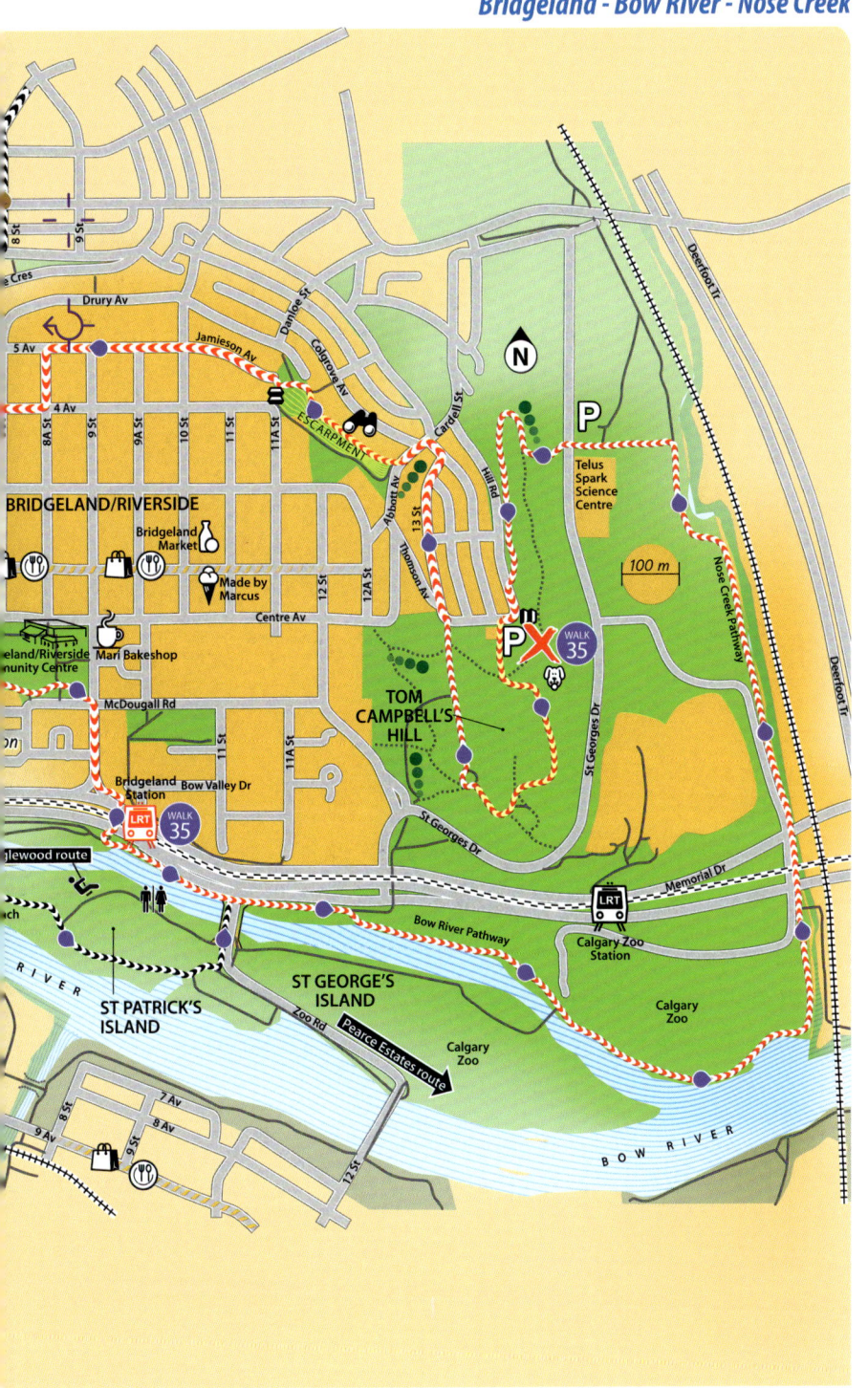

Confederation Park - Capitol Hill - Mount Pleasant - Crescent Heights - SAIT

Walks 36-39

NW

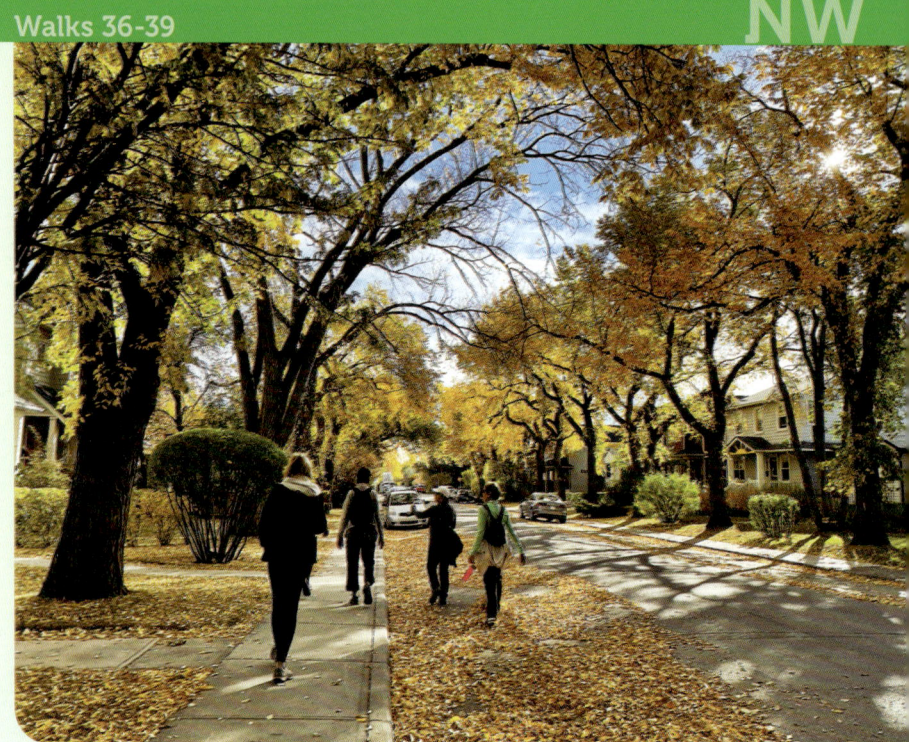

Walks at a Glance:

Paved pathways that wind beneath the poplars and alongside the creek, Confederation Park is a popular year-round destination for walking, running, and biking.

Once known as the "Coulee of the North," Confederation Park was molded and sculpted into gently sloped and contoured hillsides in celebration of Canada's Centennial in 1967. While the park's theme is oriented around the naturally occurring stream and coulee, the

Details

Categories: LRT, Café, Dog, Nature, Neighbourhood & Parks, People watch & shop, Hilly, Stroller, Historic, Vistas, Birds

Start: Walks 36, 37 and 39: The 30 Avenue parking lot, just south of 7 Street; Walk 38: Riley Park official parking lot at the end of 8 Avenue and 12 Street NW

LRT: Sunnyside or Lions Park Stations

Facilities: Bathroom at Confederation Park and seasonal bathroom at Riley Park. SAIT has bathrooms and a coffee shop

Distance & Difficulty

Walk 36: Confederation Park- Triwood- Rosemount: 7.5 km (some hills, paved paths and sidewalks)

Walk 37: Confederation Park - Capital Hill - Mount Pleasant: 8 km (mostly flat, paved pathways and sidewalks)

Walk 38: SAIT- Confederation Park- Mount Pleasant- Rosedale: 6 km (some hills, sidewalks and paved paths)

Walk 39: Confederation Park: 6 km (mostly flat, paved pathways)

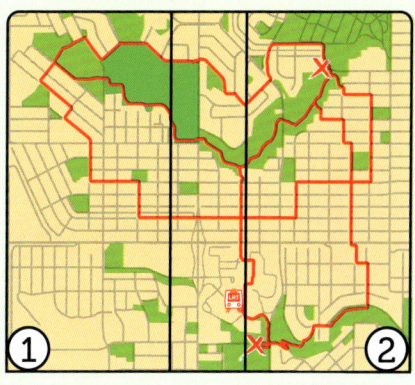

Highlights, Detours & Destinations

Christmas lights are brilliant in December at the Lion's Festival of Lights in Confederation Park Golf Course along Fourteenth Street. Bring your cross-country skis and your toboggan. Ski trails are track-set by Foothills Nordic Ski Club in Confederation Park Golf Course when snow is abundant. Check www.foothillsnordic.ca for trail and track-setting updates. Tobogganers should use the hill at the 10 Street NW parking lot, on the north side of park immediately west of Rosemont Community Centre. Confederation Park is the perfect spot for a picnic. There are picnic tables throughout the park or bring a blanket and spread out on the grass. Bring your swim gear and drop by the Mount Pleasant outdoor pool in July and August, located at 23 Avenue and 6 Street NW

park's design concept comes from a landscape style known as Picturesque, originating in England in the 18th century and still influencing the landscape architect profession today.

Serene and peaceful, all the walks travel through the park where creekside balsam poplars thrive, and shrubs like water birch, red-osier dogwood, and several species of willow provide habitat for a variety of ducks, geese, and gulls along with muskrats and many winged invertebrates like butterflies and dragonflies.

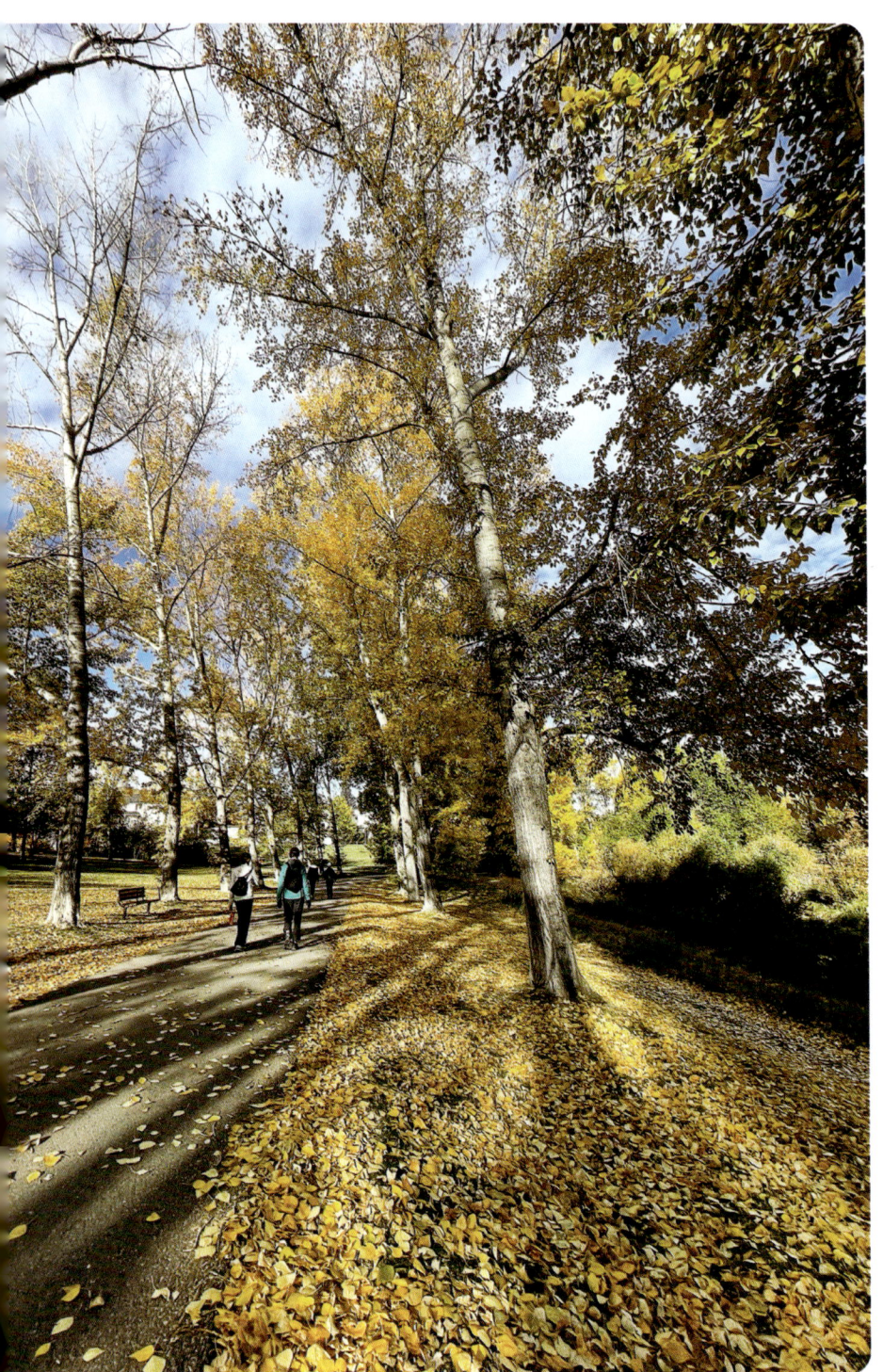

Walk 39 loops around Confederation Park, while Walks 36, 37 and 38 connect communities to the north and the south. Side street strolling leads to hidden stairways, past little libraries and past summer gardens. On Walk 37 you'll follow paved pathways along the creek, past wetlands, through a colourful mural-covered tunnel and past the Confederation golf course. Walk 38 begins in Hillhurst and travels north through the SAIT campus. For those of you who watched the HBO series "The Last of Us" you may recognize SAIT's iconic 103-year-old Heritage Hall building from episode 6 called "Kin". SAIT can now add "being featured on a record-breaking zombie show" to its rich and storied history. After a loop through Confederation Park, Walk 38 continues south to stunning views from the Crescent Heights escarpment known as McHugh Bluffs. Named after Felix McHugh, who homesteaded this property and was a prominent early entrepreneur, the bluff offers views over downtown, along the Bow River, and west to the Rockies. Continue along Crescent Road before descending into Sunnyside, a character neighbourhood. Check out Walk 41 to explore the neighbourhood and see the garage art, gargoyles in treetops, and fairy gardens—public art is everywhere in this eclectic community. Stop for some food, drinks, or some shopping in Kensington and finish off with a picnic in Riley Park. From nature to art to tasty detours, these walks have it all!

Tasty Pit Stops

There are many perfect picnic spots in Confederation Park, along the Crescent Heights escarpment, and in Riley Park, along with some tasty destinations to warm up indoors on a cooler day. Capitol Hill is home to Jimmy's A&A Mediterranean Deli known for its giant, excellent shawarma and for Jimmy himself, a friendly and colourful guy who has a loyal following. Grab and go or sit on the patio, Jimmy's has you covered. Edelweiss Village is another popular spot. Authentic European cuisine, that's what you'll find at Edelweiss. Perogies, cabbage rolls, schnitzel, bratwurst, sandwiches, and many tasty pastries, muffins, and desserts - all made fresh daily. Weeds Café is also along the route and is a perfect stop for a hot drink and some fresh baked goods.

Confederation Park - Capitol Hill - Mount Pleasant - Crescent Heights - SAIT

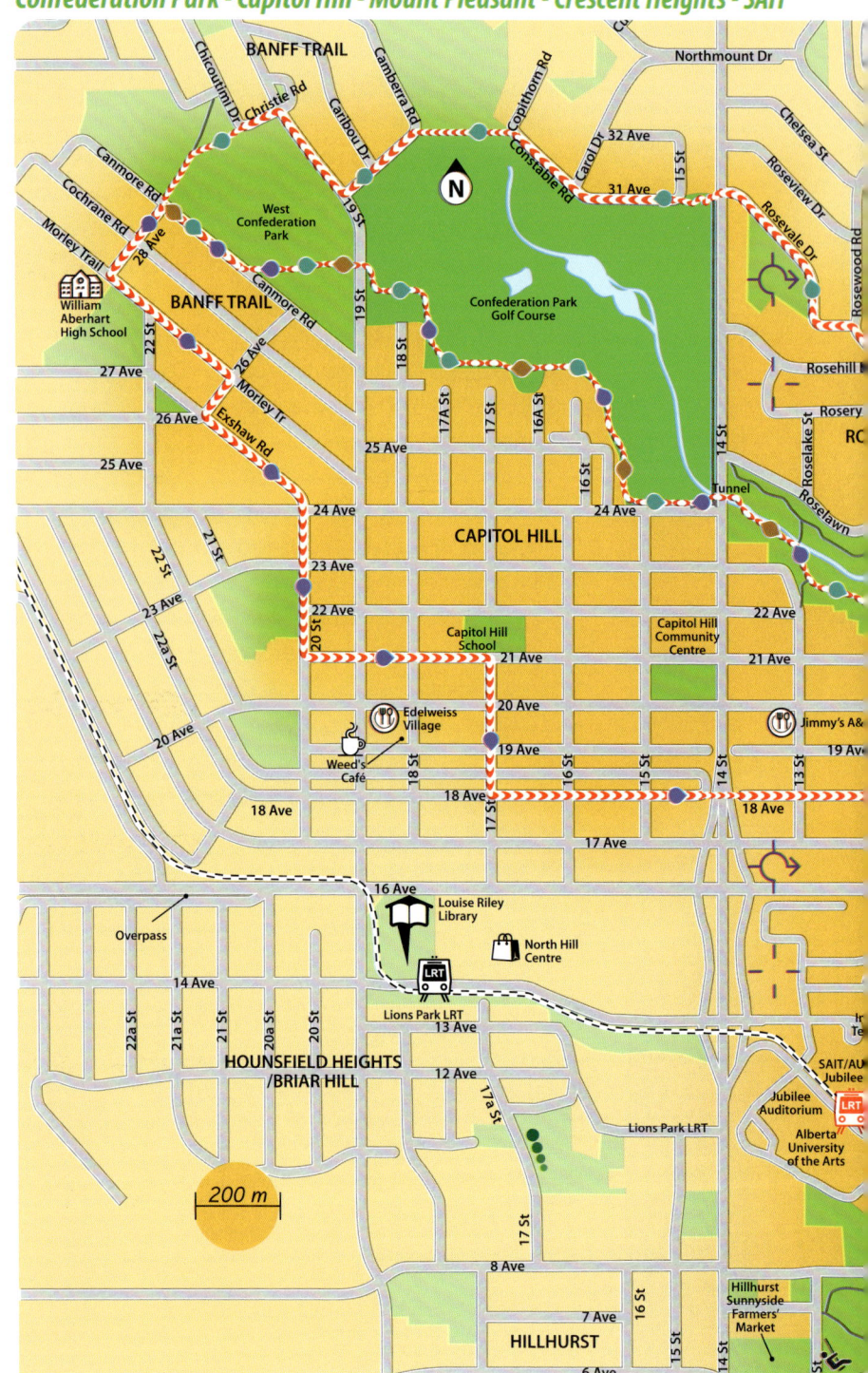

Confederation Park - Capitol Hill - Mount Pleasant - Crescent Heights - SAIT

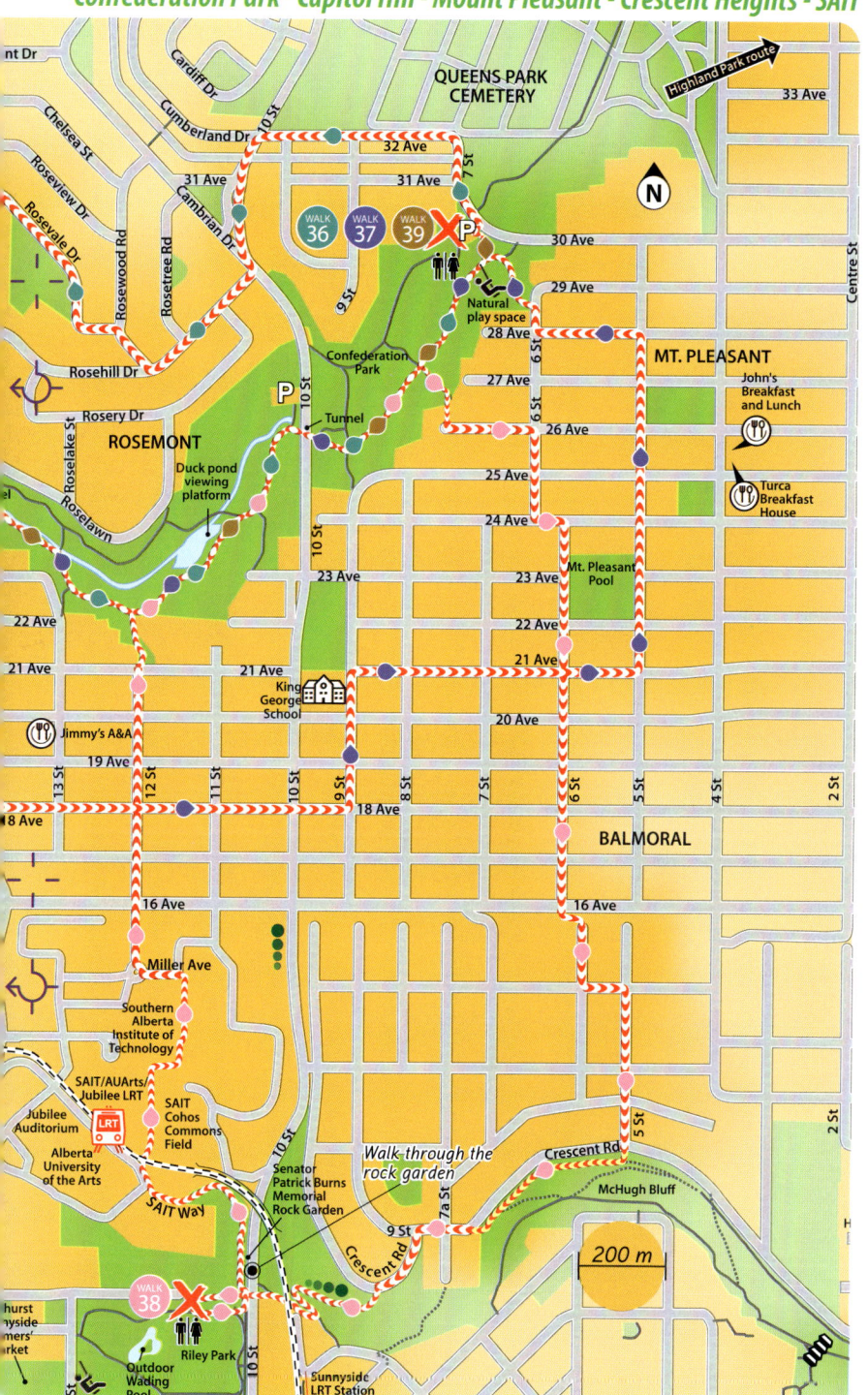

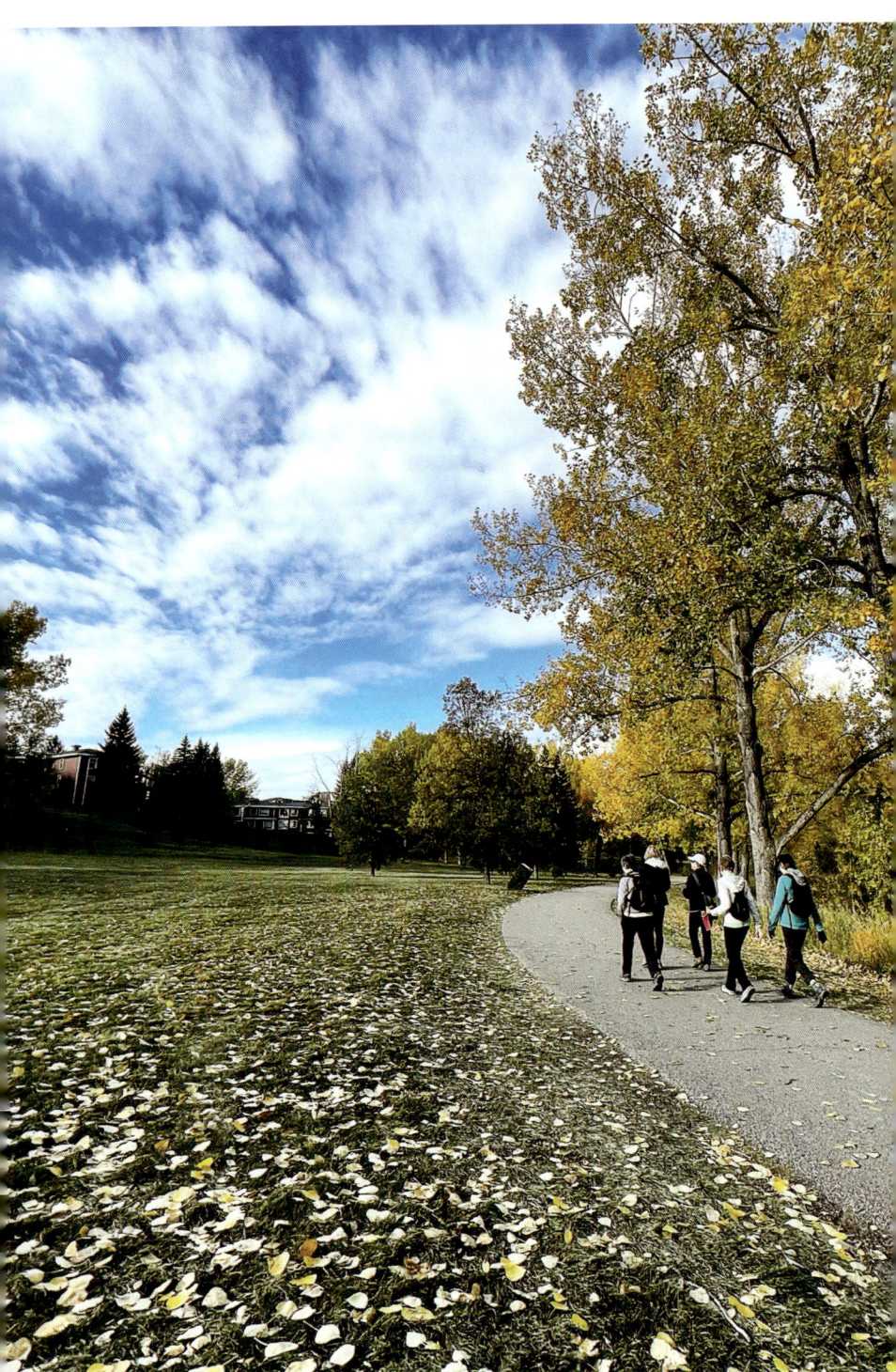

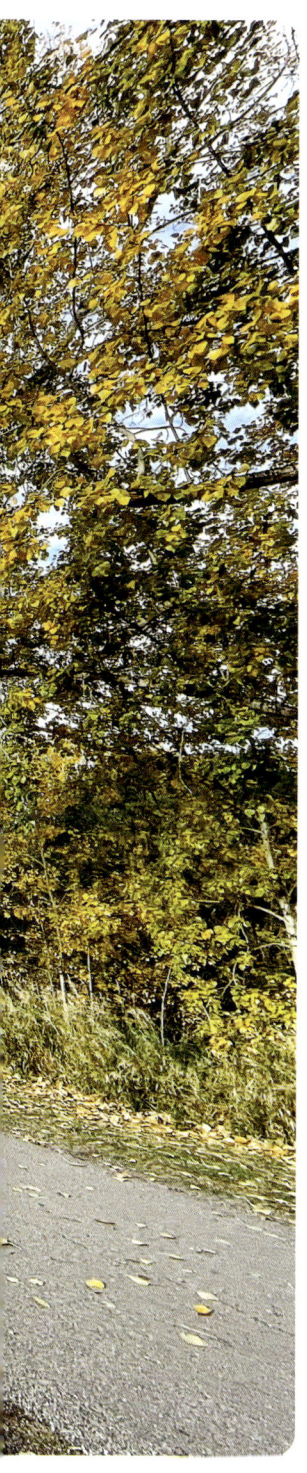

Cities That Make You Fit

It turns out that the design of your community will impact your health. Walking and biking has been engineered out of most people's lives, contributing to increasing rates of obesity, heart disease, and diabetes. Prior to the 1930s, all neighbourhoods were built on grids. With the advent of the car, this all changed. Le Corbusier, a Swiss-French architect and urban planner in the early to mid-1900s, believed that streets were no longer relevant in the era of cars and that we needed to kill the street. His work has been very influential in the creation of suburban street design. Built with the car in mind, the suburban cul-de-sac street networks funnel traffic to main arterial and collector roads. This so-called Garden City design philosophy that became popular after the Second World War creates what researchers call an "inferior pedestrian environment." The popularity of the power centre—the big box store development—is also to blame for more driving and less walking and biking. In denser, more grid-like communities, like Capital Hill and Mount Pleasant, where streets intersect, cul-de-sacs are rare, and corner stores and shops are tucked into neighbourhoods, there are lower rates of obesity, diabetes, and high blood pressure. The take-home message? In cities where self-propelled transport is safe, easy, and enjoyable, people bike and walk more and their health benefits. Calgary's 1000-km-plus paved pathway network, an abundance of ravine and slope side trails, as well as cut through paths in neighbourhoods mean many more Calgarians are excited about and enjoying active transport.

Kensington - Sunnyside Garage Art - McHugh Bluff - Princes Island Wetlands - Bow River Loop

Walks 40-42

NW

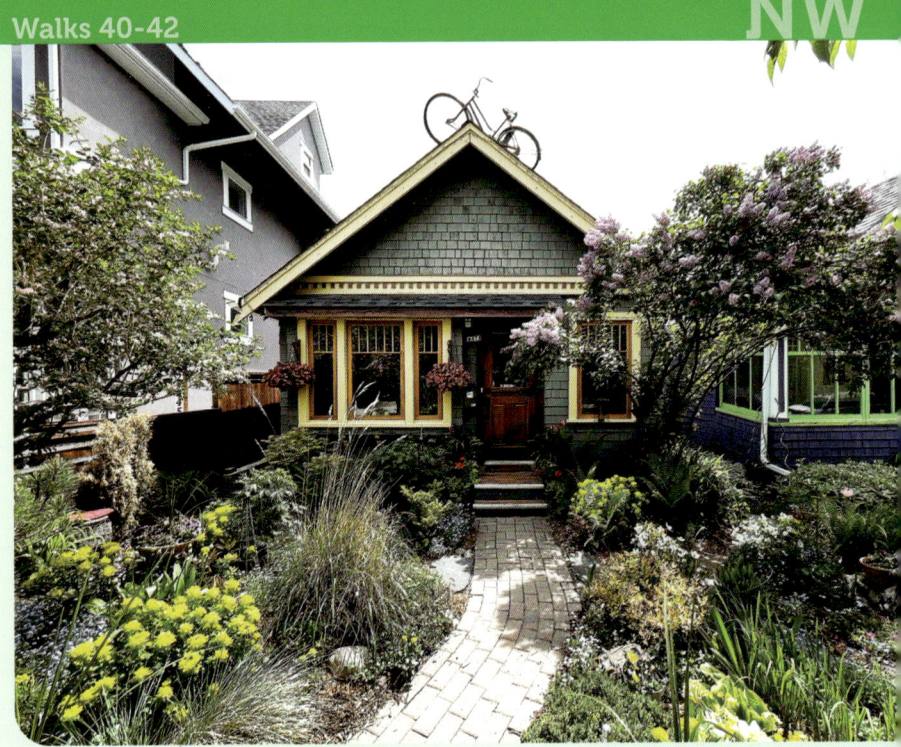

Walks at a Glance:

Explore neighbourhood side streets, the Bow River Pathway, and the best views in Calgary on these three urban hikes. Walks 40 and 41 criss-cross McHugh Bluff to views of the the Bow River Valley, Rocky Mountains, and city-centre skyscrapers reaching prominently out of the concrete. All three walks travel the Bow River Pathway and explore Sunnyside, a community with character homes, colourful displays of garage art, little libraries, and unexpected folk art perched on rooftops and treetops.

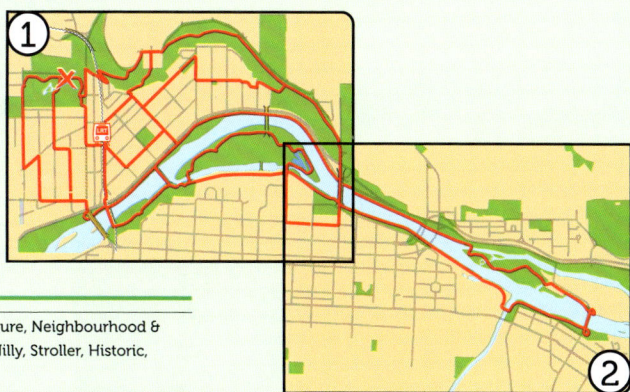

Details

Categories: LRT, Café, Dog, Nature, Neighbourhood & Parks, People watch & shop, Hilly, Stroller, Historic, Vistas, River, Birds

Start: Walks 40 and 41: Park in the official three-hour, free, Riley Park parking area. 800 12 Street NW; Walk 42: Sunnyside LRT Station

LRT: Sunnyside Station

Facilities: Seasonal bathroom (May-October) at Riley Park. Bathrooms at the bottom of the Crescent Heights stairs

Distance & Difficulty

Walk 40: Riley Park - Kensington- Princes Island Wetlands- McHugh Bluff: 7 km (hills, stairs, paved and gravel pathways)

Walk 41: Sunnyside garage art walk: 7 km (hills, stairs and paved pathways)

Walk 42: Sunnyside - Bow River Pathway- East Village- Inglewood: 10 km (mostly flat, paved pathways)

Highlights, Detours & Destinations

Dogs love the McHugh Bluff off leash. Crescent Heights Christmas lights displays are stunning in December. Bring your skates and enjoy free outdoor skating on the lagoon in Prince's Island Park. Enjoy the spectacular flower gardens in Burns Memorial Park and Riley Park in the summer. Plan to browse the Kensington shops or to take in a movie at The Plaza, Calgary's retro cinema

Walks 40 and 41 begin in Riley Park, a park that is a hive of activity in the summer, with its playground, impressive wading pool, open park space for playing Frisbee or picnicking, and colourful flower beds. And for those wanting to watch some cricket matches, visit the east end of the park where cricket has been played since 1919. Ezra Hounsfield Riley donated the park land to the city in 1910 and then secured a permit from parks superintendent William Reader to create the still-popular cricket pitch. Walk 40 climbs McHugh Bluff at the start

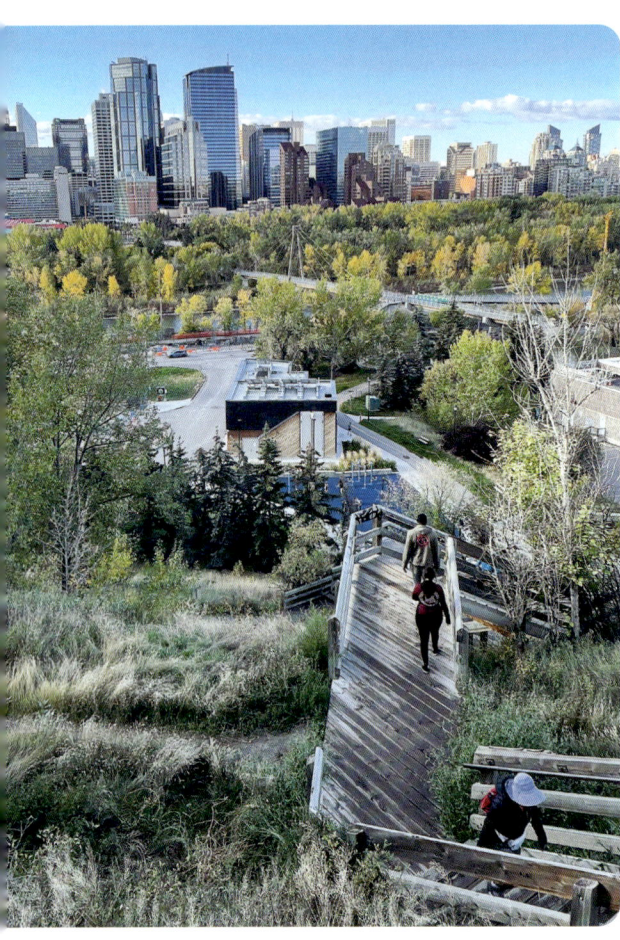

Training on the Crescent Heights Stairs

The Crescent Heights stairs and outdoor gym on McHugh Bluff have become a year-round workout destination for Calgarians in training. Climbing stairs can make your muscles burn. When the intensity of an activity increases and you stop breathing comfortably, your cells start to rely on anaerobic (oxygen-free) respiration to function. A by-product of anaerobic exercise is an accumulation of lactic acid in your muscles. That burn you feel is caused by this accumulation; slow down or stop when you feel the burn. Fitness levels determine lactate thresholds so the fitter you are the more you can climb before your legs burn. If you want an alternative to the Crescent Heights stairs, try the paved path that gradually climbs the escarpment. Gradual hills are perfect for quadriceps training. Those big muscles in at the front of your legs are used constantly when alpine skiing or climbing a hill on a bike. Build quad strength by walking uphill backward for twenty steps and then forward for twenty steps. Keep alternating until you reach the top. The bigger the step you take, the tougher the workout.

while Walk 41 and 42 travel Sunnyside side streets, past the shops and cafés of Kensington to the Bow River Pathway.

Grab a pre-hike coffee on Kensington Road before walking to the impressive Poppy Plaza war memorial at the intersection of 10 Street and Memorial Drive. A dynamic public space, the plaza is perfect place at which to sit, reflect, and watch the river flow by. Continue east along the Bow River Pathway. If you walk here during Calgary's commute –at 7:30 am or 5 pm– be prepared for an onslaught of cyclists peddling into or out of the downtown core. Cross the tubular Peace Bridge, a pedestrian bridge that accommodates both walkers and cyclists in harmony. Designed by Spanish architect Santiago Calatrava, the bridge was built to accommodate the 6,000 plus per day users who walk and bike for recreation and transport. Functional and artistic, it is a testament to the city's commitment to increasing its residents' pleasure in walking and cycling.

Continue past Prince's Island or walk the islands wetlands trails of the far east end. In the winter, the frozen pond in Prince's Island is cleared and maintained for skating. Onward to Chinatown, and depending on the walk you are following, eastward to the East village or walk north across the Bow River and up the McHugh Bluff escarpment. Named after Felix McHugh, who homesteaded this property and was a prominent early entrepreneur, the bluff host views extending downtown west to the mountains. On a winter evening, the sights are dramatic and impressive. With every step up the hillside, the downtown skyscrapers rise into view, bright, compact, and towering. In December the colourful light displays on the houses makes this area the perfect spot for a Christmas lights walk. Follow the pathway to the popular Crescent Heights stairs, where a hotbed of sweaty Calgarians regularly keep fit. Across from Prince's Island Park, these stairs are easy access for downtown office workers –or visitors staying at downtown hotels– needing a quick, outdoor, training session.

Continue to the hillside trails and walk into the trees: willows, ashes, balsam poplar, and white spruce. This off leash area is popular with pups, so you'll likely meet a furry friend or two while following these treed escarpment trails. Walk 41 loops back through Sunnyside, with side trips down back alleys in search of garage art. Walk 40 continues in the opposite direction to the top of the slope, continuing to enjoy the Rocky Mountain and Bow River vistas before descending to the Bow River Pathway for the return trip. The final part of all three walks is deciding what kind of post walk fun you want to have in Kensington; go for a coffee, visit Pages bookstore or other local shops of all sorts or go see a movie at The Plaza Theatre, a retro independent cinema that is home to a speakeasy-style cocktail bar and a patio with a food truck. And yes, there's popcorn too.

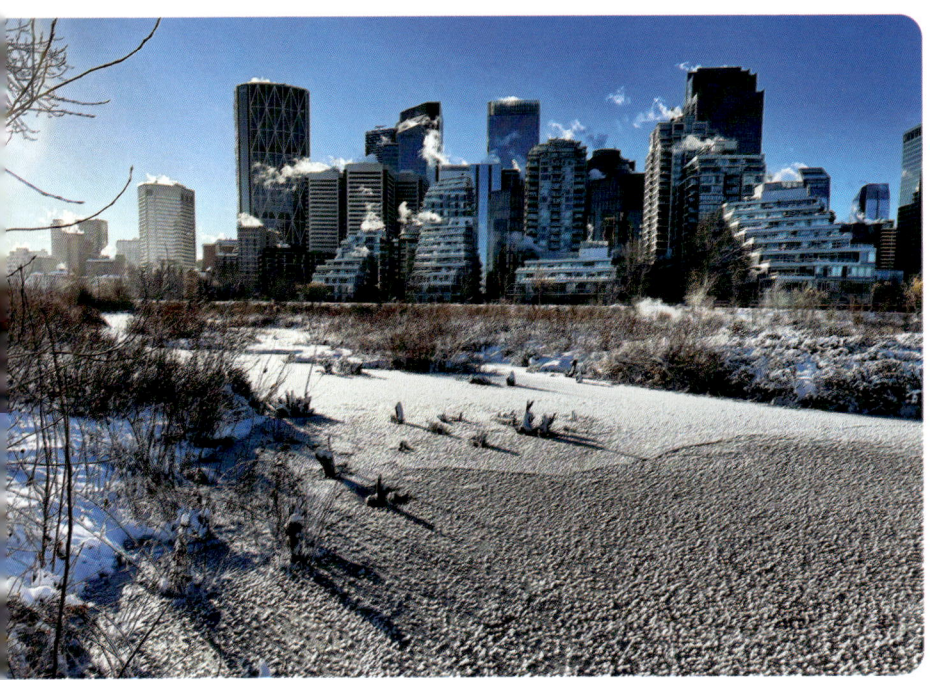

Public art surprises

Stroll Sunnyside's back lanes on Walk 41 and you'll see more than 30 bright garage door murals, depicting scenes of neighbourhood dogs, the solar system, a panda, owls, a whale, and colourful gardens. The scenes on the garage doors and fences are as varied as the people who live in Sunnyside. Collectively, they transform monotonous alleyways into a vibrant outdoor art gallery. The best approach to see them is to pick different alleys to explore each time you walk through Sunnyside as new murals continue to pop up. Follow @sunnyside_garage_art on Instagram to see the latest additions. Public art is a constant along the Bow River, beginning with the Outflow sculpture along the river near Parkdale. An inverted replica of Mount PeeChee, the third-highest peak in the Fairholme Range just north of Canmore in the Bow River watershed, the sculpture memorializes the glacial origins of the Bow and how it has shaped our city over the years. It is part of the Landscape of Memory Project that aims to keep Memorial Drive's legacy as a living memorial to the events and people that have shaped our city's landscape. Past Poppy Plaza at 10 Street is the iconic Peace Bridge that has become a Calgary landmark with 6,000 plus people crossing it daily. Continue east past the everchanging RiverWalk murals and onto St. Patrick's Island to see Bloom, a sculpture made of streetlights fused together in the shape of a flower. Detour into the East Village and you'll find Device to Root Out Evil, the upside-down church that has been no stranger to controversy as it has travelled from New York to Vancouver and Europe before finding a home in Calgary's East Village.

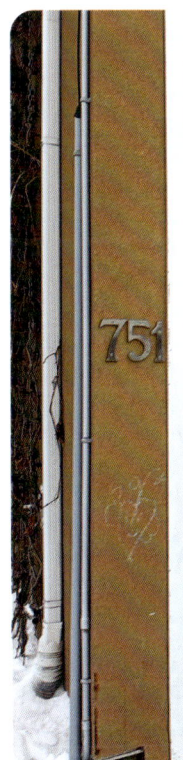

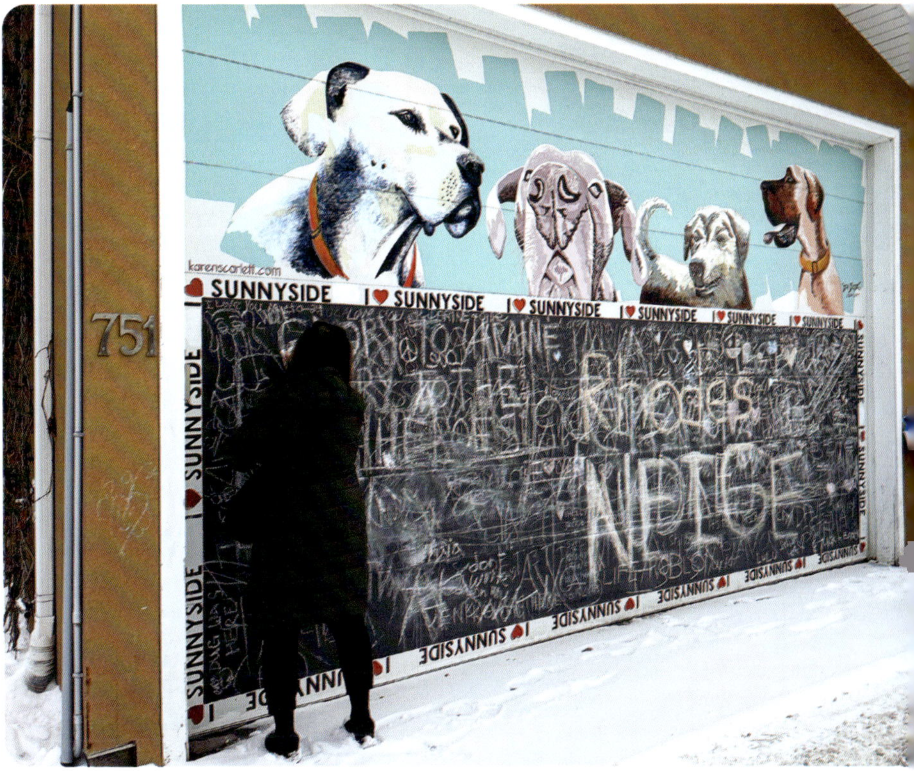

Dog mural by Karen Scarlett, karenscarlett.com

Kensington - Sunnyside Garage Art - McHugh Bluff - Princes Island Wetlands - Bow River Loop

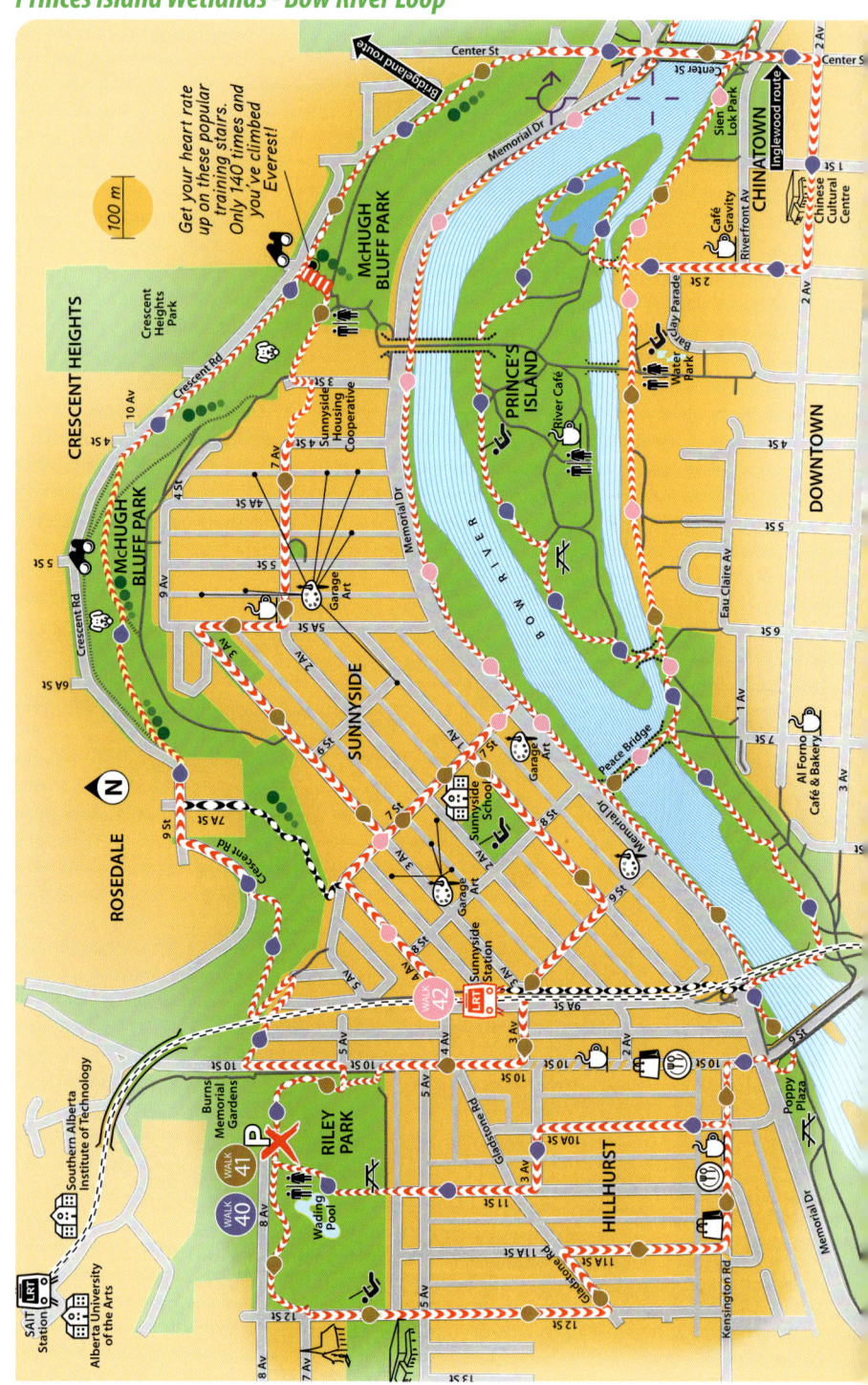

Kensington - Sunnyside Garage Art - McHugh Bluff - Princes Island Wetlands - Bow River Loop

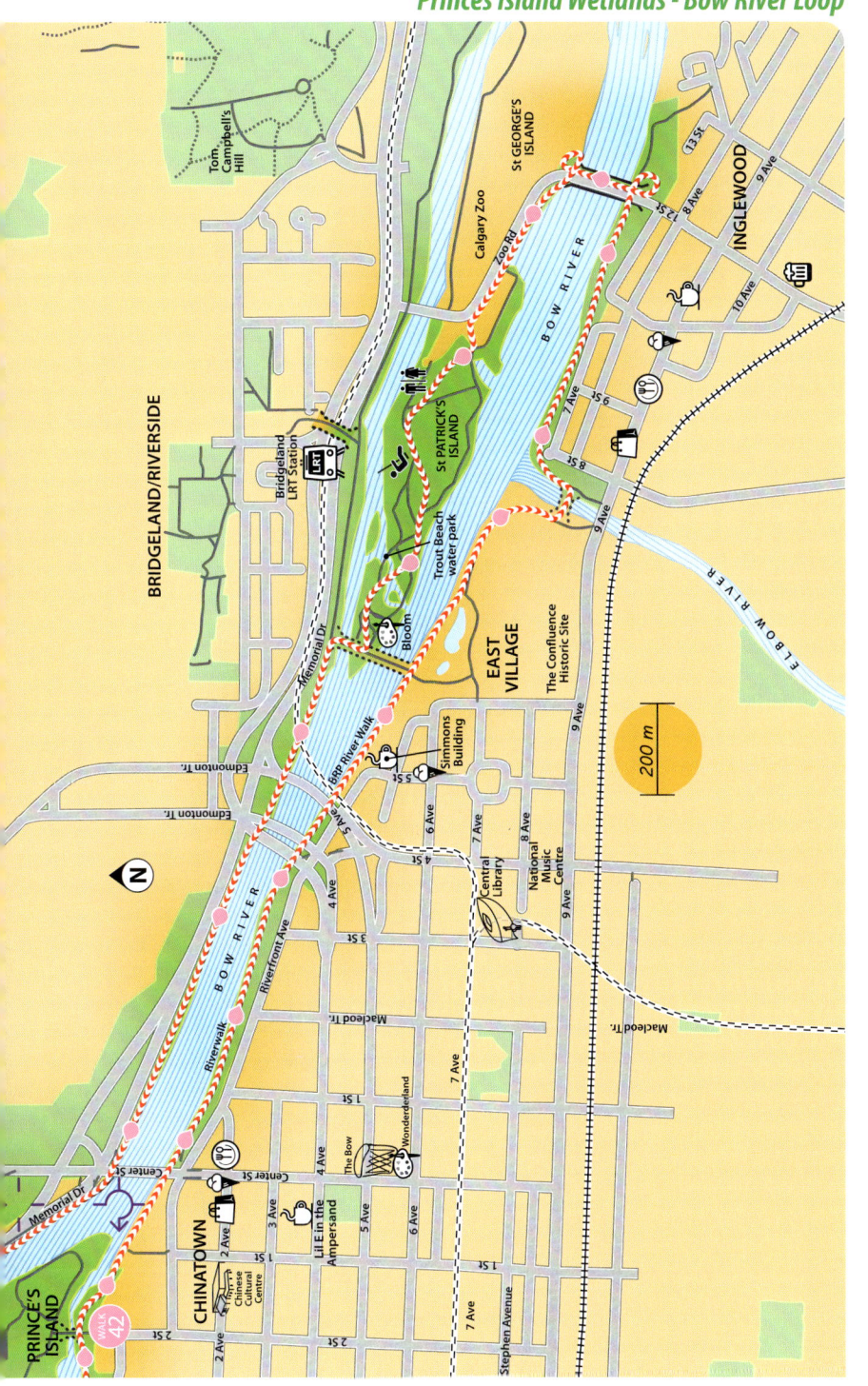

Briar Hill - Hounsfield Heights - West Hillhurst - Westmount

Walk 43 NW

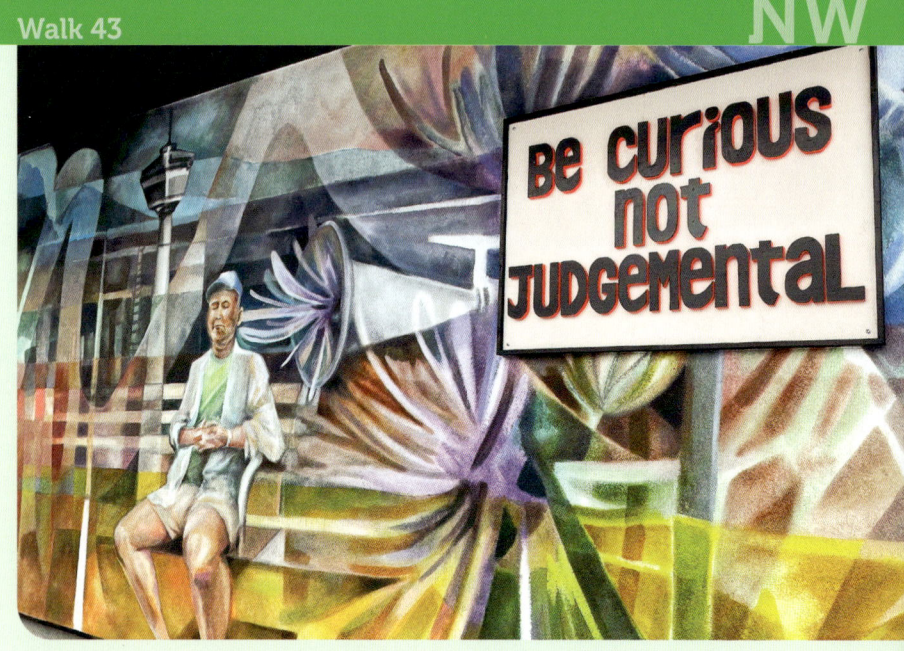

Mural by daniel j kirk, danieljkirk.ca, Intelligent Futures building

Walk at a Glance:

Grasshopper Hill, as the bluff was once known, is the off leash start and leads you to the first of many wide-open views of the downtown skyline and the communities below. Briar Hill soon becomes Hounsfield Heights, Calgary's northside Mount Royal. A quick walk south of the Lion's Park LRT Station, Hounsfield Heights is an awe-inspiring neighbourhood perched on the bluffs. The modest bungalows are slowly being transformed into palaces with boulder-terraced yards that host multitudes of flowers, waterfalls, and ponds.

Details

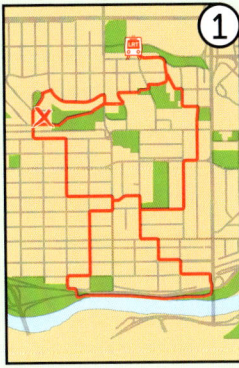

Categories: LRT, Café, Dog, Nature, Neighbourhood & Parks, People watch & shop, Hilly, Stroller, Vistas, River

Start: 9 Avenue, just east of 22 Street NW

LRT: Lions Park Station

Facilities: Cafés, restaurants and ice cream shops along the route

Distance & Difficulty

7.5 km (hills, stairs, sidewalks, paved paths and single-track trails)

Take a relaxation break in the Braun Family Park. Built to be a sanctuary in the heart of Calgary, this colourful park was designed to support youth and teen mental health recovery. With a climbing wall, basketball court, little library and so much nature, it is a beautiful addition to the community. Skirt the bluff to enjoy constant skyline views, picking a single-track trail across the wild space to descend into Hillhurst, or follow the quiet side streets to view the homes and the impressive landscaping. Walk through Hillhurst, an inner-city community that is a close walk, bike, or transit ride to the University of the Arts, Southern Alberta Institute of Technology (SAIT), and

First Settlers

Lawlessness and whisky trading in the late 1800s marked this area before the North-West Mounted Police arrived in 1875, built Fort Calgary, and helped bring some order to the chaos. The Canadian Pacific Railway arrived in 1884, and that meant Calgary had "arrived" as an urban centre. Hounsfield Lodge Farm, owned by Thomas E. Riley and Georgina Jane Hounsfield, was the original settlement in the Briar Hill and Hillhurst area. In 1890 the property extended from Sunnyside to Parkdale in the west, and from the Bow River to Sixteenth Avenue in the north. Calgary's growth by 40,000 people between 1900 and 1910 meant that this land was in demand, and the family decided to subdivide and sell.

On June 10, 1910, the Morning Albertan featured the following headline, "Hounsfield Heights; All View Lots - An Ideal Location for an Ideal Home," accompanied by a view of the subdivision of Hillhurst from the top of the bluff. Instructions on how to get there included a walk "through the park donated by Mr. E. Riley," now known as Riley Park. At substantial price tag of $800 to $1000 per 50-ft (15-m) lot meant that only the moneyed could afford to live there. Hounsfield Heights was to be the "Mount Royal of the North." In 1913 a recession hit, along with threats of war and increased unemployment. The overheated economy came to a crashing halt. When you walk through Hounsfield Heights today, you will see that it did in fact become a mini-Mount Royal of the North, one hundred years after the fact.

the University of Calgary. Take a detour to pedestrian-populated Kensington Road and walk east to shop, eat, and people watch.

Tucked in between Kensington Road and the Bow River, Westmount is easily overlooked, unless you live here. The main road in the community, Bowness Road, is incredibility wide, parts of it with a tree-lined median. The road was built wide to accommodate a streetcar route to the town of Bowness, before 1964, when Bowness was annexed to the City of Calgary. Impressive properties with character share the street with older homes and beautiful new ones. The architectural variety keeps things interesting and attractive. Cross the Bow River and follow the Bow River Pathway. The city zips along Memorial Drive as you walk beneath the poplar trees along the river. Calgary's well-used 1000 km+ pathway system –the most extensive urban pathway and bikeway in North America– is such a wonderful way to link communities. And even in the winter these paths are well used since the city of Calgary clears the snow off 500 km of trails so Calgarians can walk and bike year-round. Bravo Calgary!

Continue over the pedestrian overpass and walk back through the community. On a hot day, make a motivational stop for some ice cream or warm up in the colder months with a coffee or diner meal along 19 Street before zigzagging back to your starting point.

Tasty Pit Stops

Amato Gelato along Kensington Road and Made by Marcus Ice Cream Shop on 19 Street will make your walk even better in the summer months or during those wonderful warm chinook days in February. Once on 19 Street your options are many. Warm up with a hot drink and tasty baked goods at Vintage Caffeine or Pocket Coffee. And for a healthy and tasty hit, stop by Kosa, a health food store and café that serves up smoothies, coffees and prepared lunches to go. Or if a burger, fries and a beer are just what the doctor ordered, plan a stop at Dairy Lane.

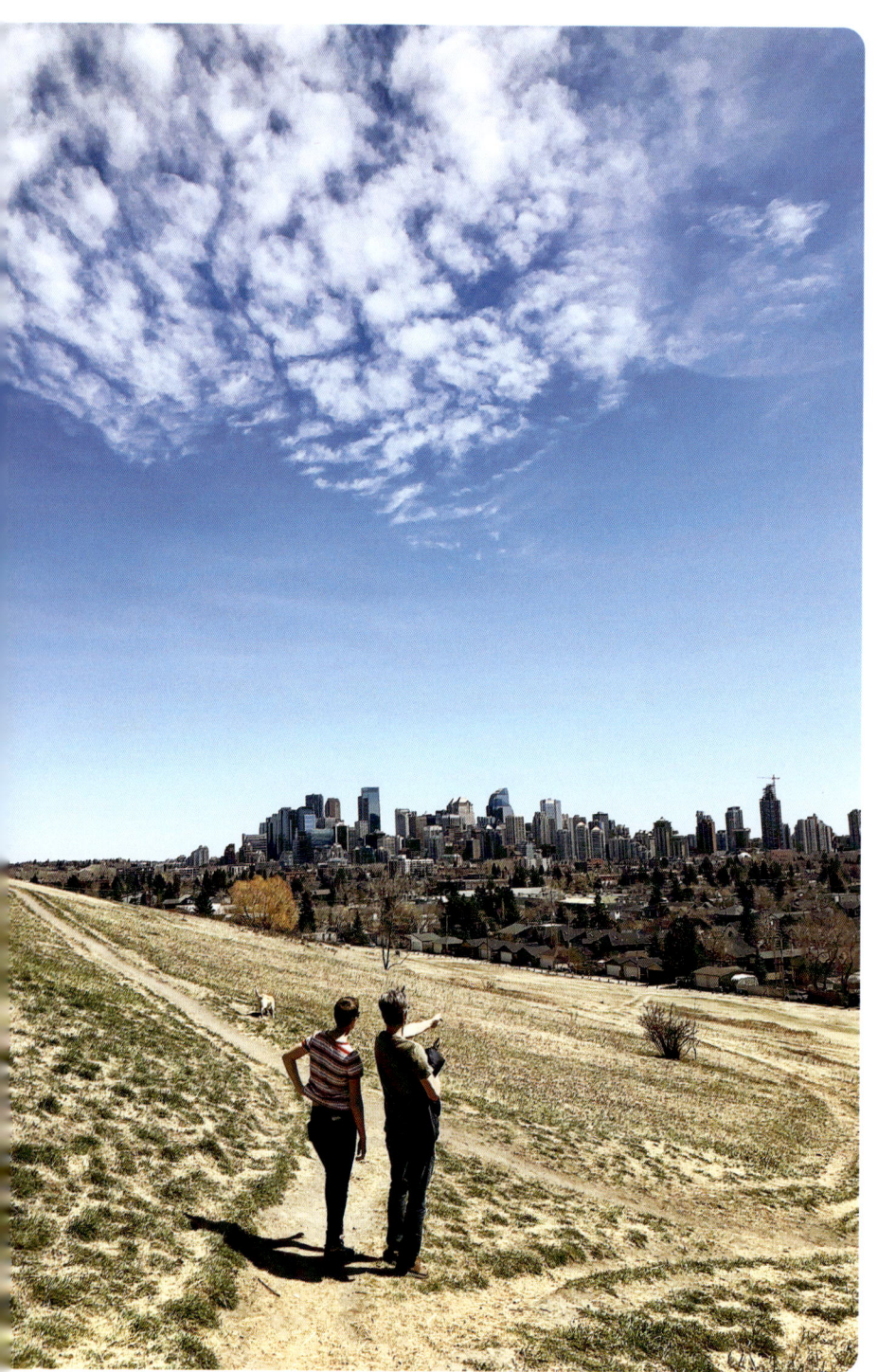

Briar Hill - Hounsfield Heights - West Hillhurst - Westmount

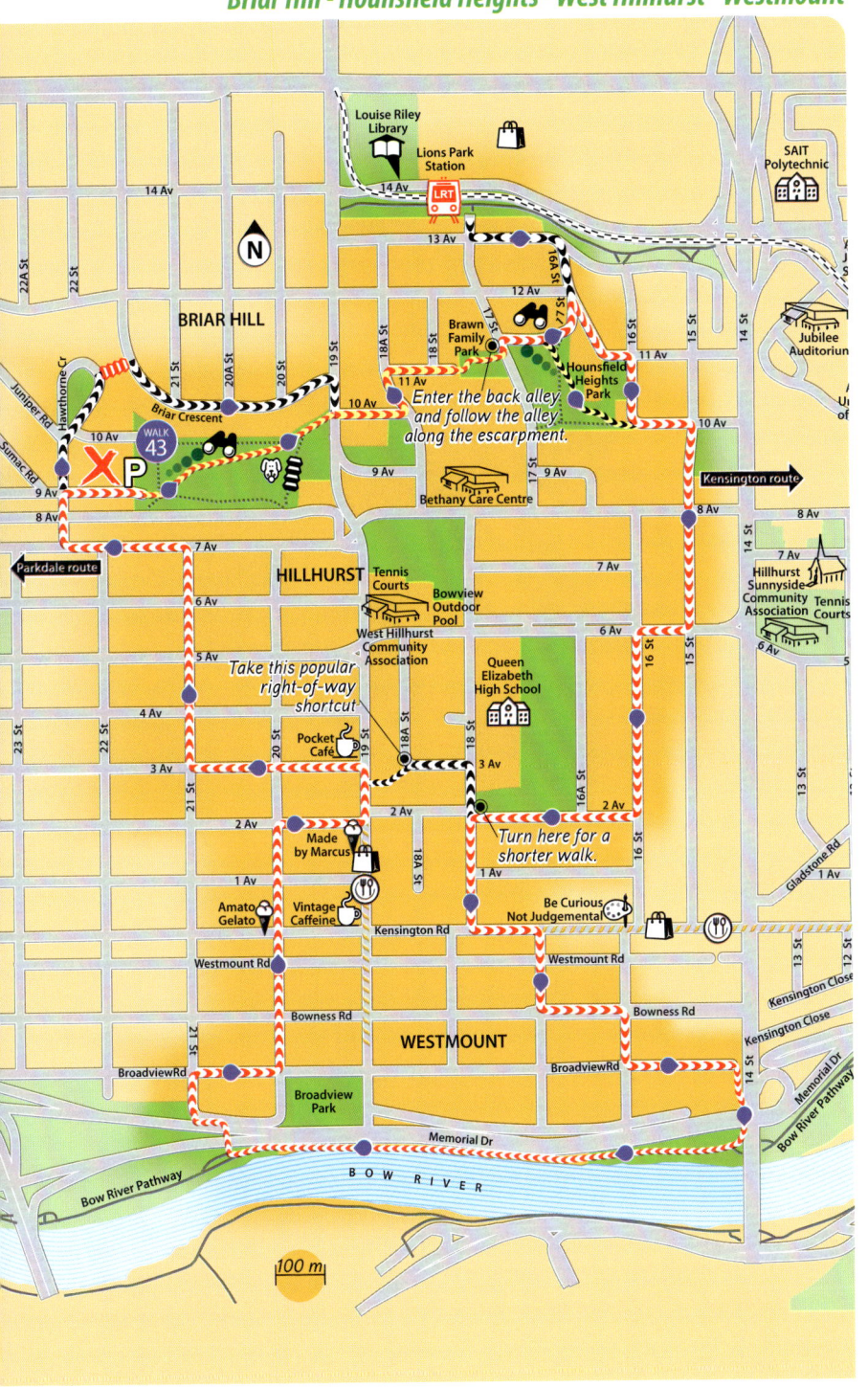

Parkdale - St. Andrews Heights - University District - Montgomery

Walks 44 - 46

NW

Walks at a Glance:

These walkabouts connect four Calgary neighbourhoods, and they all offer up views of the Rockies and the Bow River. From Edworthy and Shouldice Parks, Walks 44 and 45 begin with a Bow River Pathway stroll before cutting into the neighbourhoods of Montgomery or Parkdale.

Developed in the mid nineteen hundreds, these neighbourhoods were once considered suburbs, but now are a central location for Calgarians who want shorter commutes and especially for those who work at one of the hospitals up the hill.

Details

Categories: LRT, Café, Dog, Nature, Neighbourhood & Parks, People watch & shop, Hilly, Stroller, Vistas, River

Start: Walk 44: Edworthy Park, Bowness Road and Shaganappi Trail NW

Walk 45: Shouldice Park, Bowness Road and Montserrat Drive NW

Walk 46: Montalban Park, 23 Avenue and 47 Street NW

LRT: University Station

Facilities: Year-round bathrooms at Edworthy Park and Central Commons Park, University District. Seasonal bathrooms at Shouldice Park. Cafés, restaurants, shops and a free outdoor skating rink in the University District. Skate, helmet and skating aid rentals at Central Commons Park, University District

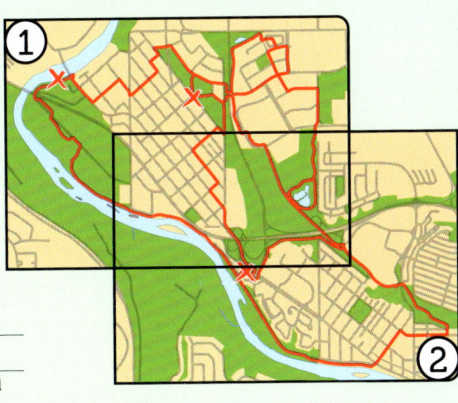

Distance & Difficulty

Walk 44: Parkdale-St. Andrews Heights- University District- Montgomery: 7 km (hills, paved paths, sidewalks, and single-track trails)

Walk 45: Shouldice Park- Bow River Pathway- Montgomery- University District: 9 km (hills, paved paths, sidewalks, and single-track trails)

Walk 46: University District Loop: 5 km (one hill, paved paths)

Highlights, Detours & Destinations

The University District has a leisure (no hockey) skating rink that is temperature regulated so the ice will be available all winter long

---

Walk 44 climbs the escarpment green space along shaded pathways to St. Andrews Heights. Enjoy the views from the hilltop as you venture west, skirting the escarpment, past the Foothills Medical Centre. Along with views of the Rockies, the colourful Alberta Children's Hospital stands out. Children were asked how they would like the hospital to look, inside and out, and with their input; the multi-coloured, Lego-like structure was built. The building's colourful design, the multitude of windows bringing natural light to all rooms, and beds for family members, is meant to help reduce stress and promote healing. Walks 45 and 46 lead you west through the University District. Dubbed a multi-generational community built to encourage cross-generational connectivity, the neighbourhood hosts the Commons Park near University Avenue, 12 km of pathways that connect ponds, parks and off leash area park and a main street, with local café's, shops and restaurants. Night markets happen throughout the summer and the Central Commons Park has a free outdoor skating rink with fire pits that brings energy and fun to the area in the darker months.

Walk 46 follows the paved pathway to the University of Calgary West Campus Park wetlands. Listen for the red-winged blackbirds and watch for the abundance hawks; they swoop, sometimes too close, to cyclists and walkers. If a post walk lunch is on your agenda, continue to Bowness Road to find some tasty treats or settle in at a picnic table in Edworthy or Shouldice Parks for a peaceful picnic along the Bow River.

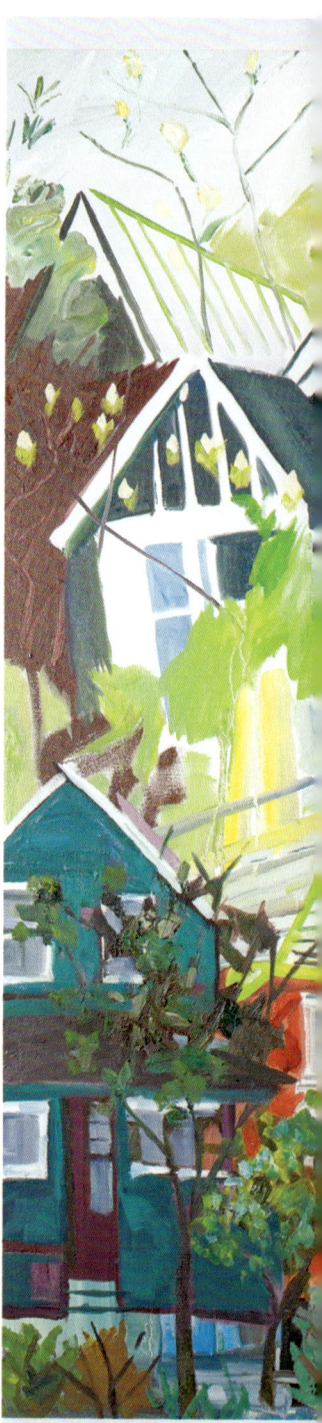

> ## The power of noticing what was always there
>
> When you step out on your walkabout, be sure to get lost sometimes. I mean, not really lost, but also, maybe not completely sure of where you are. Change your route mid stride and turn down an alley or take that cut through path or set of stairs just to see where it goes. Research shows that disrupting our well-worn routines, both good and bad, can rejuvenate and reset our brains for the better. In the book, "Look Again", authors Tali Sharot and Cass Sunstein explain how our lives become so routine that we become habituated to the things around us, and we stop noticing what is most wonderful in our lives. We also stop noticing what is terrible and we become unconcerned by our own misconduct, blind to inequality, and are more liable to believe misinformation. By noticing what is around us we can reignite the sparks of joy, innovate, and recognize where improvements urgently need to be made. The key to this disruption—to seeing, feeling, and noticing again—is change. By temporarily changing your environment, changing the rules, changing how you interact with the city you see things anew, allowing you to more deeply appreciate the good around you. Left right left right, exploring Calgary on foot is a reset for our brains which leads to fresh ideas, new perspectives and insights. Let's walk!

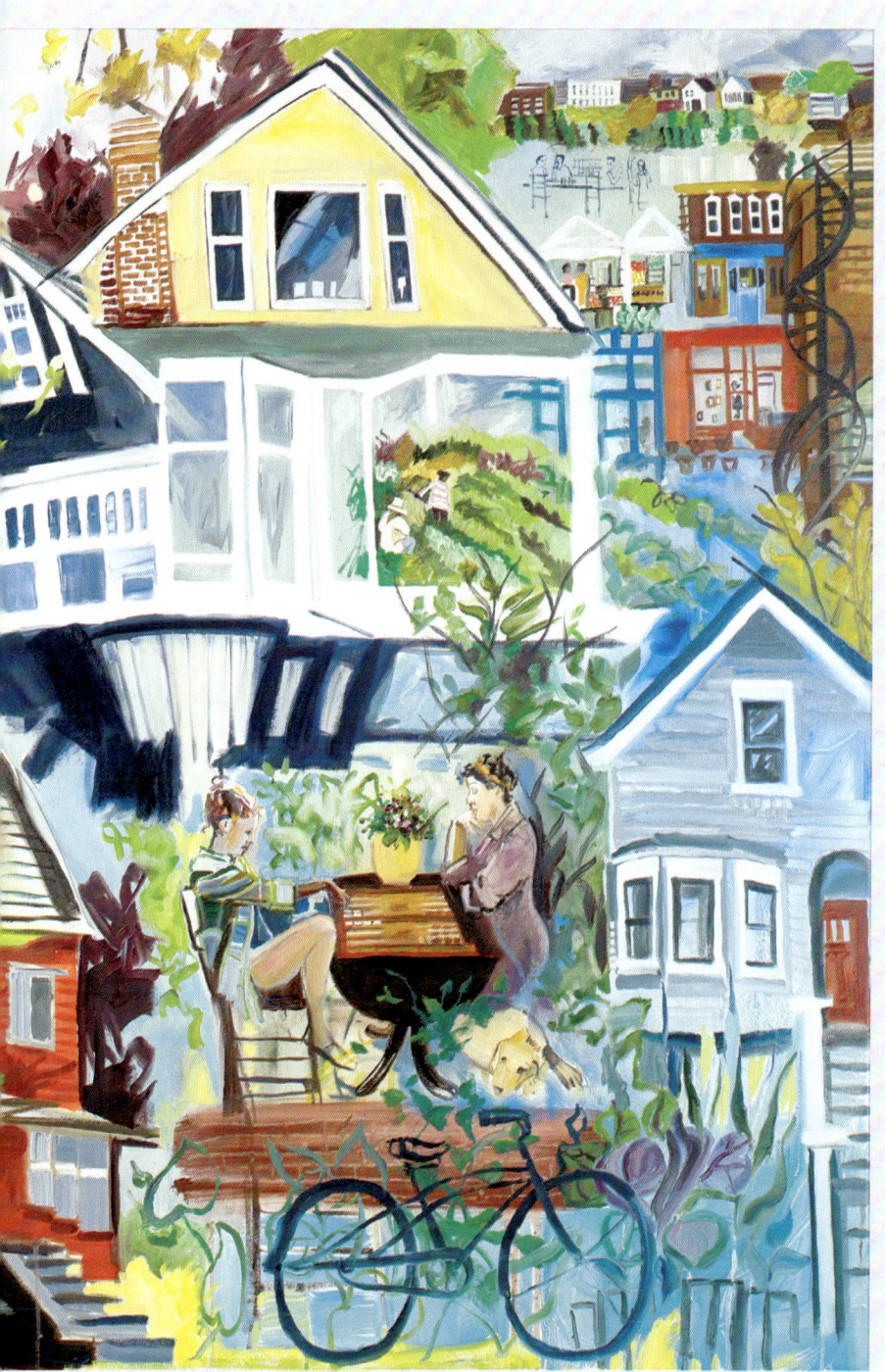

Garden Board Game Backgammon, Urban Garden Series by Jill Thomson

Parkdale - St. Andrews Heights - University District - Montgomery

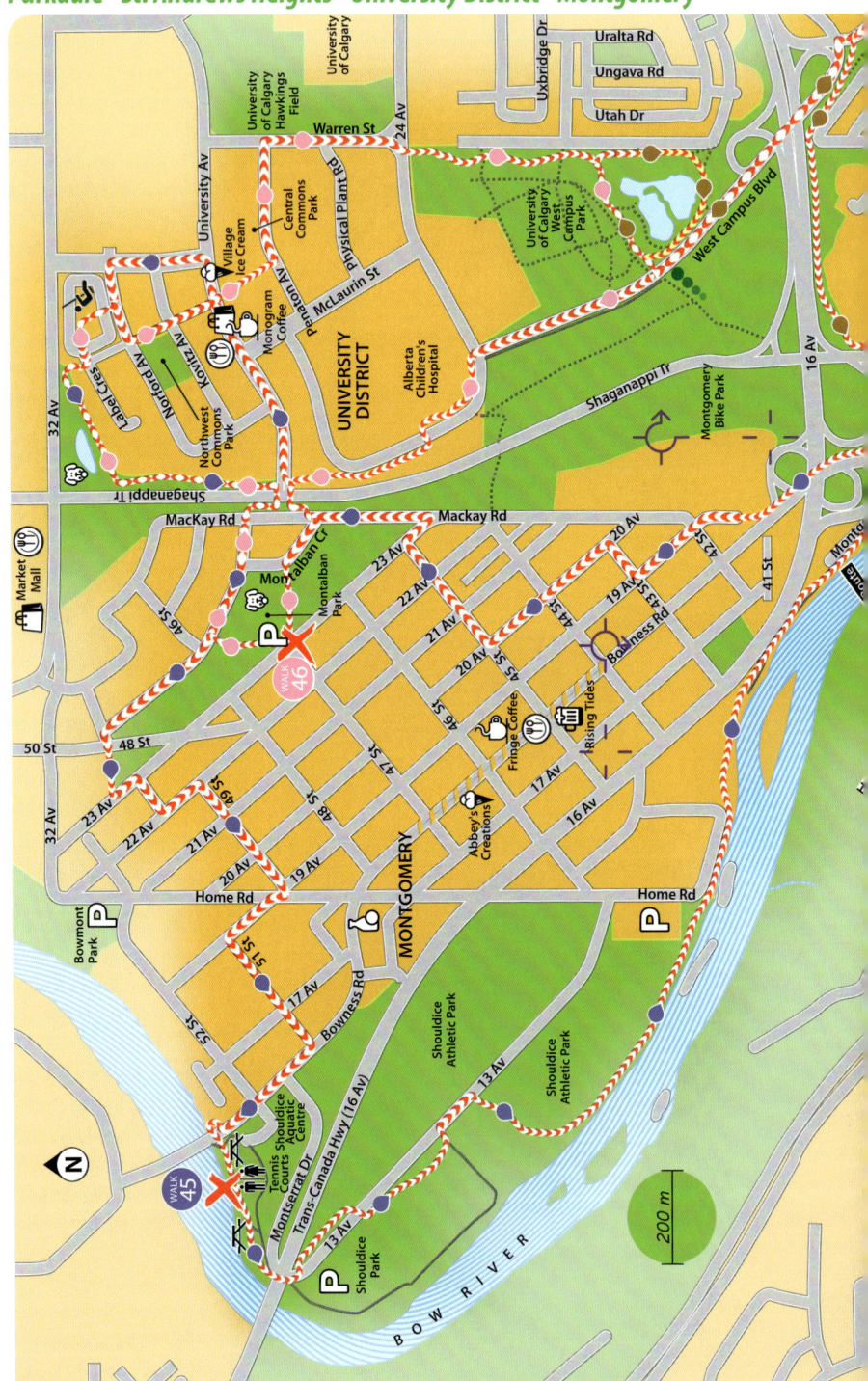

Parkdale - St. Andrews Heights - University District - Montgomery

Douglas Fir Trail - Wildwood - Quarry Road Trail - Edworthy West

Walks 47 and 48

SW

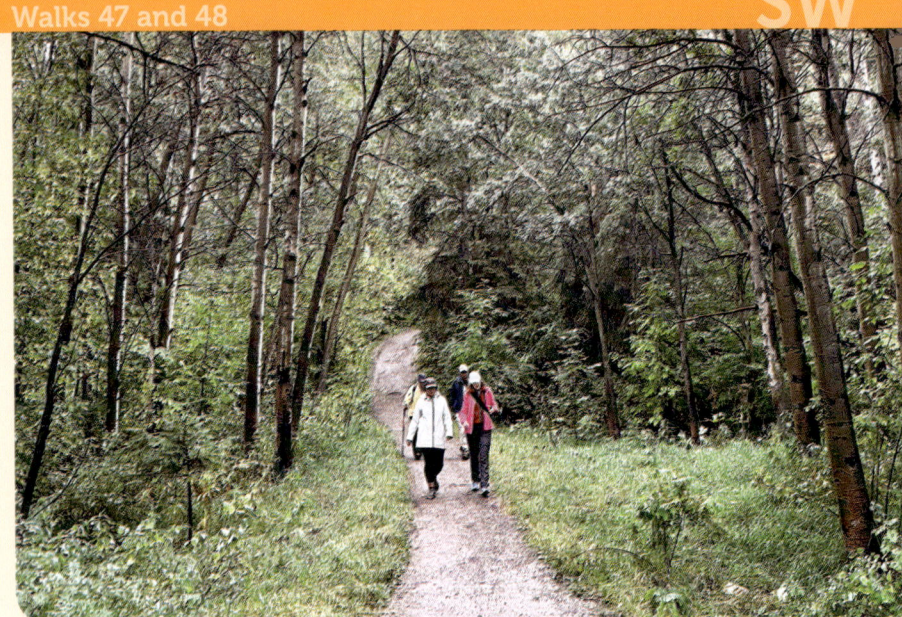

Walks at a Glance:

Hidden amongst the most easterly stand of Douglas fir trees that tower above the Bow River is the Douglas Fir Trail. Stairs, bridges, creeks, and narrow winding paths dip and climb 60 m from the river valley to the lookout point is the start of Walk 47.

A fantastic trail for physical training, it is also a shaded wilderness oasis in the height of the summer. Trees, some more than 2 m in diameter, and multitudes of western Canada violets line the trail.

The Douglas Fir Trail is often closed east of the lookout due to slope erosion. If it is open, take it, but if not, follow the route thorough Wildwood and observe the

Details

Categories: Café, Dog, Nature, Neighbourhood & Parks, Hilly, Vistas, River, Birds

Start: Walks 47 and 48: Edworthy Park, north or south side meet place. North: 4105 Montgomery View NW; South: start at the bottom of the Edworthy Street hill

Walk 48: Edworthy off leash parking at the end of Spruce Drive SW

Facilities: Year-round bathrooms in Edworthy Park. Cafés along the walk on the north side

Highlights, Detours & Destinations

The Douglas Fir Trail escarpment has many springs that are causing the hillside to slide and the bridges to tip so the trail may be closed east of the lookout. An ice flow covers part of the Douglas Fir Trail and Bow River Pathway below from December through May so bring traction devices. The trail gets very muddy and slippery after a rain and bridges can be slippery with frost on late-fall and early-spring mornings

Distance & Difficulty

Walk 47: Douglas Fir Trail- Wildwood- Quarry Road Trail: 7.5 km (Challenging, steep and uneven with many stairs and hills. The Douglas Fir Trail can be muddy, slippery and icy)

Walk 48: Edworthy Off Leash - West Trails: 3 km (single track trails, hills, sidewalks)

Alternate return route Walk 47: The Quarry Road Trail and Bow River Pathway (gravel and paved paths)

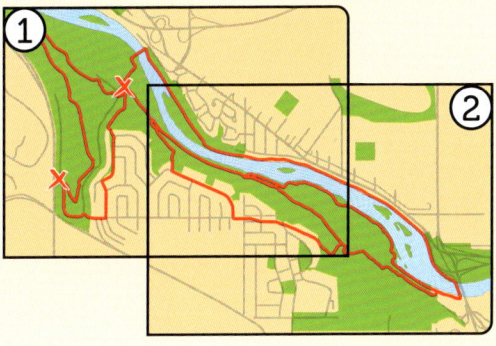

magnificent homes perched on the escarpment. Travel off the beaten path through green space trails tucked behind homes to reconnect with the Douglas Fir Trail and the Bow River Pathway below. Follow the Quarry Road Trail and return along the Bow River Pathway on the north or south side or descend along the western end of the Douglas Fir Trail to the marsh trail along the railway and listen for the chorus of frogs. Move slowly to sneak a peek before they stop croaking and dive for cover. At dusk, tip you head back and watch for the great horned owls on this same open flat stretch of the trail. These magnificent birds fly low over the open areas near the railway tracks when the natural light fades.

Walk 48 begins in the Edworthy Off Leash and travels the Edworthy west trails. Starting in the off-leash dog you can pick your path from many options as you walk west. You soon leave behind most of the people and pups as you connect to a series of interconnecting pathways that parallel the train tracks from on high. These single-track wilderness trails offer up stunning views of the Bow River Valley and Calgary's downtown.

The Drunken Forest

If the Douglas Fir Trail is open, you'll pass by a sign that reads "Slide Area No Stopping". This marks the spot where a landslide swept twenty-eight rail cars off the tracks in 1956. The instability of the slope is due partly to the number of springs in the area. The escarpment is 200 feet high and very steep. Natural springs, plus water draining from the communities above result in a very unstable slope. Continued "creeping" leads to trees leaning at odd angles. The tipsy condition of the trees has led to an alternative name, the "the drunken forest". The slope is being monitored by the city and at one time the trail was being repaired by volunteers, but Mother Nature is powerful and every year the trail continues to be affected by a sliding slope. I hope that the trail east of the lookout can be saved but at the time of writing its future remains uncertain.

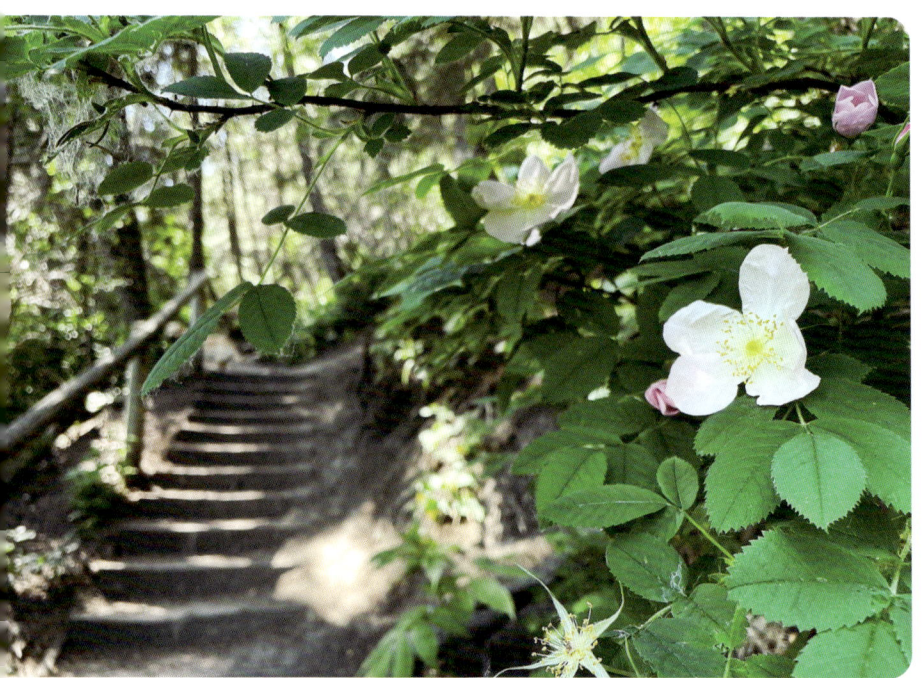

Loop back down the slope to the parking lot below the popular training hill. If you need a cardio challenge, do a hill a few times before continuing into Wildwood.

Keep your wallet ready for an ice-cream stop or a hot drink on a cold day. A few tasty eateries are along the route or not far from it. This wonderful wild walkabout has a very civilized café ending.

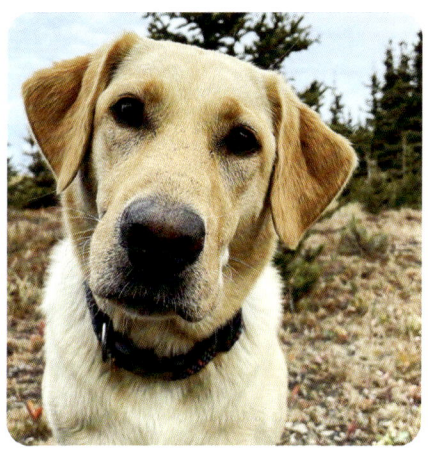

Picnic Planning Pit Stops

At the top of the Quarry Road Trail, near Walk 47, is Pie Junkie in Spruce Cliff. This is the perfect spot to grab your picnic lunch. Walk back to the route to enjoy downtown views with your savory or sweet pie (or both!). Plan a pre walk visit to the Shaganappi Mediterranean Market, on 17 Avenue just west of 37 Street SW. This hidden gem has the best value produce so plan to stock up on tomatoes, lemons, and parsley for your Middle Eastern feast while you shop for picnic supplies. I recommend the baba ganoush and some fresh pita bread along with a meat pie, some olives and cheeses for a tasty picnic. Return on the north side of the Bow River to visit the Caspian Bakery and Supermarket for all things Persian. They make taftoon, leavened flour bread from Iran, as well as Ghormah sabzi (lamb stew) and bastani sunati, decadent saffron and pistachio ice cream.

Location:
Caspian Bakery & Supermarket: 3403 3 Avenue NW
Pie Junkie: Spruce Centre, Cedar Crescent and Spruce Drive SW
Shaganappi Mediterranean Market: 3919 17 Avenue SW

Douglas Fir Trail - Wildwood - Quarry Road Trail - Edworthy West

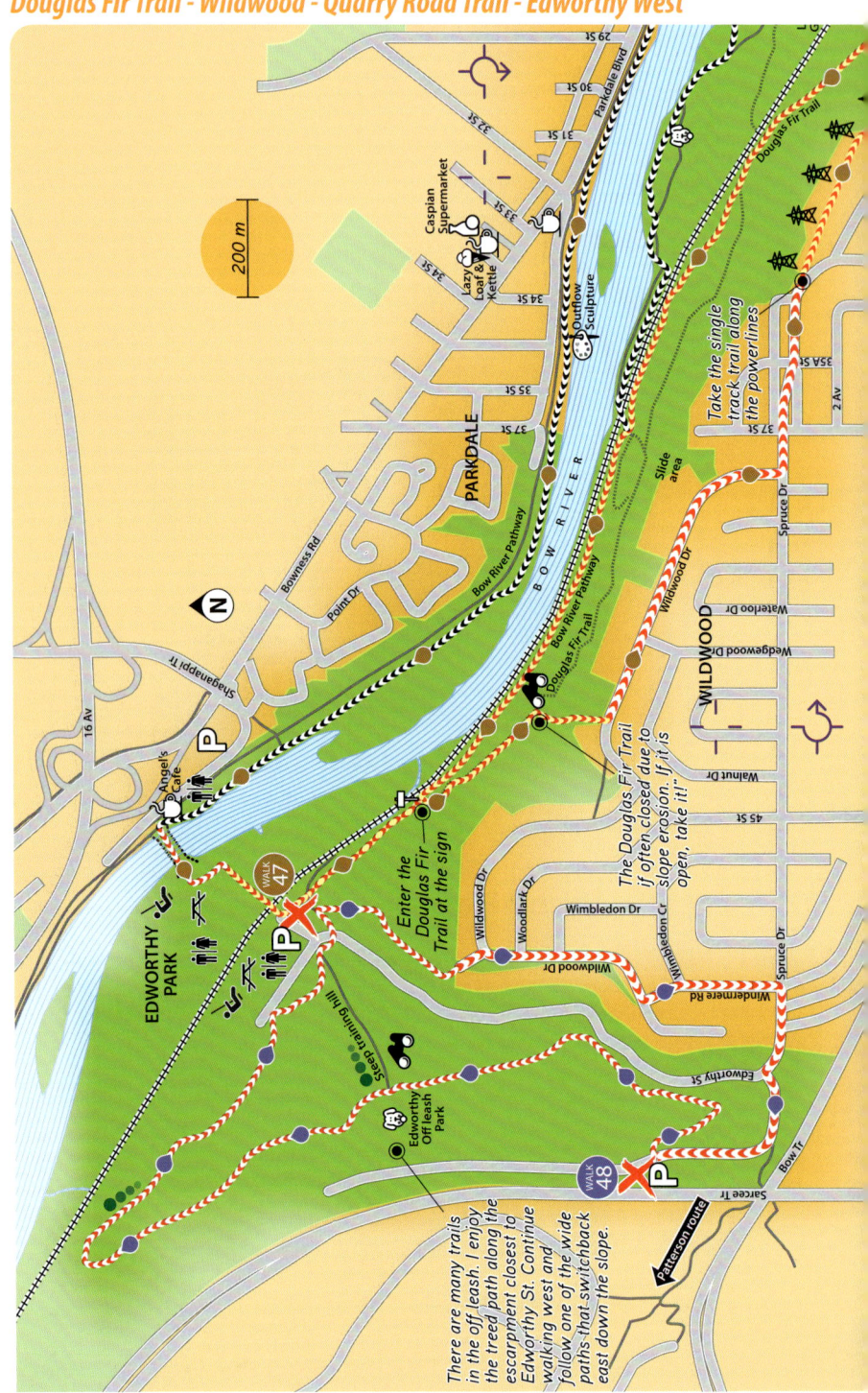

Douglas Fir Trail - Wildwood - Quarry Road Trail - Edworthy West

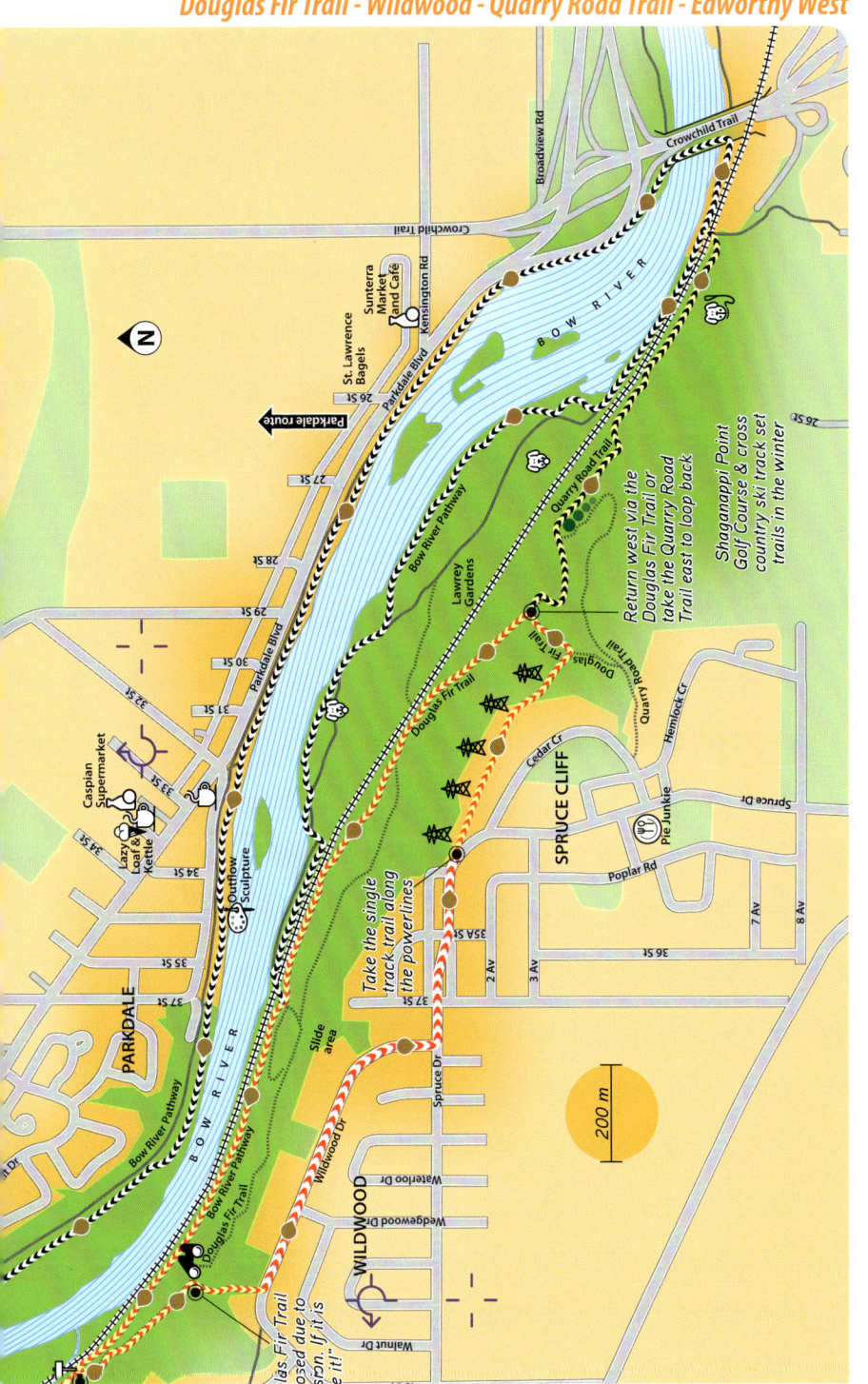

Patterson - Coach Hill - Paskapoo Slopes

Walk 49 SW

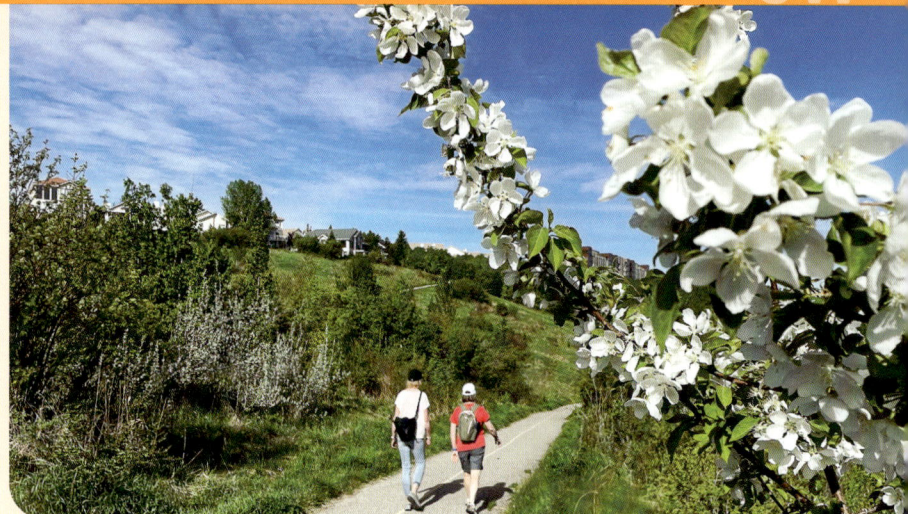

Walk at a Glance:

Offering unobstructed views of the Bow River Valley and the prairies beyond, this urban walkabout offers the perfect vantage point to get the lay of the land in Calgary. Navigating a mix of forested singletrack trails, quiet side streets and paved pathways, walkers soak up spectacular vistas while imaging that, 8,500 years ago, the cliffs along the escarpment were used extensively by Indigenous peoples as a buffalo jump, a unique method of hunting bison. In fact, archeologists have uncovered kill and processing sites, sweat pits and camps slope-side.

Back to present day, continue along paved pathways through saskatoon filled ravines that open up to the community of Patterson. This hilly neighbourhood offers the perfect view of Calgary's compact downtown reaching skyward. Connect to earthy pathways along

Details

Categories: Café, Dog, Nature, Neighbourhood & Parks, Vistas, Birds

Start: 77 Street and Cougar Ridge Drive SW, near the Calgary French School

Facilities: None

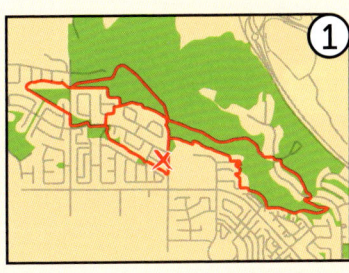

Distance & Difficulty

5.5 km (hilly, paved paths and single-track trails)

Highlights, Detours & Destinations

The Paskapoo Slopes are covered in delicious saskatoons in August and wildflowers all summer long

the slopes, stopping to smell the wildflowers or snack on some saskatoons in the summertime. Continue along one of the Eastlands trails, a popular mountain biking trail network that twist and turns on the Paskapoo Slopes below Cougar Ridge. Walkers are welcome to explore the area while keeping an eye open for speedy cyclists enjoying the network of steep single-track trails that make for fun and sometimes challenging descents, as well as cardio-intensive climbs. The top of the slopes is heavily treed, but as you descend, the trees open into grassland and big views of the city. As you navigate the slopes, watch for old cars, a glacial erratic, and a Buddist Stupa, an unexpected shine in the forest that is used for meditation.

Patterson - Coach Hill - Paskapoo Slopes

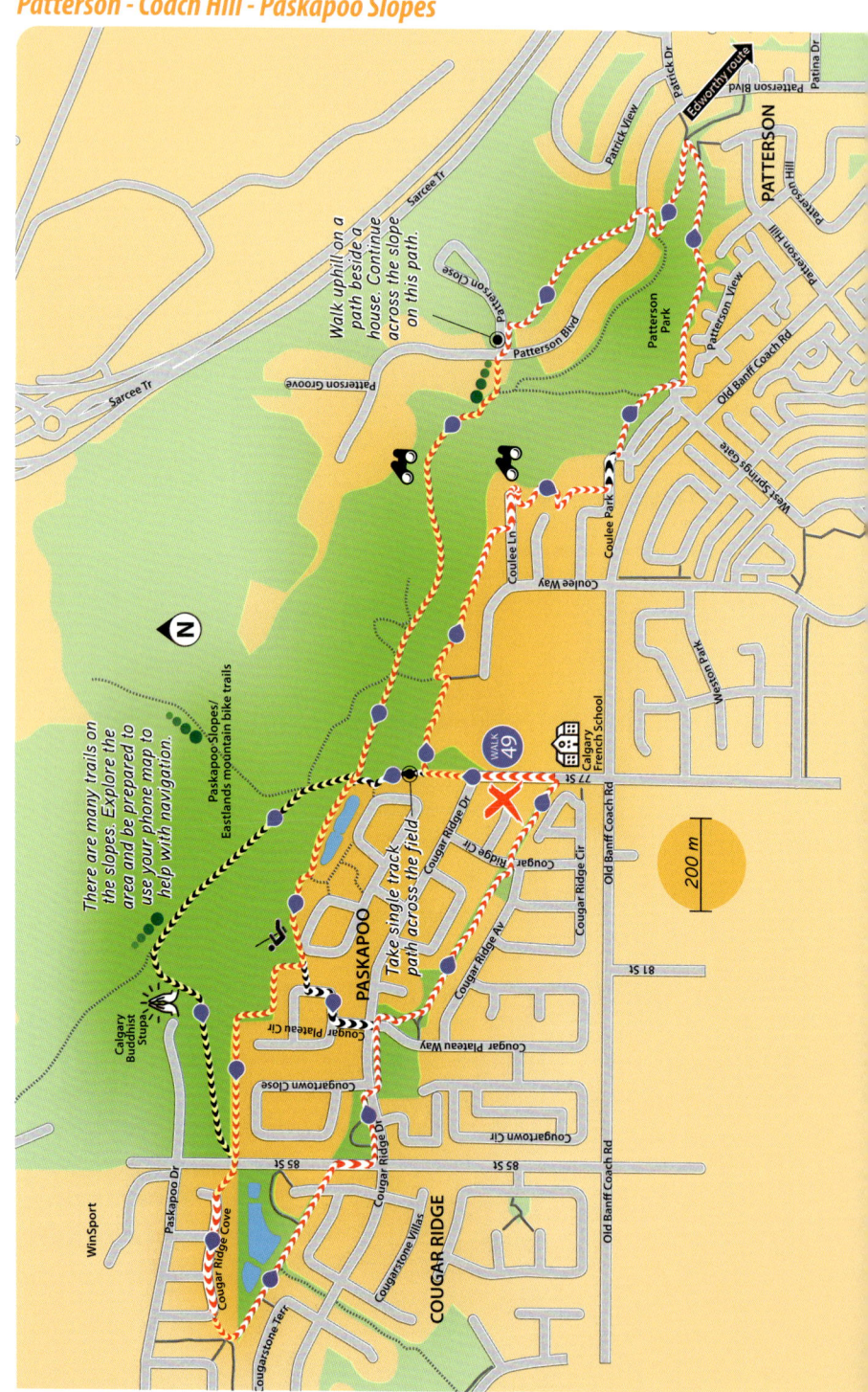

Back into the neighbourhood, walk past ponds and some impressive Cougar Ridge homes and gardens. Continue to the wetland that sits above Canada Olympic Park and WinSport. Circumnavigate the pond, enjoy a picnic lunch, and then continue eastward along paved paths and sidewalks, back to your starting point.

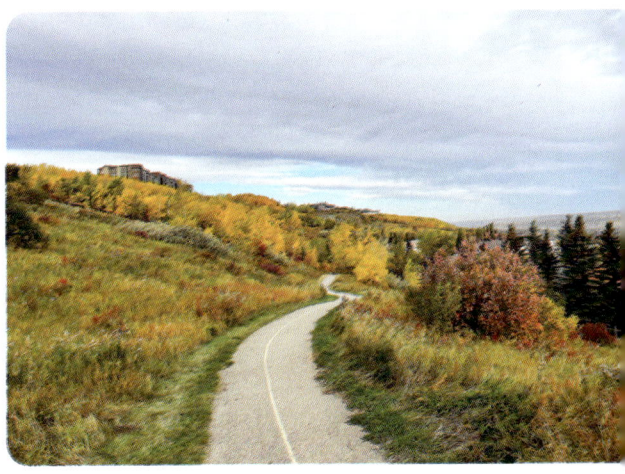

Tasty Pit Stops

Not far from the Paskapoo Slopes are many options to recharge with picnic supplies, hot drinks and ice cream. On 85 Street, just south of Old Banff Coach Road you will find Deville Coffee for your caffeine fix. If brunch is what you need then swing by Morning Brunch Co. or Brekkie. Ice Cream is served up at La Diperie and My Favourite Ice Cream Shop. Or travel south of Bow Trail and visit The Good Earth Café in Strathcona Square.

Paskapoo Slopes Buffalo Jump

Imagine that 8,500 years ago, Indigenous Peoples used the cliffs along the escarpment as a buffalo jump, a unique method of hunting bison. In fact, archeologists have uncovered kill and processing sites, sweat pits, and camps slope-side. Archeological evidence shows that the Indigenous Peoples, including the Stoney, Cree, Tsuut'ina, and Blackfoot, have lived in and visited the Bow Valley for over 10,000 years. The cliffs and steep slopes of the area made it a good spot for the Plains Peoples to stampede buffalo. One bull might supply 500 lb (227 kg) of meat. This meat was dried and made into pemmican, a mixture of dried meat, berries, and bone marrow stored in buffalo skin bags. Pemmican was the main source of nutrients for the peoples of the plains throughout the winter. European explorers also used it as a nutritious and long-lasting food source.

Strathcona and Aspen Ravines, Springbank Hill and Signal Hill

Walks 50, 51, 52

SW

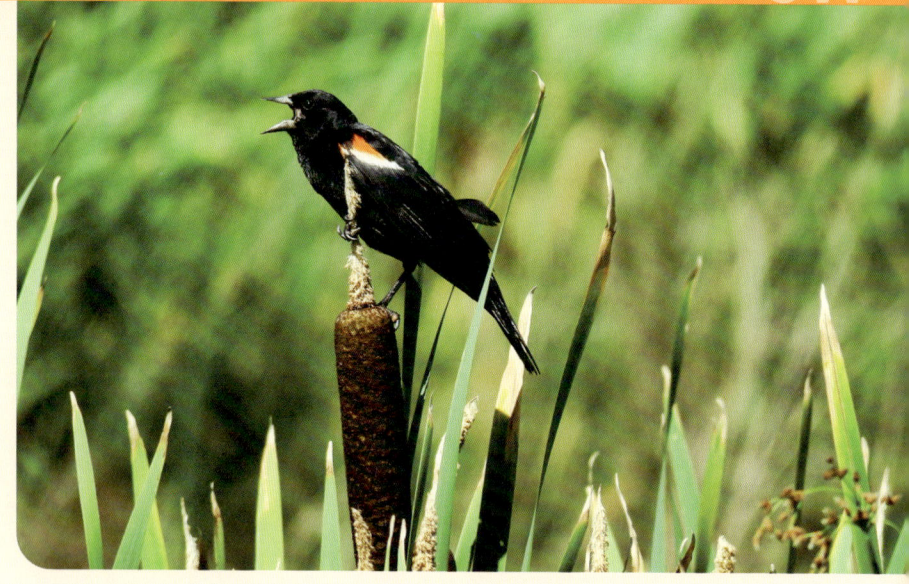

Red-winged blackbird by Sara Tehranian

Walks at a Glance:

Tucked into Calgary's southwest suburbs are a series of ravines that offer the urban explorer a wilderness immersion alongside the cul-de-sacs. Step out on Walk 50 into Strathcona Ravines Park, an environmental reserve that offers a break from the energy of the city, giving walkers a chance to slow the pace amongst the poplars and trembling aspens.

A boardwalk at the west end of the ravine crosses a seasonal stream and wetland; it's an excellent area in which to look for birds such as flycatchers and waxwings. Birds of prey such as great horned and great gray owls have also been spotted in this park. And you might see moose and deer as they prefer the ravine wilds to the side streets.

Details

Categories: LRT, Café, Dog, Nature, Neighbourhood & Parks, Hilly, Vistas, Birds

Start: Walks 50 and Walk 52: Optimist Athletic Park, 5020 26 Avenue SW; Walk 51: A Ladybug Bakery & Café, 10 Aspen Stone Boulevard SW; Walk 52: Signal Hill Park, 2972 Signal Hill Drive or Signal Hill Library, 5994 Signal Hill Centre SW

LRT: Sirocco and 69 Street Stations

Facilities: All the walks pass by cafés. Walk 52 passes by the library

Distance & Difficulty

Walk 50: Strathcona and Aspen Ravines: 6.5-7.5 km (hills, paved paths and sidewalks)

Walk 51: Aspen Landing- Aspen Woods: 6 km (hills, paved paths and sidewalks)

Walk 52: Signal Hill- Springbank Hill: 7.5-8.5 km (paved paths, sidewalks, and stairs)

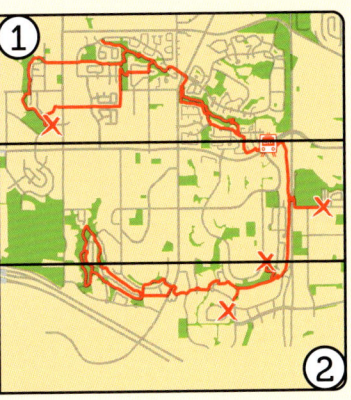

Highlights, Detours & Destinations

Bring traction devices for your shoes in the winter as the ravine trails can be icy and slippery after Chinooks

Aspen Woods and its ravines pathways is the setting for Walk 51. Starting near Aspen Landing, this walk is perfect for those who want a mix of environments, from the ravine wilds to connector paths that lead to suburban side streets. I recommend this walk for all those walkers who have a hankering for pastries and coffee, which is everyone isn't it?

Glenbrook is the starting point for Walk 52 which travels up, over and alongside Sarcee Trail on a paved pathway before climbing to Battalion Park where expansive views of the Tsuut'ina Nation, the foothills, and the Rocky Mountains are a constant. This area was a military reserve prior to the First World War for the Canadian forces. There are 16,000 stones hauled by soldiers and arranged to form four numbers (137, 113, 151, and 51) on the hillside. The numbers correspond to the four battalions of the Canadian Expeditionary Force that trained in that area before leaving to fight in the war.

Continuing along a mix of quiet side-streets and paved paths, Walk 52 leads you into Springbank Hill with its maze of regional pathways and stairway connectors that travel between houses and connect to wilder, tree canopied ravines with wetlands. The big surprise is the colourful birdhouse alley in one of the ravines. Loop back on single track trails alongside the wetlands where red-winged blackbirds will be your walking companions. Keep a close eye for birds of all types, including the tiny Northern Saw-Whet Owl that is featured and was photographed in Calgary. At 20 cm high, it is the second smallest owl in Alberta next to the Northern Pygmy Owl, which measures 16 cm in length. Once back in the neighbourhood, navigate side streets, pathways and stairs to where you began.

Signal Hill Geoglyphs

What are those large white numbers on Signal Hill you ask? They have separate yet similar stories originating in Albertan military history. The 113 is the oldest of the four and was put together by the 113th Canadian Expeditionary Force known as the Lethbridge Highlanders, one of many battalions that made up the Canadian Expeditionary Force (C.E.F.) that fought in the trenches of the First World War. In 1916, the group trained at Sarcee Camp, a section of the former Sarcee Indian reserve (now Tsuut'ina Nation) near Calgary. It was during the five months spent there that the battalion placed the painted stones that formed the 113 geoglyph on or nearby Signal Hill before shipping off to Europe. In Europe, the battalion was split up to serve as replacements for other battalions, with some 300 of them heading to Le Havre, France, to join up with the 16th Battalion, one of the most famous Canadian battalions of the war. The other numbers, though they have been moved slightly from their original locations, were all formed in the area by subsequent battalions of the C.E.F. that trained at Sarcee Camp during the First World War, including the 137th Infantry Battalion of Calgary, the 151st Central Alberta Battalion, and the 51st Canadian Infantry Battalion

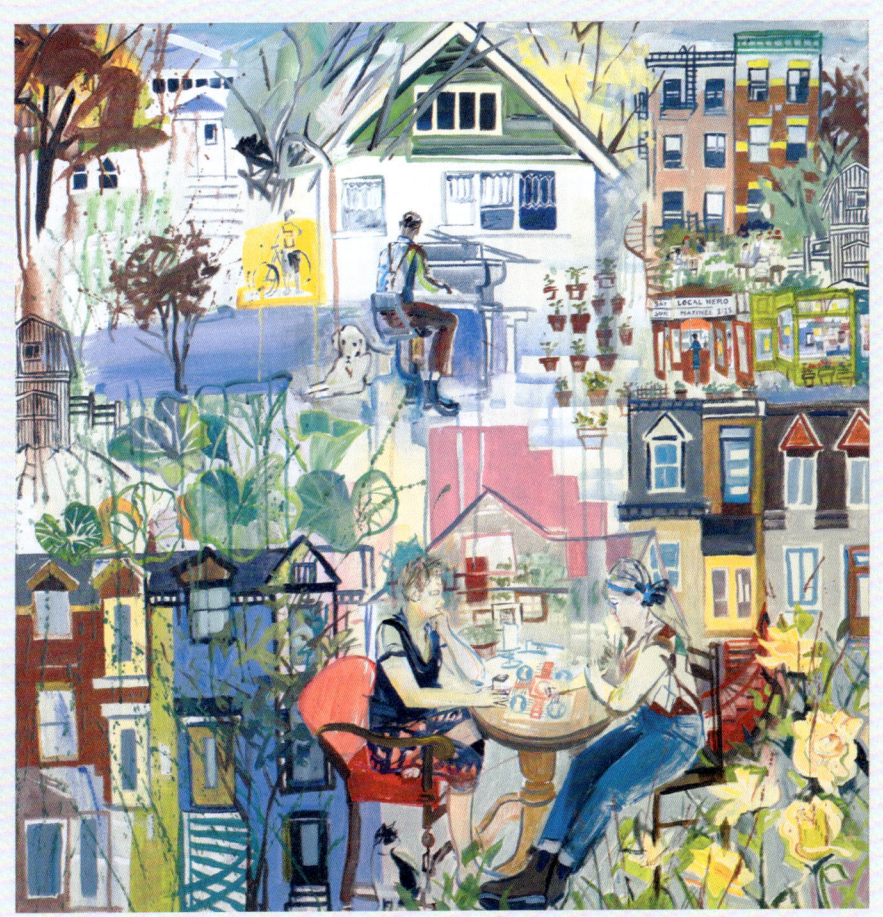

Garden Board Game Parcheesi, Urban Garden Series by Jill Thomson

Tasty Pit Stops

Sunterra Market in West Market Square is the perfect stop pre or post walk. Grab a picnic lunch from the supermarket before your walk or stop by the café after your trek for a drink and some baked goods, made fresh daily. The Good Earth Café at Strathcona Square makes a nice mid walk stop. Hearty lunches and baked goods are their specialty. And for those urban trekkers who want to increase their distance, navigate the side streets to the Ladybug Bakery and Café in Aspen where mouth-watering brunch, fresh bread, desserts and melt-in-your-mouth pastries await.

Location:
Sunterra market: West Market Square: 1851 Sirocco Drive SW
Good Earth Café: Strathcona Square: 555 Strathcona Boulevard SW
A Ladybug Bakery & Café: 2132-10 Aspen Stone Blvd SW

Trembling Aspen Clones

Groves of trembling aspen, native trees with round leaves that are easily coerced into movement by the wind, cover the slopes throughout Calgary. Trembling aspen leaves are a fresh green in the spring and turn a vibrant yellow in the fall. All aspens within a grove are genetically identical. The original tree clones itself by sending out suckers from underground roots, each of which becomes a new aspen. Some trembling aspen colonies in Alberta are over six thousand years old. All clones within a colony change colour at the same time in the fall. Trembling aspen groves make great hiding spots for animals and add sparkling slopeside colour to these walkabouts.

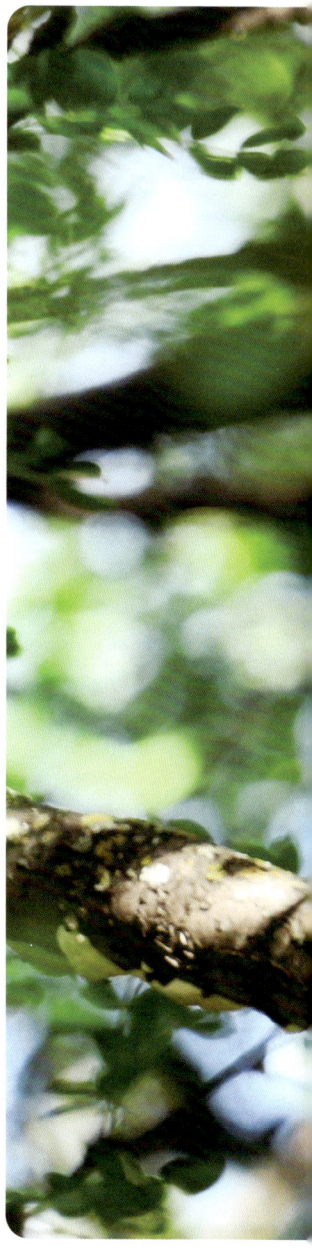

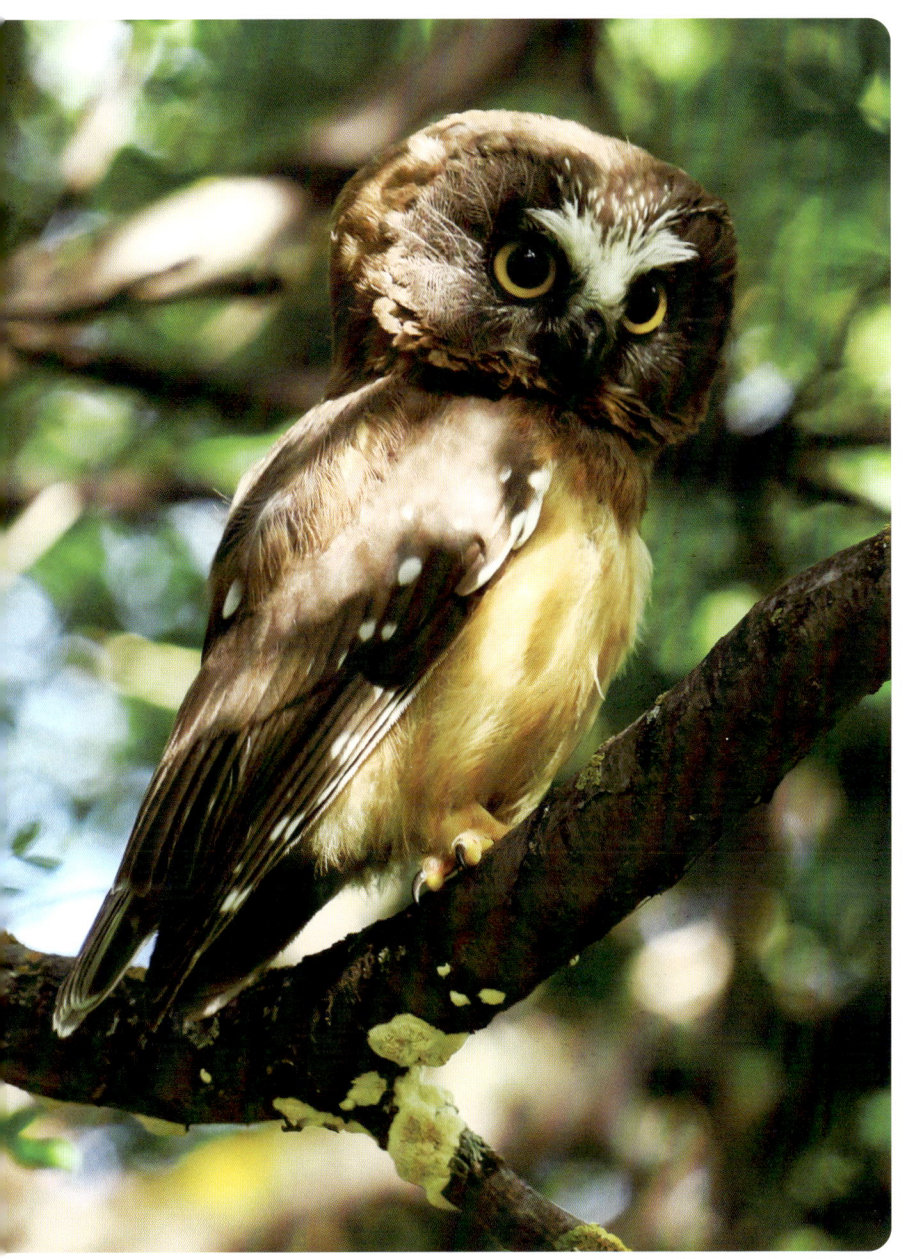
Northern Saw-Whet Owl by Sara Tehranian

Strathcona and Aspen Ravines, Springbank Hill and Signal Hill

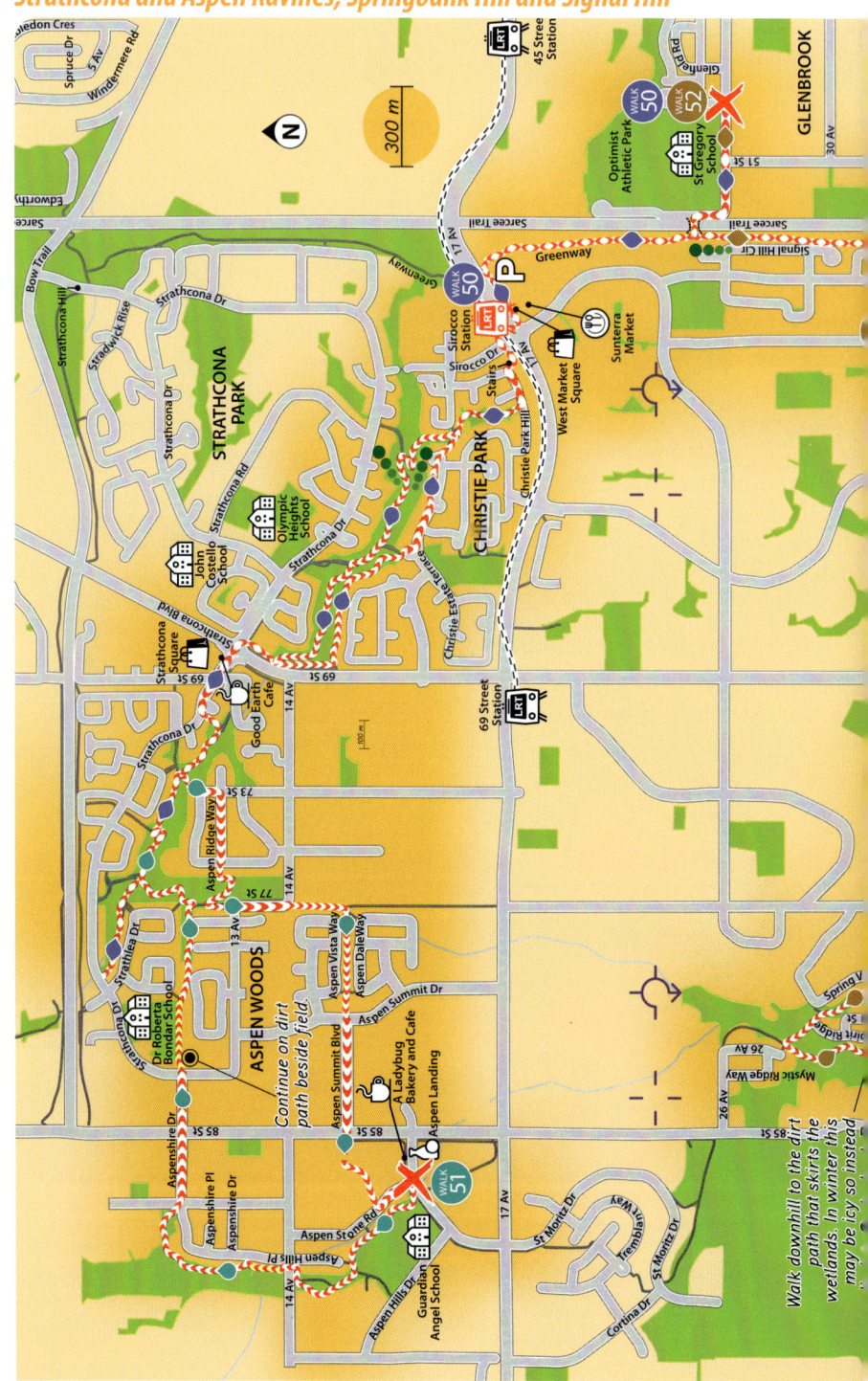

Strathcona and Aspen Ravines, Springbank Hill and Signal Hill

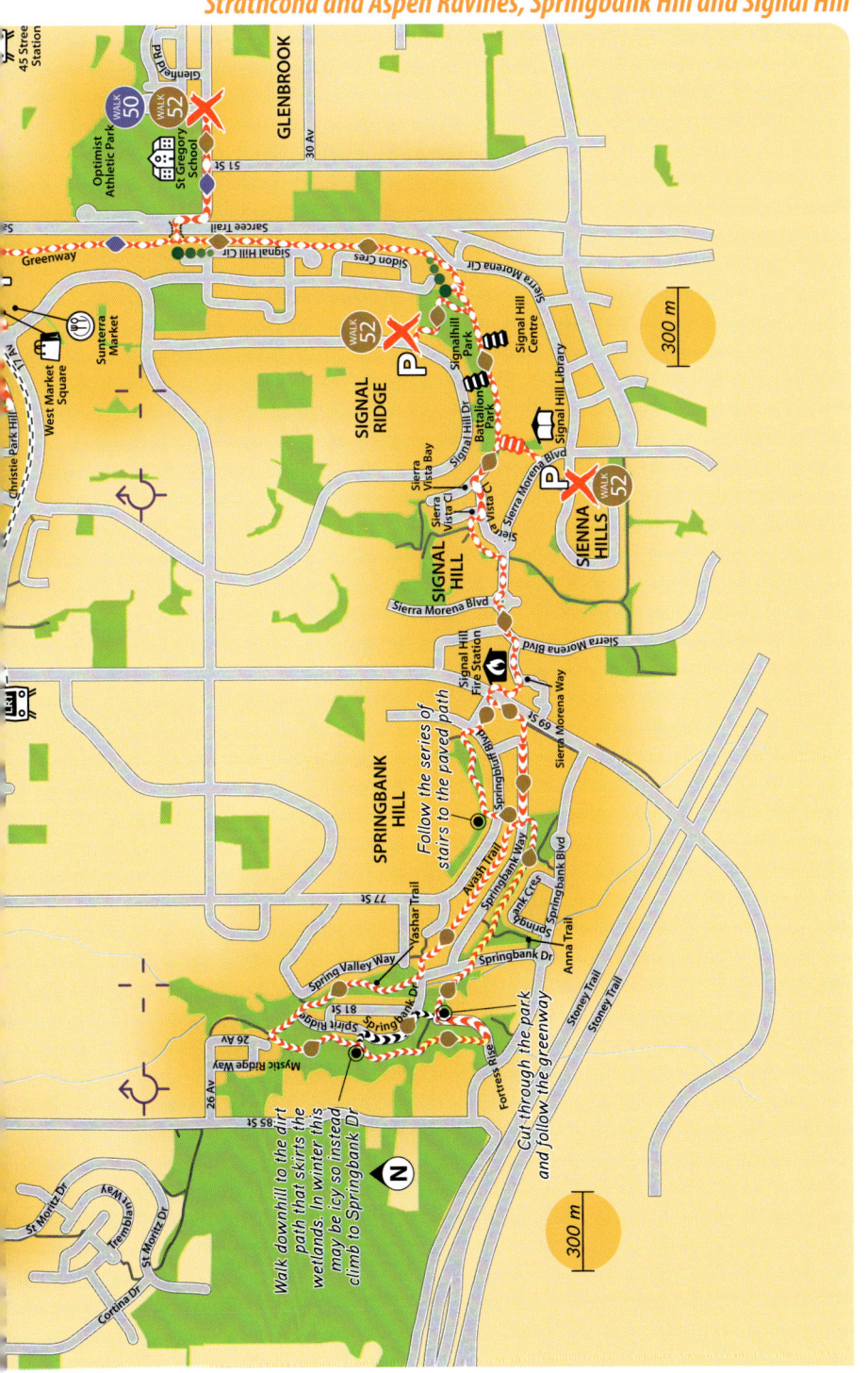

STRATHCONA AND ASPEN RAVINES, SPRINGBANK HILL AND SIGNAL HILL

Sunalta - Beltline - Mount Royal - Bankview - Scarboro - Kilarney

Walks 53-55

SW

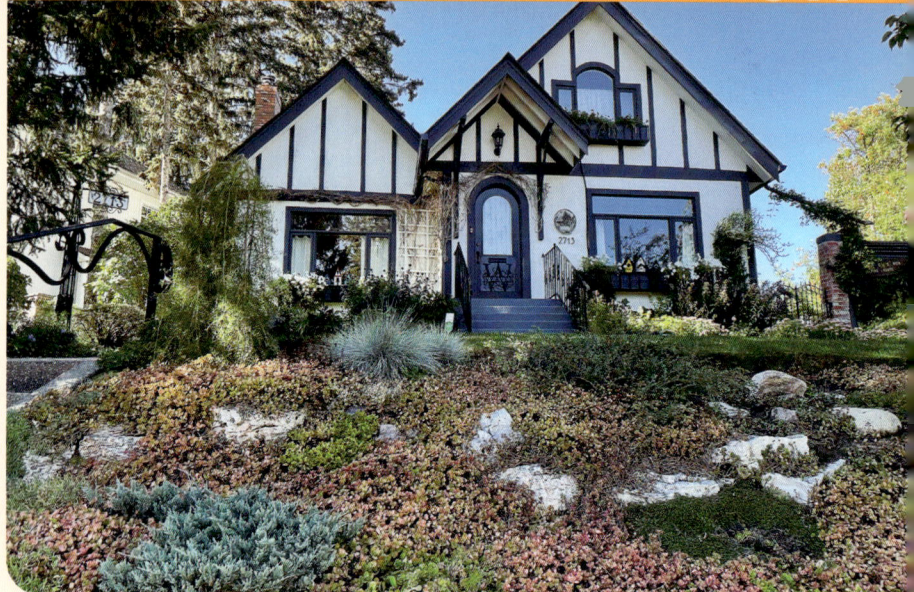

Walks at a Glance:

Bankview is Calgary's mini-San Francisco with its steep streets and high density. The area has undergone many changes since its ranching beginnings in 1882. Now jam-packed with life, the neighbourhood's mix of apartment complexes, condos, 1900s bungalows, and new multi-million-dollar escarpment homes create a vibrant and varied community.

Continue north across 17 Avenue and enter Scarboro, one of Calgary's more affluent neighbourhoods. Unlike most Calgary communities, Scarboro is not on a grid. The leafy streets curve, dip, and climb past well-kept homes with varying square footage. Walk 54 continues west over Crowchild Trail and into the neighbourhoods of

Details

Categories: LRT, Café, DoWg, Nature, Neighbourhood & Parks, People watch & shop, Hilly, Stroller, Historic, Vistas, River

Start: Walks 53 and 55: Scarboro Community Association, 1747 14 Avenue SW; Walk 54: Bankview Community Association: 2418 17 Street SW

LRT: Sunalta and Shaganappi Point Stations

Facilities: Cafés and libraries along the routes

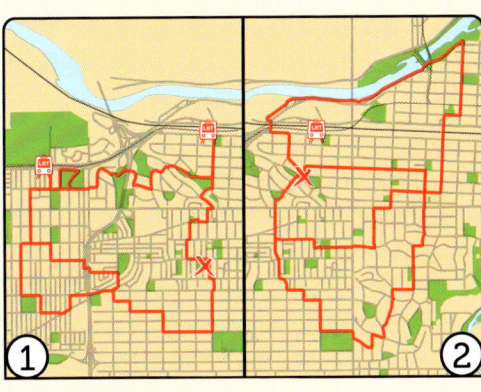

Distance & Difficulty

Walk 53: Sunalta - Beltline- Mount Royal - Bankview- Scarboro: 5.5 km (hilly, sidewalks)

Walk 54: Bankview – Scarboro – Kilarney - South Calgary: 7.5 km (hilly, sidewalks)

Walk 55: Scarboro - Bow River – Downtown - Beltline: 8 km (sidewalks, paved paths)

Highlights, Detours & Destinations

Christmas lights and a café or restaurant stop make for a nice evening walk in December. People watching on 17 Avenue is in full swing in April when spring-happy Calgarians stroll the streets, embracing the above-zero temperatures and sunlit evenings. In May and June the blossoming apple and cherry trees, as well as purple lilacs, are a feast for the senses. Gardens are in full bloom from mid-July through to October

Shaganappi, Killarney and South Calgary where pleasant streets host a mix of 1950 bungalows and newer builds along with many parks scattered throughout. Take a detour to cSPACE King Edward, the arts hub in South Calgary. Grab a gift from the Alberta Craft Council, a coffee or visit one of the many artists that have open studios, offer courses and sell their creations.

Walks 53 and 55 continue through Sunalta, past well-placed pocket parks that increase the neighbourhood's green-space quotient. Density increases with every street as you move toward 14 Street and the bustle of the city. Connaught is in the Beltline, a condo populated inner-city area. No need for a car if you live here.

Tasty pit stops, cafés to craft beer

As an urban walker, you may walk alone through green, lush, and peaceful landscapes, or amongst busy streets surrounded by other people. Seventeenth Avenue is a pedestrian-friendly shopping area that is worth a detour if you are in the mood for the latter. During the warm months, enjoy people watching on a patio while sipping a glass of wine and enjoying a meal. Walks 53 and 55 pass by Kalamata Grocery, a landmark in the Beltline and the best spot to pick up picnic supplies. Shelves and rows are stacked full of Greek specialties, but it's the 16 types of fresh olives, multiple varieties of feta, and the different kinds of sesame-based halva that will "make a Greek out of ya," as the owner once said after he handed me a spicy green olive to taste. Walk 55 passes by Loophole Coffee, a downtown café known for its good coffee and live music and the popular local spot that makes the best cappuccinos, Gravity Café on 8 Street. Back on 17 Avenue, decide between locally made ice cream from Made by Marcus or continue east to the local favourites, Caffé Beano and Analog Café. Both locations have outdoor seating with a unique perspective on the people populated Beltline. If you are walking routes 53 or 54, then plan a stop at Our Daily Brett for a hot drink, a full meal or to grab some tasty items to go or continue to the cSPACE, the arts hub where Aroma Café serves up coffee, pastries and authentic Mexican food. Detour just south of Walk 54 to 34 Avenue in Marda Loop for many cafés, wine bars, sandwich and ice cream options or keep walking to the Coffee Cats Café in Killarney. For craft beer fans, swing by Buffalo Brewing in Killarney, Two House Brewing or to my favourite spot, Tailgunner Brewing where you can enjoy the delicious Acme pizza at long tables that are perfect for chatting with new to you friends. If you want to grab some craft beer to go, visit the Alberta Beer Exchange where you'll find a huge variety of single cans from around Canada. The perfect ending to your urban trek.

Location:
Kalamata Grocery: 1421 11 Street SW
Loophole Coffee: 1040 8 Avenue SW
Gravity Café: CBE building, 12 Avenue and 8 Street SW
Made by Marcus: 1013 17 Avenue SW
Caffe Beano and Analog Café: 9 Street and 7 Street 17 Avenue SW
Our Daily Brett: 1507 29 Avenue SW
Aroma Café at cSPACE: 1721 29 Avenue SW Buffalo Brewing: 2801 24a Street SW
Coffee Cats Café: 2765 17 Avenue SW
The Alberta Beer Exchange: 1642 10 Avenue SW
Two House Brewing & Tailgunner Brewing: 10 Avenue SW

All services and transit are just a walk away; this area is the perfect place to stop for lunch or a coffee. And keep an eye out for murals. Since 2017 the Beltline Urban Murals Project (BUMP) has hosted mural artists every summer to bring the Beltline walls to life. Check out the updated mural map at www.yycbump.ca. Take a detour and walk along 17 Avenue for a bit of people watching and window shopping.

If you are following Walk 53 you will climb into the community of Mount Royal and soak up the city's wealth. During the early 1900s Mount Royal was promoted by the Canadian Pacific Railway as the exclusive neighbourhood for Calgary's most affluent citizens and it continues as such today. The residents share their riches with the urban walker in the form of well-kept homes, varied in their design, and expansive gardens.

Walk 55 continues north through the west end of downtown and back along the Bow River Pathway. There are so many interesting walk combinations in these inner-city communities. Be sure to take many detours down back alleys and leafy side-streets. Switching up your route mid stride is the best part of urban exploration.

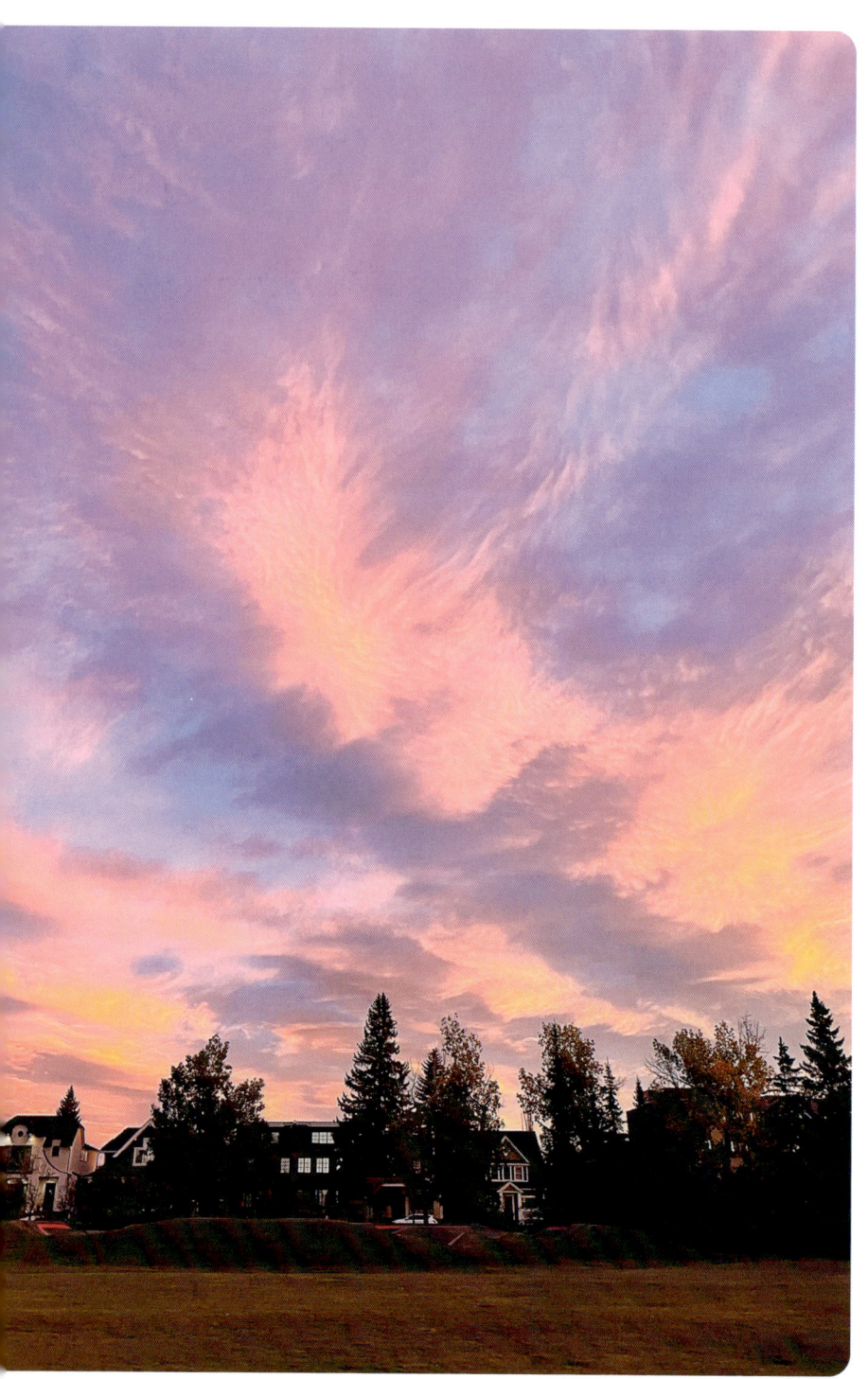

Tyndall Stone Fossils

Walks 53 and 55 passes by some fossils hiding in the Tyndall Stone on the CBE building on 8 Street at 12 Avenue. Tyndall Stone is a limestone that was deposited 450 million years ago in what is now known as the Selkirk Member of the Red River Formation. Back then, what is now southern Saskatchewan and southern Manitoba was covered in a warm and shallow sea just south of the equator. A diverse community of animals and algae lived at the bottom of this sea in a muddy carbonate platform like the Bahamas today. After they died, they were buried in the sediment and over time, they were fossilized. The stone is grey to tan in colour and mottled or blotchy. The mottling is the preserved tunnels made by burrowing marine animals looking for food or refuge from predators, probably a kind of arthropod like an ancient shrimp while others were ancient worms. Probably due to slight differences in porosity and permeability, the sediment in the tunnels got replaced by dolomite crystals whereas the surrounding rock is made of calcite. Get up close to the CBE building and look for fossils that could include nautiloids, corals, stromatoporoids, gastropods, receptaculites, brachiopods, bryozoans, crinoids, and trilobites.

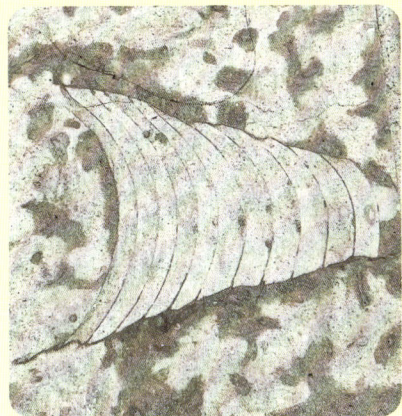

Nautiloid Fossil in Tyndall Stone

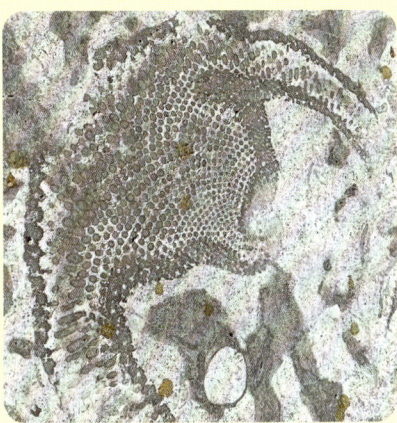

Fossil Algae in Tyndall Stone

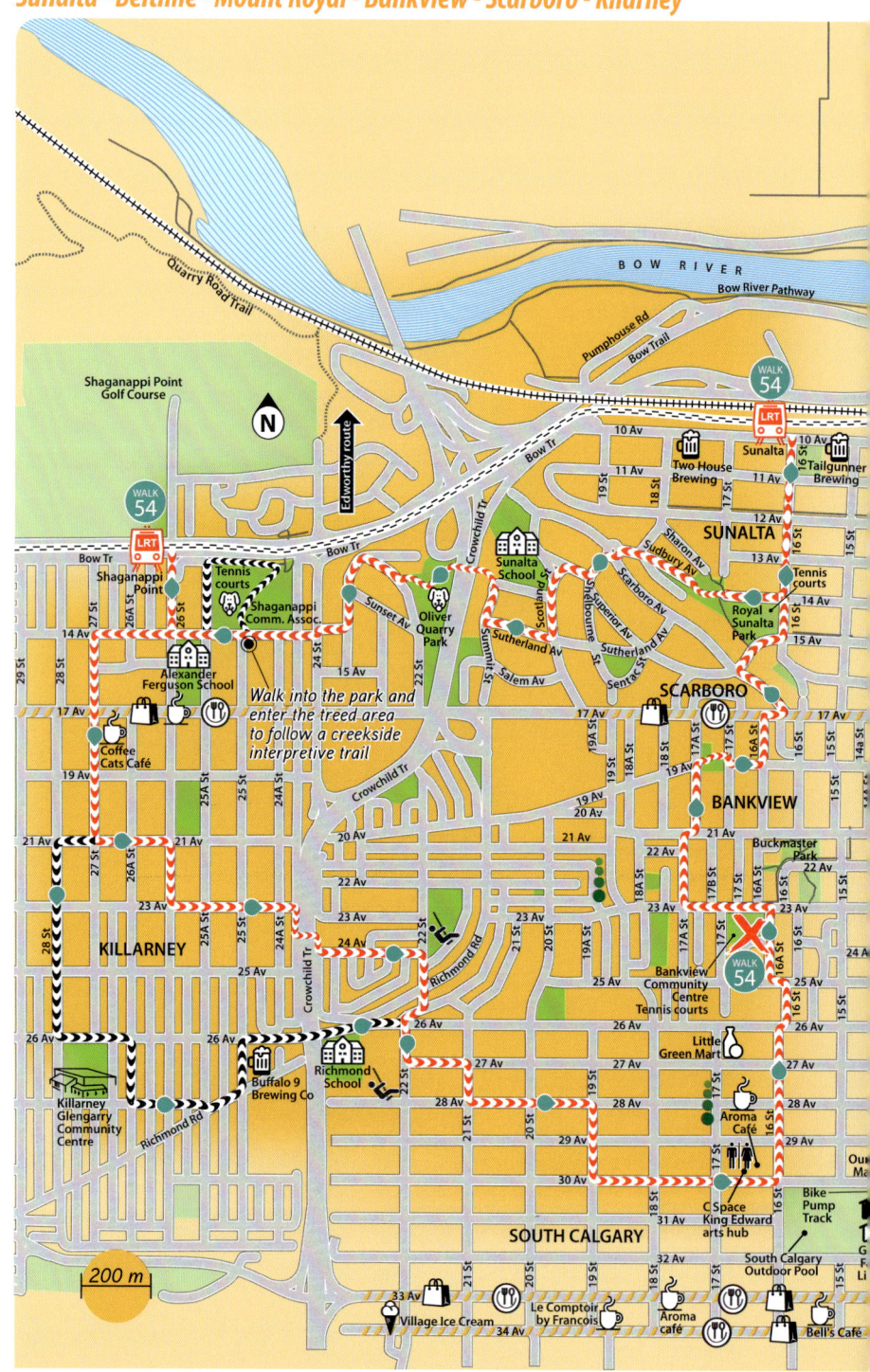

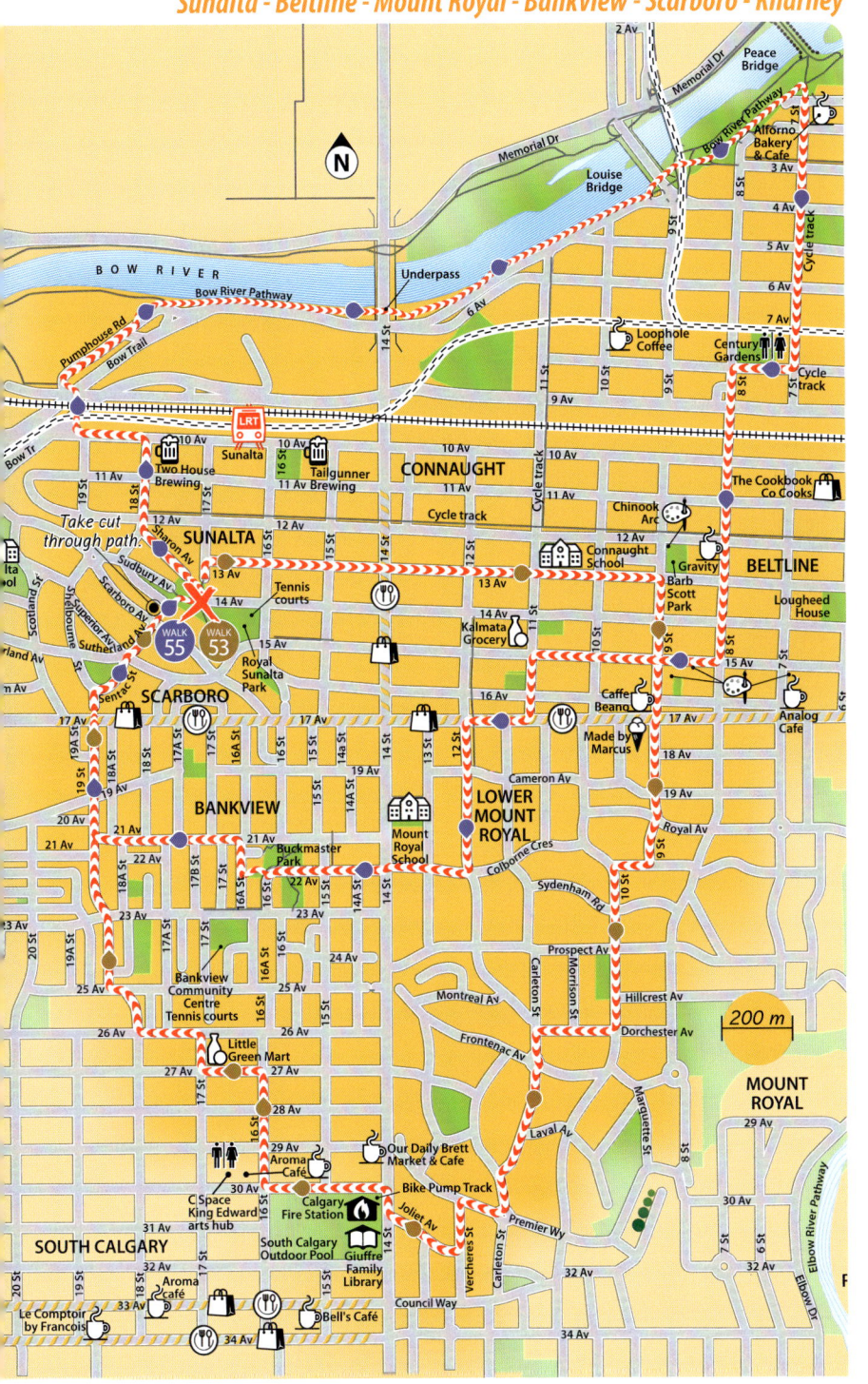

Downtown and Beltline Murals and Art

Walks 56 and 57

SW

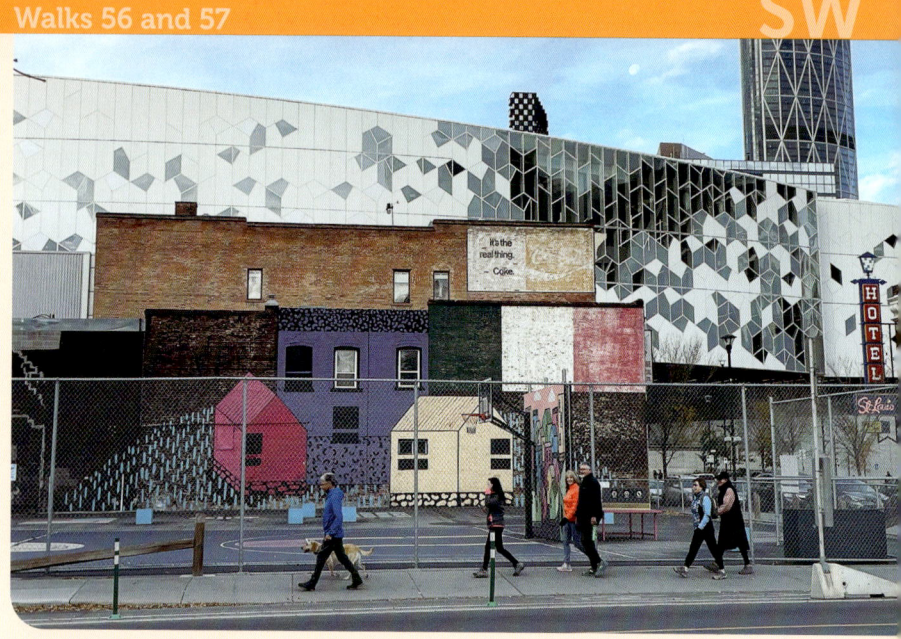

Walks at a Glance:

Engage in this public-art and mural treasure hunt through the downtown core, East Village and the Beltline. Public art is always a surprise, a distraction from the business towers above you and the cars, people, and sidewalks surrounding you.

Modern-day urban planners design streetscapes for the benefit of pedestrians, integrating the unexpected into the everyday built environment. The unpredictable is what makes walking in the city so enjoyable.

Starting at the glassy, swirling, sloping masterpiece that is the Calgary Central Library, walk back in time into Calgary's historic heart along Stephen Avenue (8 Avenue). Named after Lord Mount Stephen, the first

Details

Categories: LRT, Café, Dog, Nature, Neighbourhood & Parks, People watch & shop, Stroller, Historic, River, Birds

Start: Walks 56 and 57: Calgary Central Library, 800 3 Street SE

LRT: City Hall Station, Victoria Park Station or any downtown station

Facilities: Calgary Central Library has bathrooms. Coffee shops are along both routes

Distance & Difficulty

Walk 56: Downtown - Princes Island - East Village: 6 km (mostly flat on sidewalks, paved and gravel paths)

Walk 57: Downtown and Beltline Murals and Art: 6km (mostly flat on paved pathways, sidewalks)

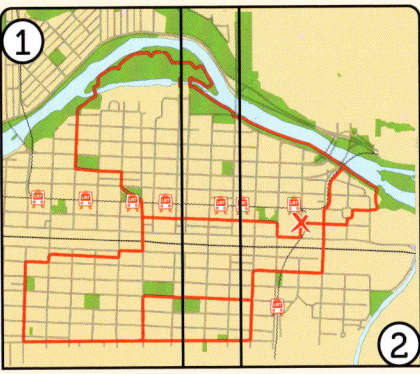

Highlights, Detours & Destinations

Christmas lights on Stephen Avenue Mall, 8 Avenue, make this a festive walk from the end of November through Christmas. Bring your skates and enjoy the ice rink at Olympic Plaza. How about a night skate under the city lights? A Zamboni keeps the ice in perfect condition. The BUMP mural festival happens in August. Check www.yycbump.ca for the details

president of the Canadian Pacific Railway, 8 Avenue hosts many of the sandstone buildings from Calgary's early days. After the fire of 1886, local Paskapoo Sandstone became the material of choice for schools, Calgary's first library (Memorial Park) and the old City Hall.

Walk 56 heads north to the Bow River Pathway and Prince's Island Park. Immerse yourself in some wetland wilds before connecting to RiverWalk and the East Village. Walk 57 travels along the people-populated streets of the Beltline, a community where the walls have become canvasses thanks to the Beltline Urban Murals Project (BUMP). Every August since 2017, mural artists

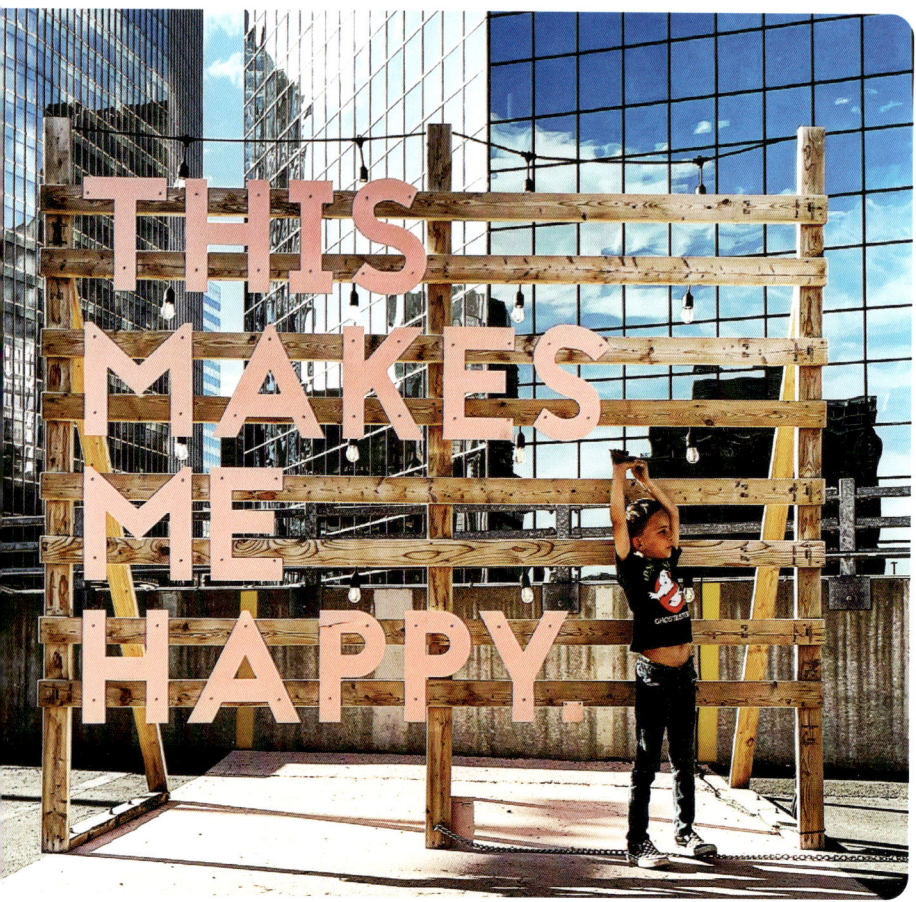

High Park by Cody Stuart

The Last Free Space: Libraries are for Everyone

As you start your walk at Calgary's newest library, the Central Library, and walk by Memorial Park Library, Alberta's first major public library which opened in 1912, consider the role that libraries play in our city. Libraries are the last place in every town and city that people can simply exist. In a library, no one is asked to pay anything simply to sit. Modern libraries have books of course, but they also offer free classes, guided walks (by me!), book groups, Internet access, resume and tax help, tutoring, and multimedia resources for anyone who might wander in. Libraries, as they exist in the twenty-first century, are the only remaining public domain. In a library, anyone of any walk of life can come and go as they choose, and so long as they remain respectful of the space they can remain as long as they wish. Libraries welcome everyone, offering a place to be and easily accessible resources to the most vulnerable populations. Libraries are the last bastions of quiet and calm where nothing is asked of one but to exist. Hooray for libraries!

descend with paints in hand to colour up the walls. Walk through Memorial Park and enjoy a picnic at one of the many outdoor tables just outside the historic Memorial Park Library. Built in 1912, it is Alberta's first public library. Stroll farther south to 17 Avenue, the popular walking, shopping, and dining street, or walk west along the 13 Avenue greenway followed by a visit to Barb Scott Park and an intriguing public sculpture called "Chinook Arc." It comes alive with colour at night. Explore the mural covered back alleys and be sure to climb to the top of High Park on 10 Avenue where the views and the murals takes centre stage.

Downtown Calgary is on track to become an urban walking destination as the city transitions beyond a traditional 9 to 5 business district towards a vibrant city centre where people live, and the arts thrive. Office towers are being converted to residential and there is an expansion and modernization of Arts Commons at Olympic Plaza as well as a redevelopment of Stephen Avenue in the works. The Glenbow Museum is getting a facelift and Victoria Park in the greater downtown area is home to the up-and-coming culture and entertainment district at Stampede Park. Slow your pace and appreciate walking for walking's sake, to simply experience the urban cityscape, alleyways, and hidden corners and surprises.

Downtown and Beltline Murals and Art

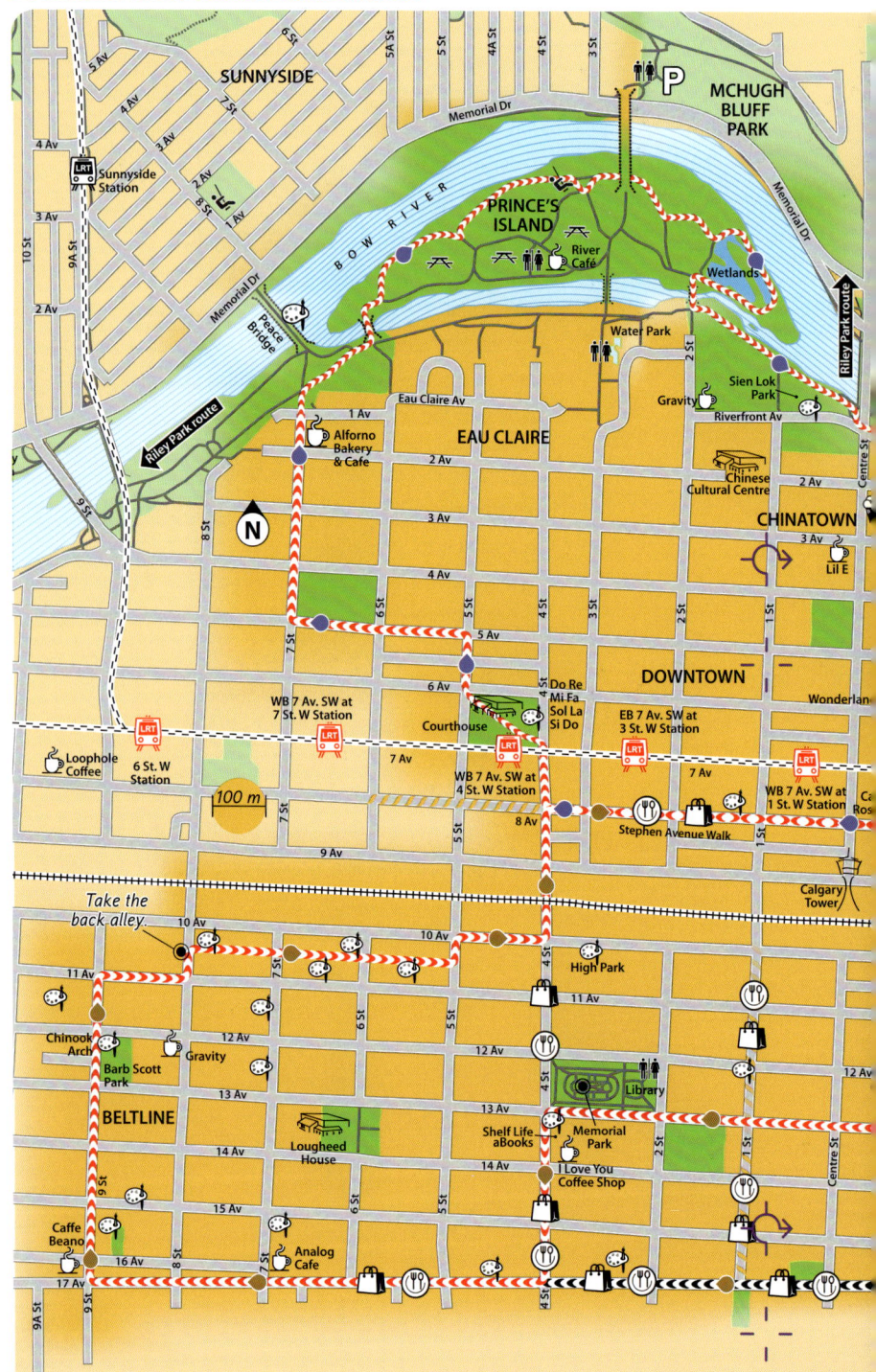

Downtown and Beltline Murals and Art

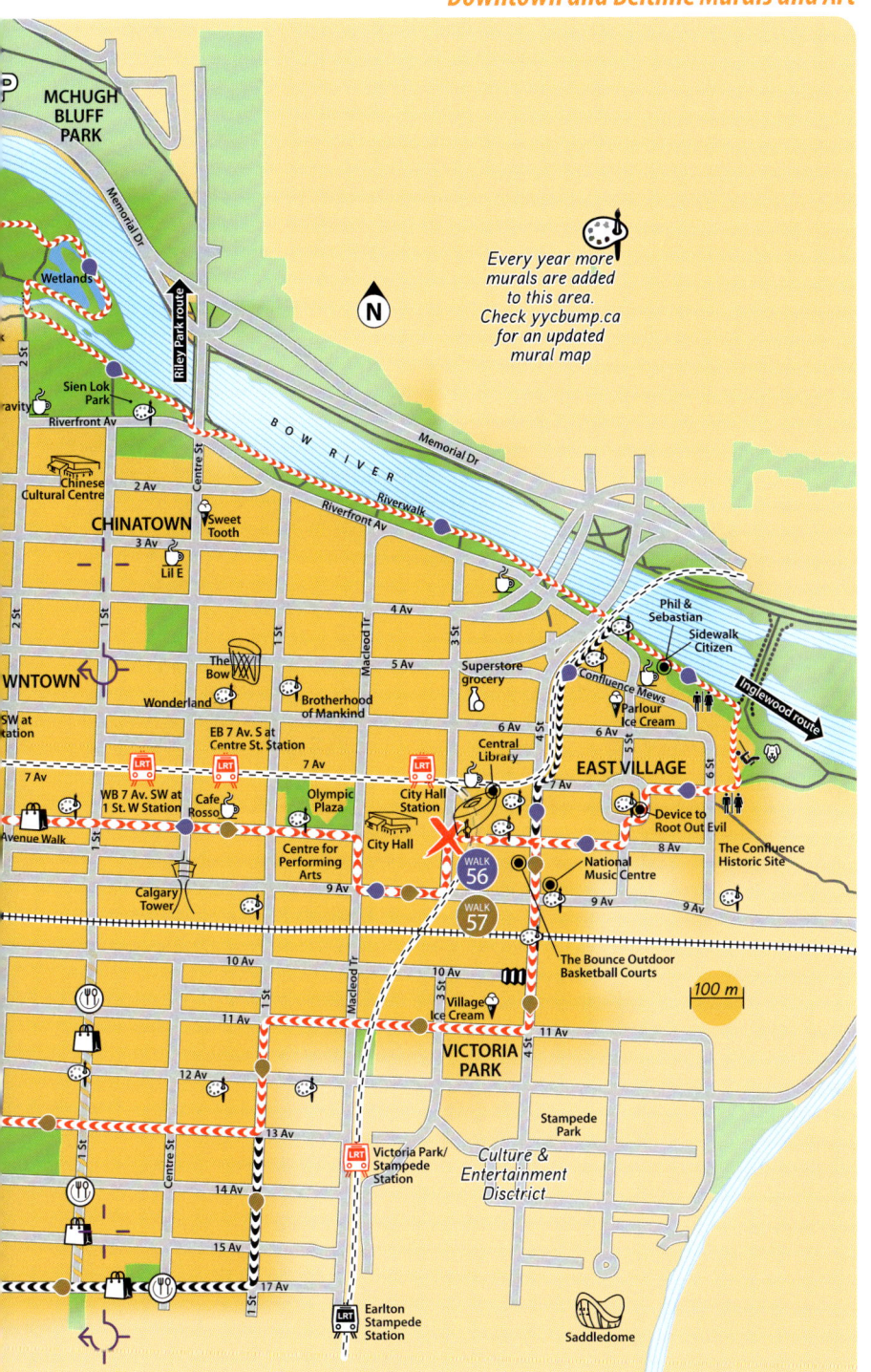

Downtown Destinations

Art, pocket parks, wetlands, and spectacular public spaces with cool cafés are scattered throughout downtown Calgary. Here are a few favourites to check out:

Century Gardens: Originally developed in 1975 for Calgary's Centennial, this park was built in the Brutalist style with lots of concrete. Redesigned in 2018 and opened in 2021, the new park is stunning and open and perfect for picnics. It hosts two park pavilion buildings, waterfalls, public art, an amphitheatre, and a central water feature splash pad. A large grassy area is welcoming and there are even public washrooms.

Location: 826 8th Avenue SW

Tasty Pit Stops: Lil E Coffee and the Ampersand Building: "What makes us different, makes us great." Lil E Coffee is inside the spectacular Ampersand building, an inviting public space that encourages visitors to settle in at one of the comfy spots provided for people to sit, plug in and work, or just watch the world go by. Get in line and grab a coffee at Lil E, where greatness is brewed and served by individuals with intellectual and developmental disabilities. Greatness starts with a belief that each person has what it takes. And if wonderful breads and pastries is what you need (yes, sometimes it is a need), then detour to Manuel Latruwe Bakery Café in Victoria Park. I have been buying my bread here for 20+ years and their pastries, quiches and mini desserts are simply wonderful. I Love You Coffee Shop is a cozy little spot in a reinvented basement in the Beltline. This popular record store café is a quirky and unexpected spot where you can listen to jazz, browse the record store and enjoy a hot or cold drink.

Location: The Ampersand, 140 4th Avenue SW; Manuel Latruwe, 1333 1 Street SE; I Love You Coffee Shop, 348b 14 Avenue SW

Courthouse Park: This wonderful little park beside the historic Sandstone Courthouse is a great place to settle in with a snack or lunch and to check out the running horses art piece Do Re Mi Fa Sol La Si Do, by Canadian artist Joe Fafard.

Location: Corner of Sixth Avenue and 4th Street SW

Prince's Island's Festivals and Wetlands: Prince's Island was named after Peter Anthony Prince, a lumberman from Quebec who came to Calgary in 1886 and founded the Eau Claire Lumber Mill. The Eau Claire and Bow River Lumber Company dug a channel (now the lagoon) to get logs from Kananaskis closer to the Calgary sawmill, resulting in an island. The island is now one of Calgary's top spots for summer festivals and picnics. In the east end of the island there is a wetland park and pathway that offers up urban wilds backdropped by downtown towers. Bird life is abundant, and beavers also call the wetland home. Take a break on your bike ride to stroll the pathway and soak up some urban nature.

Location: Prince's Island Park, 4th Street and 1st Avenue SW

Public Art: A piece that I love is The Van Gogh Monumental on 10th Avenue at 1st Street SW. The painted bronze statue stands larger than life at four metres tall and depicts a young Vincent van Gogh walking with bag in hand and a painting strapped to his back. This statue is part of Bruno Catalano's Les Voyageurs series, which is known for striding characters somehow defying physics with a distinctive gap mid-statue. The artist describes the statue: "Defragmented man, destabilized, stripped of his bearings, he walks towards his salvation as much as towards his loss. Everything will now have to be reinvented." And be sure to make a detour to see Wonderland, the 3.5-metre-high, wire-frame sculpture of a giant girl's head standing guard at the outdoor plaza at the Bow building. You can find a map of all of Calgary's public art at maps.calgary.ca/PublicArt/

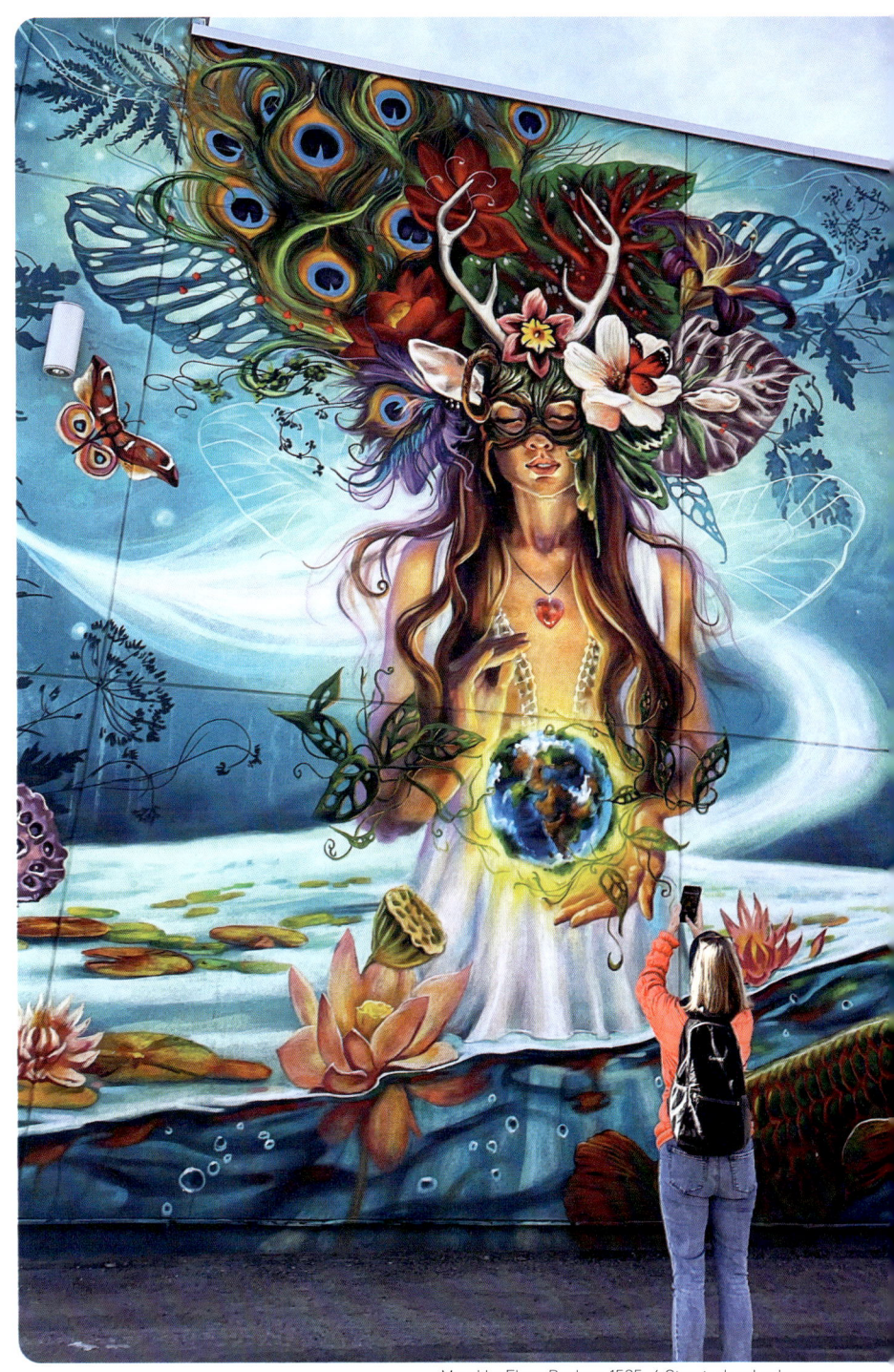

Mural by Elena Bushan, 1525, 4 Street, elenabushan.ca

Roxboro - Erlton - Ramsay

Walk 58

SW

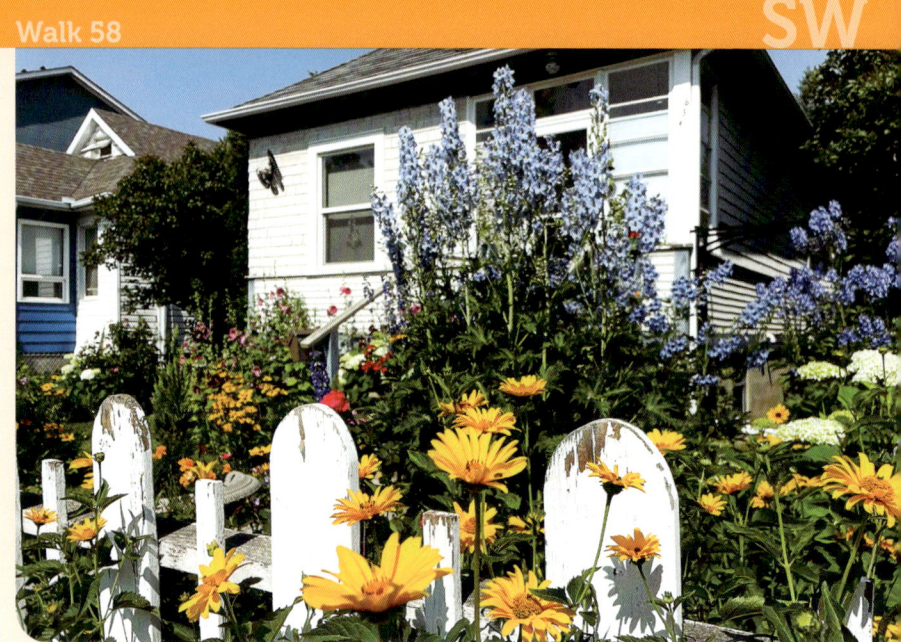

Walk at a Glance:

Connecting five communities, this route sheds light on the kind of diversity Calgary can pack into a 5-km radius. Climb the dirt path into Roxboro Natural Park, an escarpment green space. The views from the top of the bluff are expansive, taking in the tree-canopied streets of Roxboro and the money-making business core beyond.

Connect through the St Mary's cemetery in Erlton and continue up and over Macleod Trail. You'll get a glimpse of the treadmill of life, the cars whizzing below, before you descend into the calm of Union Cemetery. Reader Rock Garden is the next detour, a wonderful, inner-city,

Details

Categories: LRT, Café, Dog, Nature, Neighbourhood & Parks, People watch & shop, Hilly, Historic, Vistas, River

Start: Roxboro, 30 Avenue and 2 Street SW

LRT: Erlton Station

Facilities: Cafés along the route. See Walk 59 for tasty stops along 4 Street SW

Distance & Difficulty

7.5 km or 8 km via alternate route (Hills, stairs, sidewalks, paved paths and single-track trails)

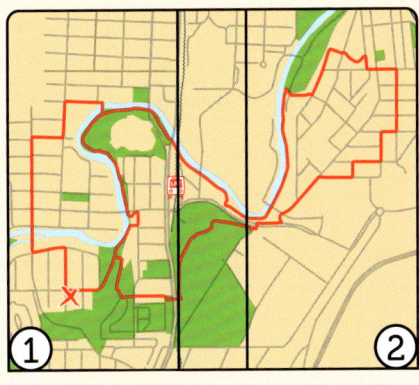

Highlights, Detours & Destinations

Learn all out Calgary Stampede history at the SAM Centre Stampede museum where interactive exhibits bring the history of the Stampede to life. The Centre is also home to the beautiful Maisie's Eatery. I suggest that you walk every street in Ramsay and Mission as there is character and colour throughout these neighbourhoods

perennial garden that sits below the cemetery, on the south side of the Stampede grounds. The garden is named after creator William Roland Reader, the City of Calgary parks superintendent from 1913 to 1942. In the early 1900s, Reader collected alpine plants while hiking in the mountains. He introduced them to this formerly bare hillside. Over thirty years he continued to develop his garden, testing the abilities of over four thousand plants in the prairie climate. The now-reconstructed garden blooms from mid-March through October. It is a mini oasis, a nice spot for a picnic or just a wander.

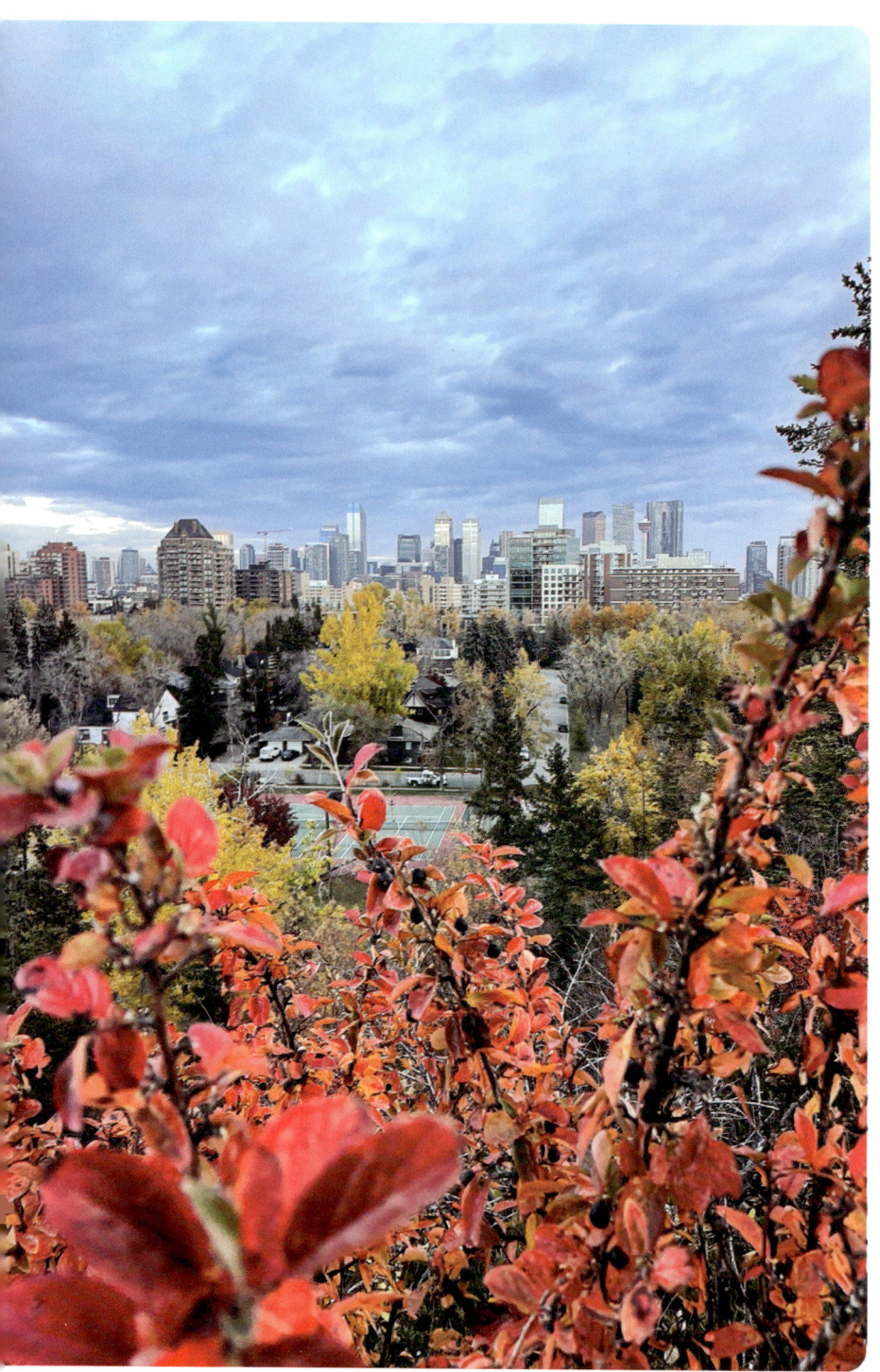

Walk east past the Reader house, now a restaurant, and set your sights on Ramsay and Inglewood, Calgary's first communities. Variety is the spice of life, and not knowing what you might find around the next corner is what makes for a fun urban walkabout. Ramsay is a neighbourhood wherein residents' interests, and thus their characters, are visible to all who pass by. An art installation, a colourful house, the little free library on a front lawn; I always have my camera at the ready for the unexpected. Plan to graze as you walk. A warm microclimate and rich soil bring early blooms, as well as a multitude of pears and apples falling from trees throughout the fall.

Climb to Scotsman's Hill, the place to watch the Stampede fireworks in early July and snap a photo of the iconic view over Stampede Park: city towers reach skyward, and the Rocky Mountains stretch out across the horizon. Find the escarpment staircase and drop down to the RiverWalk pathway and Stampede extension. Follow the Elbow River Pathway south along the Stampede grounds to Lindsay Park. Walk through the side streets of Mission and along popular forth Street for a coffee or some shopping or continue along the Elbow River Pathway to the hidden pathway that leads you back to your starting point.

Reader Rock Garden

As you walk through Reader Rock Garden, imagine that in 1913 the site was nothing more than a dusty barren bit of land. Thanks to William Reader, an Englishman who brought his love of gardening to Calgary in 1908, the site was transformed. In April 1913 Reader became the parks superintendent for Calgary, and during his twenty-nine-year career, he helped develop many of Calgary's parks, cemeteries, and civic nurseries. Between 1922 and 1929, thousands of tons of boulders, originating from Banff to Drumheller, were brought to the garden site to create an alpine rock garden. Reader's passion for gardening led him to collect plants from around the world. He introduced many of these into the rock garden, and at one time, up to 850 varieties of seeds were documented in the Reader Rock Garden. Reader taught Calgarians that it is possible to have a beautiful garden in Calgary, despite our tough growing conditions.

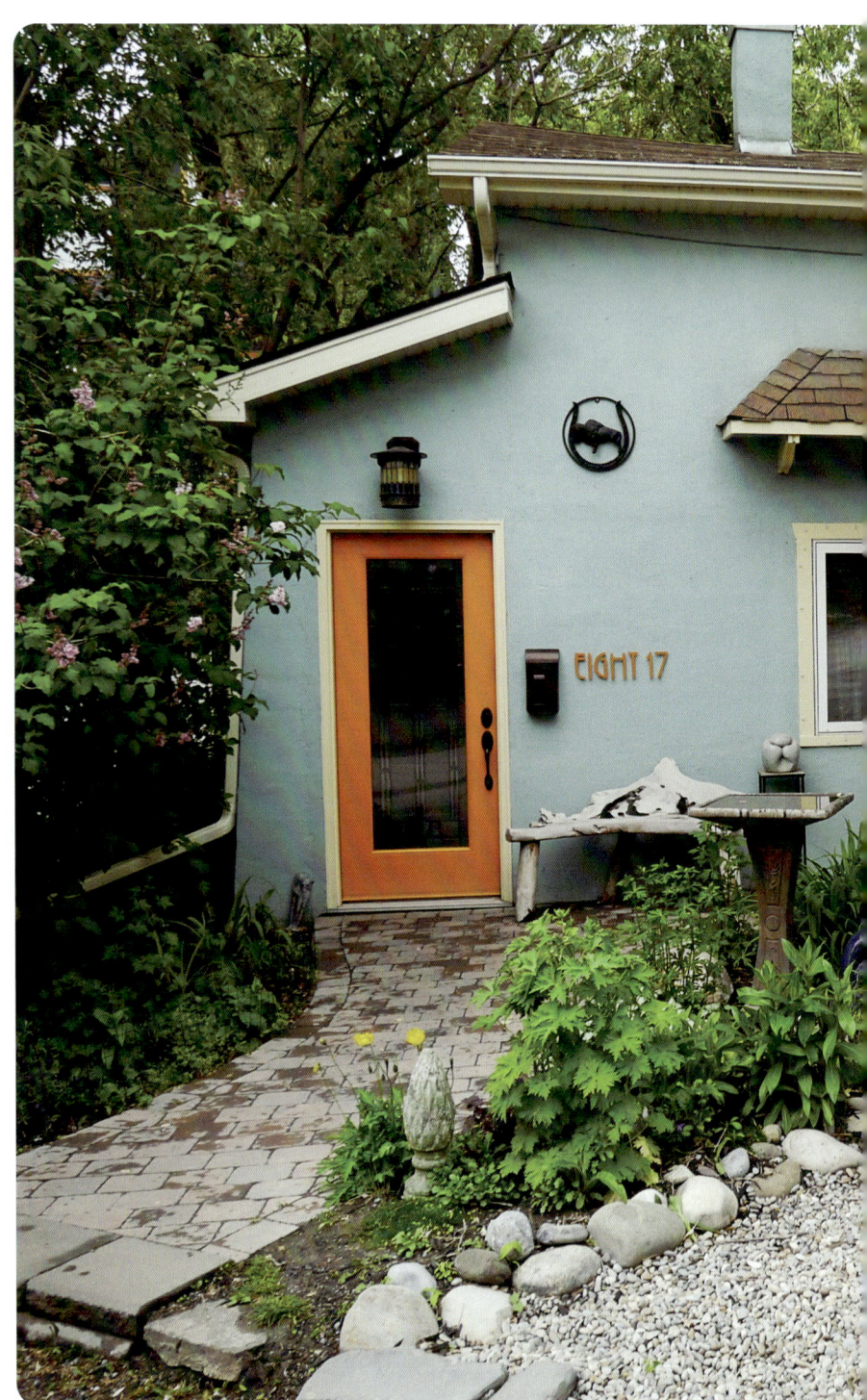

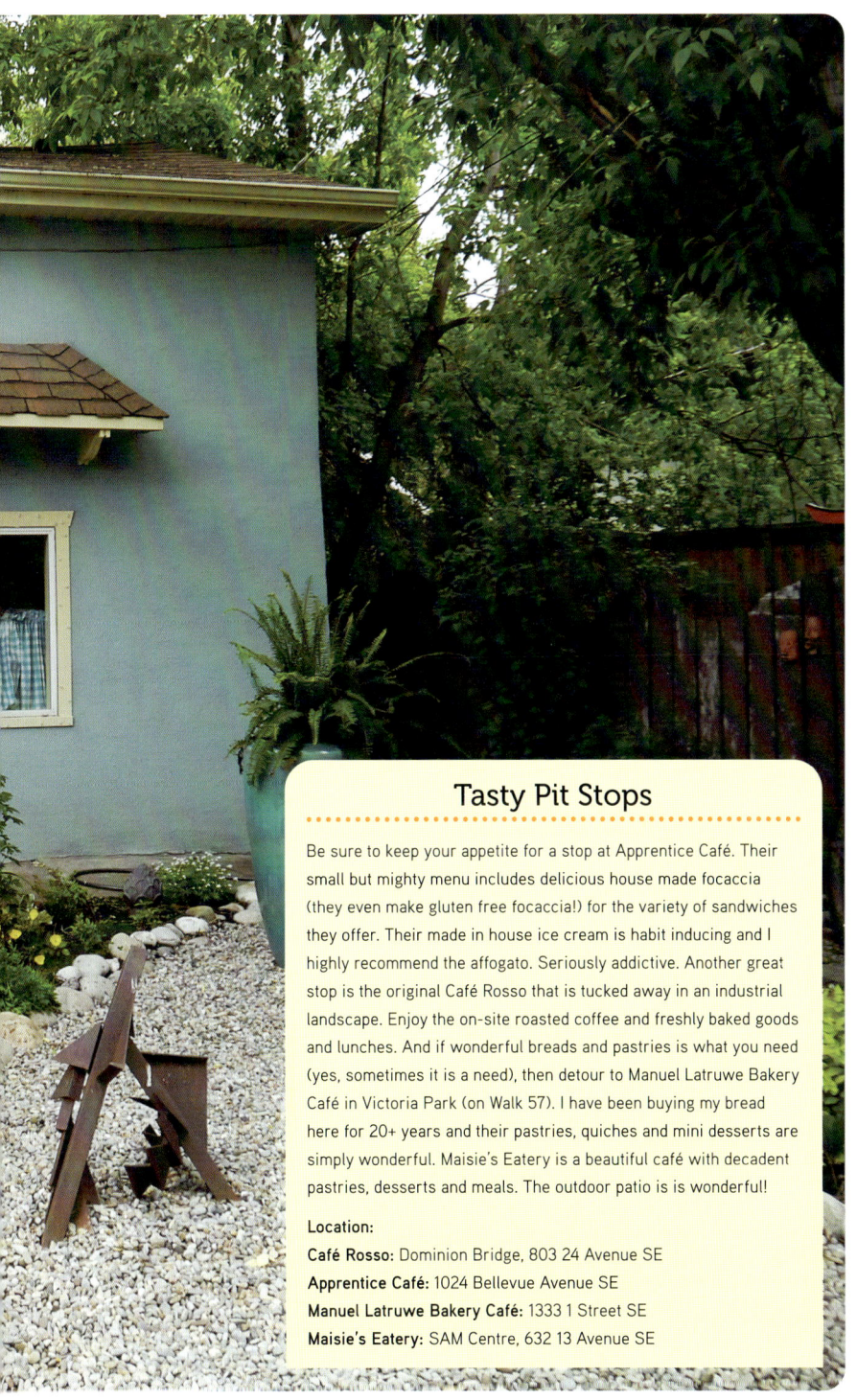

Tasty Pit Stops

Be sure to keep your appetite for a stop at Apprentice Café. Their small but mighty menu includes delicious house made focaccia (they even make gluten free focaccia!) for the variety of sandwiches they offer. Their made in house ice cream is habit inducing and I highly recommend the affogato. Seriously addictive. Another great stop is the original Café Rosso that is tucked away in an industrial landscape. Enjoy the on-site roasted coffee and freshly baked goods and lunches. And if wonderful breads and pastries is what you need (yes, sometimes it is a need), then detour to Manuel Latruwe Bakery Café in Victoria Park (on Walk 57). I have been buying my bread here for 20+ years and their pastries, quiches and mini desserts are simply wonderful. Maisie's Eatery is a beautiful café with decadent pastries, desserts and meals. The outdoor patio is is wonderful!

Location:
Café Rosso: Dominion Bridge, 803 24 Avenue SE
Apprentice Café: 1024 Bellevue Avenue SE
Manuel Latruwe Bakery Café: 1333 1 Street SE
Maisie's Eatery: SAM Centre, 632 13 Avenue SE

Roxboro - Erlton - Ramsay

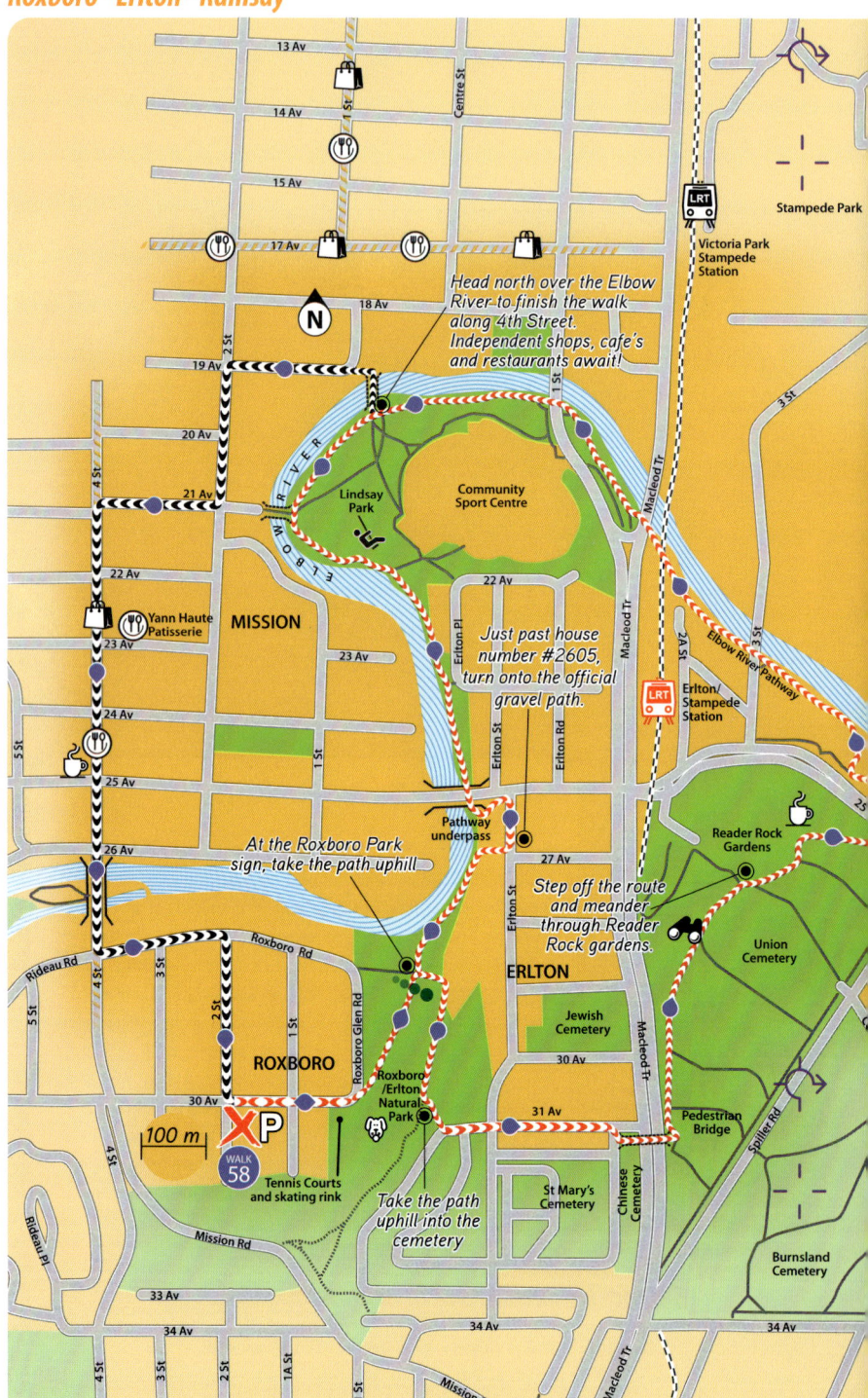

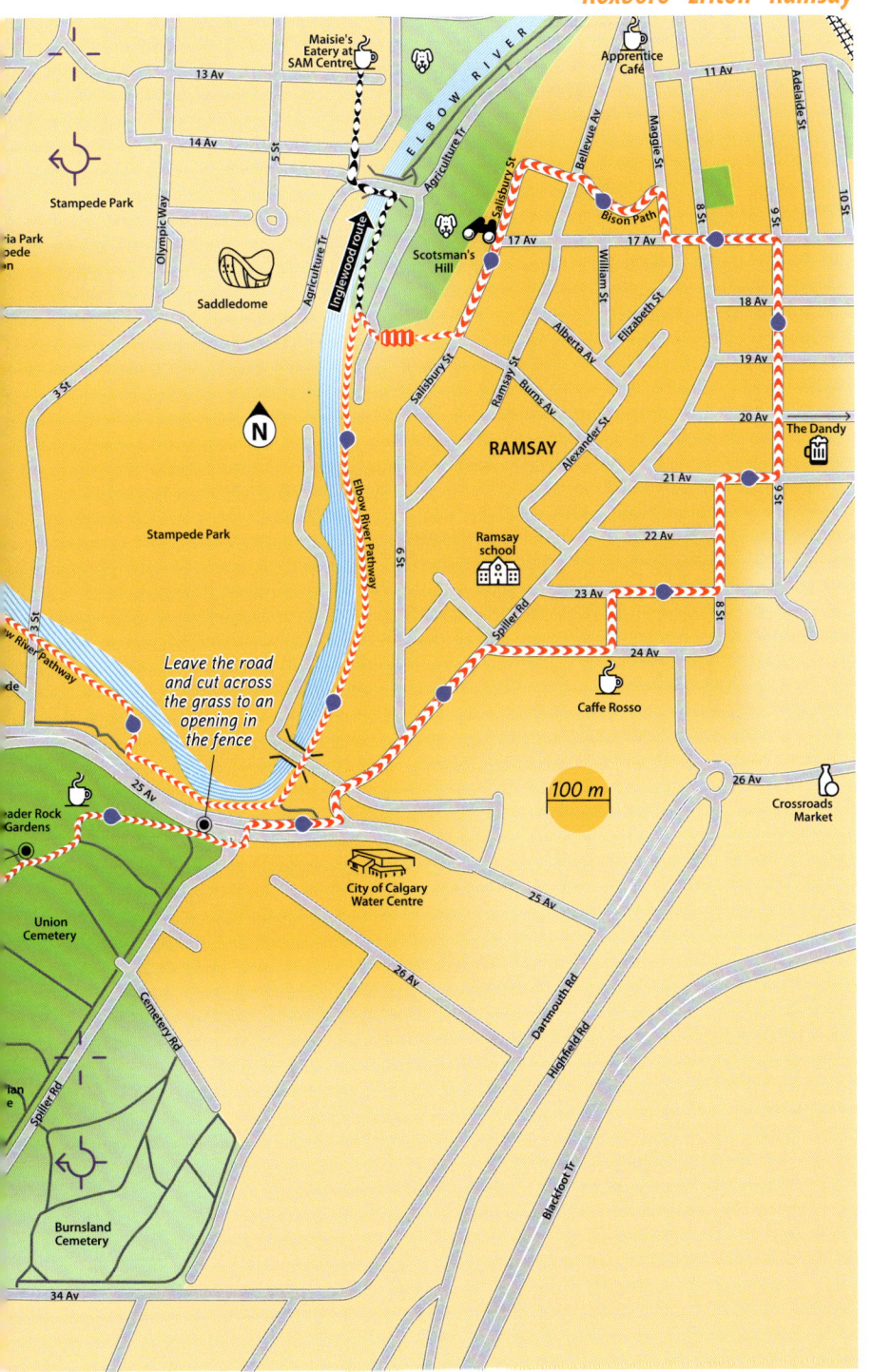

Stanley Park - Roxboro - Mount Royal - East Elbow

Walk 59   SW

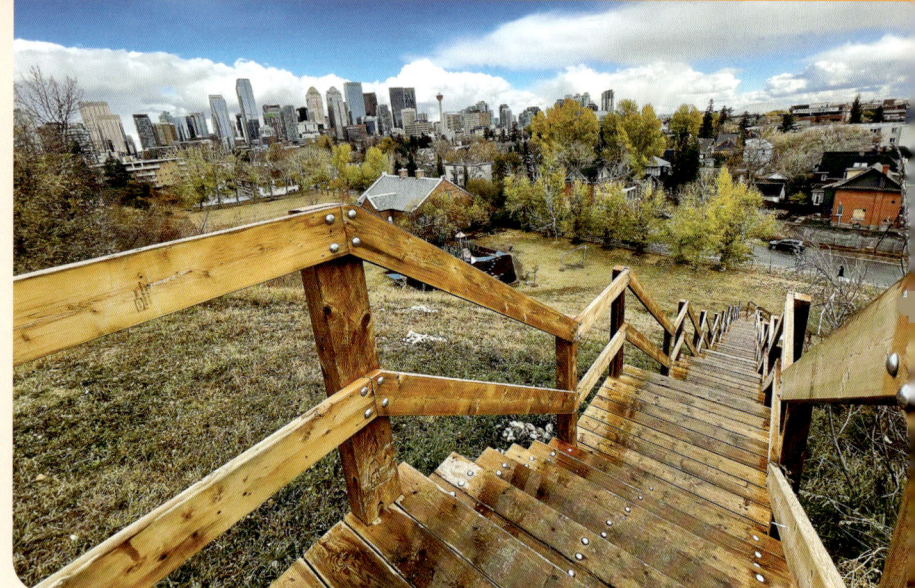

Walk at a Glance:

Walk from Stanley Park uphill to Parkhill, a neighbourhood with unique architecture, where contemporary houses are replacing the original modest homes. The elementary school - turned condos on 2 Street mixes the old with the varied infill designs. Skirt the escarpment along grass paths and soak up big views of the Rockies beyond and the community of East Elbow below.

A set of stairs leads you to the next green-space gem: Roxboro/Erlton Natural Park. Calgary has an abundance of off-the-sidewalk trails that give the urban hiker the feeling they are walking in a remote wilderness area. Wolf willow shrubs are in full bloom in June as you climb from Mission Road into the park space. The scent of their yellow flowers is pungent - a prairie trademark. Descend

Details

Categories: LRT, Café, Dog, Nature, Neighbourhood & Parks, People watch & shop, Hilly, Stroller, Vistas, River

Start: Stanley Park official parking lot on 42 Avenue just west of 1A Street SW

LRT: 39 Avenue Station

Facilities: Bathrooms at Stanley Park are open year round

Distance & Difficulty

10.5 km (hills, sidewalks, paved paths and stairs)

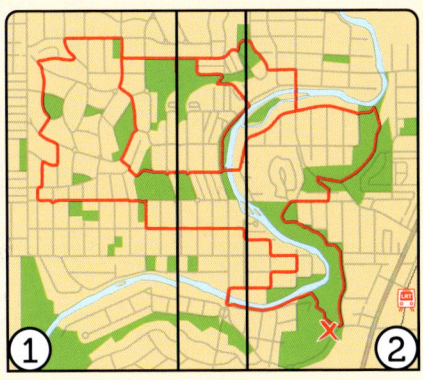

Highlights, Detours & Destinations

Skate on the phenomenal outdoor rink and oval at the Elboya Heights Community Centre on Park Avenue. Check out the Christmas Lights Displays in December. Plan a summer swim at the outdoor pool in Stanley Park

the slope and travel through Roxboro and Rideau and keep an eye out for the gorgeous private garden across from the Rideau pedestrian bridge.

Cross the Elbow River on one of the many pedestrian bridges that allow self-propelled folks to efficiently connect communities. Continue through the streets of Elbow Park before climbing up the green-space slopes that are covered in saskatoon shrubs. Stop for a saskatoon snack in August before continuing between houses on the cut-through pathway. Mount Royal is the next community on your urban hike bucket list. This neighbourhood is pleasant to walk through year-round, and at Christmastime, the colourful light displays are festive. A nighttime, full moon, winter walk is fun in this

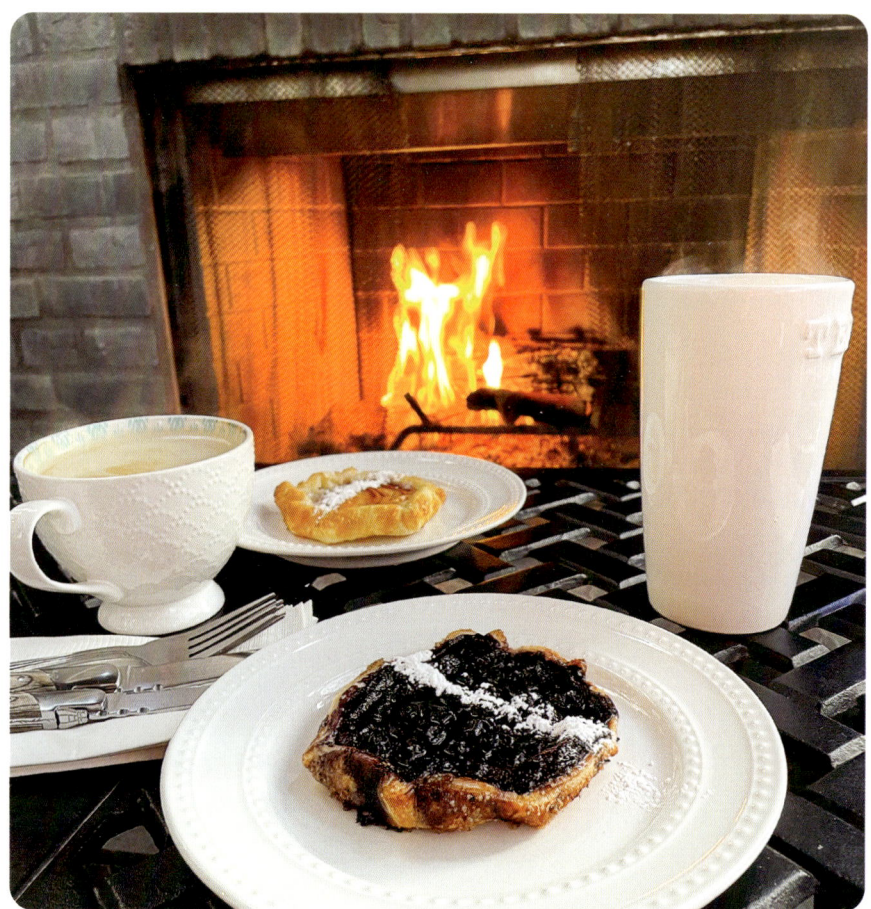
Le Comptoir by Francois

community: the moon is bright enough to allow you to walk confidently through the quiet residential streets. Sometimes nighttime walks allow you to catch glimpses of the lit-up interiors giving walkers a chance to assess paint colours and enjoy some artwork. Take the alternate route along Hillcrest Avenue to stunning downtown views from Evamy Ridge. Take the stairs into Cliff Bungalow and connect back to the main route.

Venturing onward, the route crosses Elbow Drive into East Elbow Park, a hidden gem tucked away in the heart of the inner city. The walker experiences a peaceful jaunt in this community, enjoying a landscape of well-tended gardens and a mix of older modest homes and grand new abodes. Connect to the Elbow River Pathway once again and continue back to Stanley Park. A large leafy green space, this is the perfect stop for a post-hike picnic, a swim in the outdoor pool in the summer, or in the winter a skate at Calgary's nicest volunteer managed outdoor rink and perhaps some tobogganing on the hill above. Enjoy a mini-skating oval, curling area, two hockey rinks, and bonfires to keep you warm.

Tasty Pit Stops

Take a detour north along 4 Street SW to find a host of restaurants, cafés and shops. Yann Haute Patisserie occupies a yellow house tucked off Fourth Street. Pastries, a few breads and baguettes, and colourful macarons are house specialties. My favourite is the almond croissant that melts in your mouth. There is no sit-down service at Yann's, so plan on packing your treat with you to enjoy post-walk at a picnic table along the river in Stanley Park or on Elbow Island Park, off the Mission Bridge. Just around the corner from Yann's is Phil & Sebastian, where coffee is the specialty. For a mid-walk treat, venture off the route onto 34 Avenue SW. Bell's Café is the first stop and the made in house muffins here are legendary! Continue further west to the year-round dog friendly patio at Le Comptoir by Francois.

A fireplace and heat lamps keep is toasty warm in the cold months and the house made pastries, quiches, cakes and decadent grill cheese are outstanding. For those looking for a cold one, the Marda Brewing is just the ticket! Check out every expanding selection of little local shops and eats on 34 Avenue, a destination in the making for all things cozy and delicious.

Location:
Yann Haute Patisserie: 329 23 Avenue SW
Phil & Sebastian: 2207 4 Street SW
Bell's Café: 34 Avenue and 14 Street SW
Le Comptoir by Francois & shops on 34: 1928 34 Avenue SW
Marda Brewing: 3528 18 Street SW

Stanley Park - Roxboro - Mount Royal - East Elbow

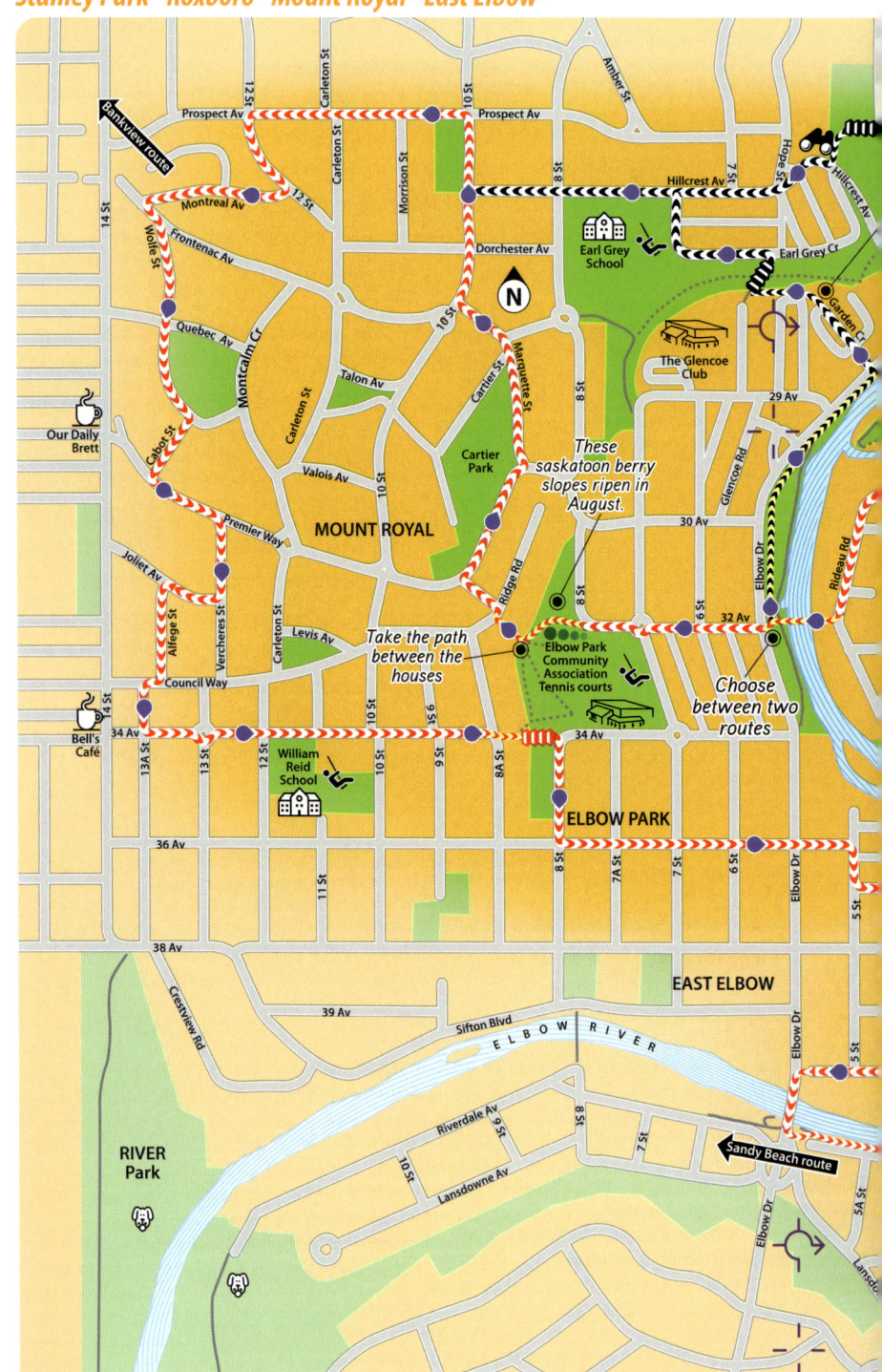

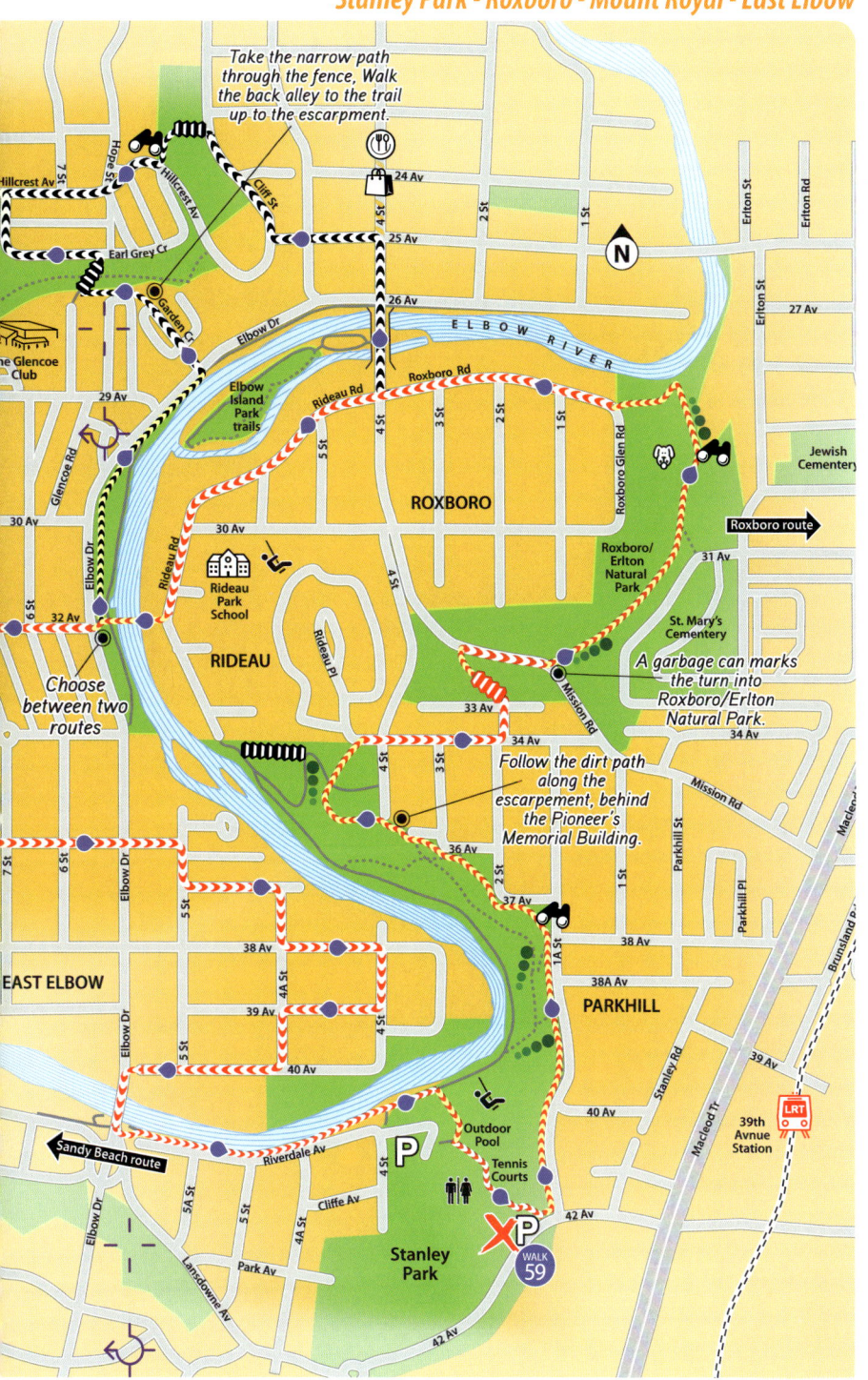

Sandy Beach - Elbow Park - Britannia

Walk 60   SW

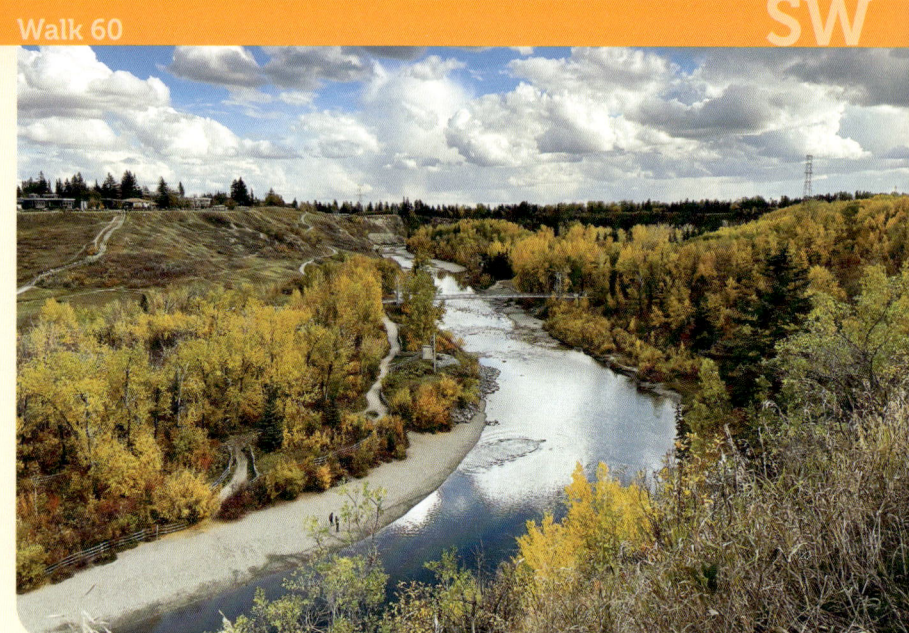

Walk at a Glance:

Connecting neighbourhoods on foot is my favourite way to get to know a city. This route travels across pedestrian bridges, along regional pathways, and then detours on short-cut community pathways and stairways tucked in between houses.

From Sandy Beach Park, an earthy stairway leads into the trees and exits into the River Park off-leash area, where enthusiastic pups and breathtaking views of the Elbow River Valley and the downtown core are your reward. Chinook arches are a spectacular, and very welcome, sight from the River Park escarpment. The warm winds that blow in from the West Coast, over the Rocky Mountains, melt Calgarians' frosty faces.

Details

Categories: Café, Dog, Nature, Neighbourhood & Parks, Hilly, Stroller, Vistas, River, Birds

Start: Sandy Beach Park, 4500 14a Street SW

Facilities: Sandy Beach has seasonal indoor bathrooms and port-a-potties year round

Distance & Difficulty

8 km (paved and gravel paths, stairs and hills)

Highlights, Detours & Destinations

Saskatoon berries are abundant on the Britannia Slopes in early August. Check out the Saskatoon pie recipe in Walk 12. Magical early-morning hoar frost covers trees surrounding the Elbow River on frigid days

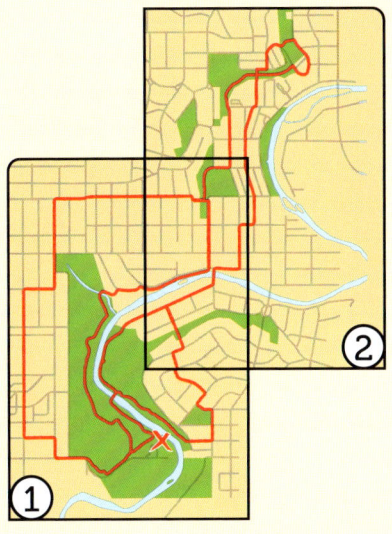

Continuing through River Park, you'll cross a couple of small bridges and climb through the trees to the community of Elbow Park. One of Calgary's oldest communities, Elbow Park was an upper middle-class suburb of Calgary shortly before World War One. It is hard to believe that in 1909, Elbow Park was considered a suburb, but it now sits in the heart of the inner city; a city that is now home to over one million people. Walking this route in May and June is guaranteed to lift winter-weary spirits as the neighbourhood comes alive with a palette of purple, pink, and white: blossoming lilac, apple, crab-apple, and cherry trees. The sweet smell of these blossoms is sure proof that summer is near.

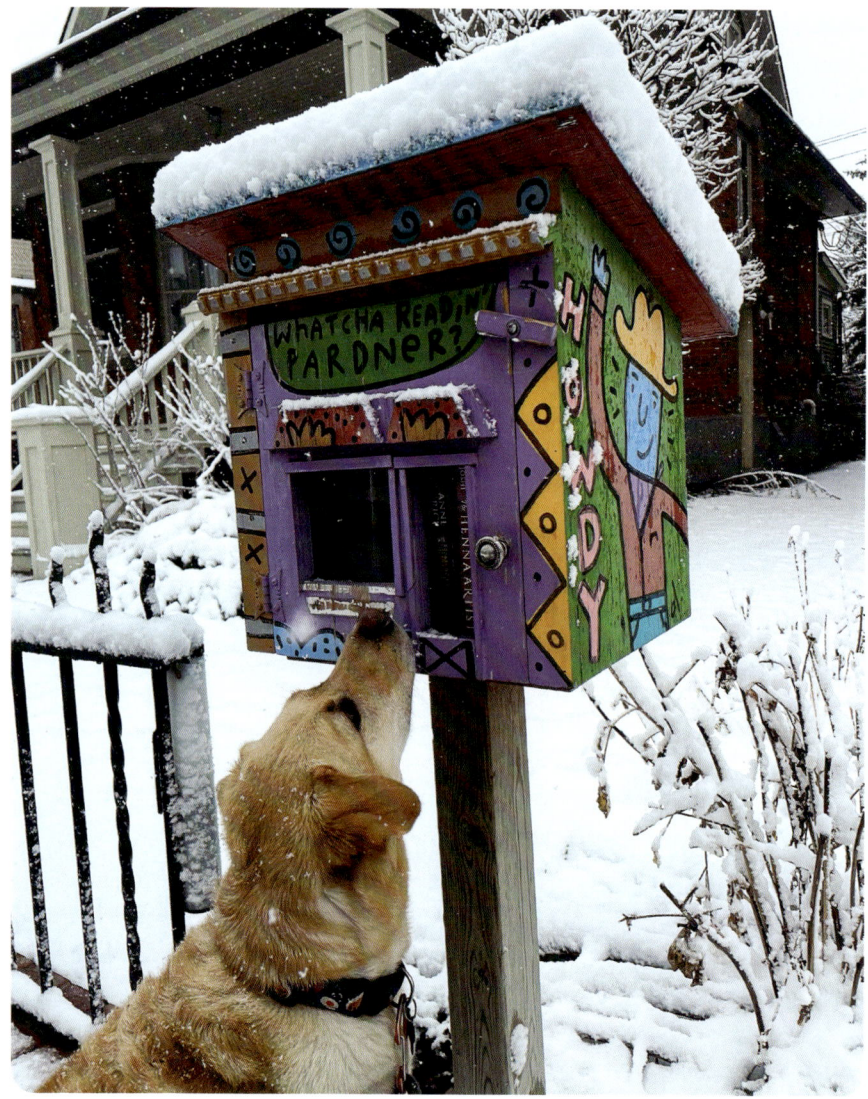

Tasty Pit Stops & Shops

Britannia Plaza is a great place to grab some food, a coffee, or some locally made ice cream. Sunterra and Lina's Italian Market have hot food to go, sandwiches, paninis and all sorts of baked goods and fresh produce. Stop by Village Ice Cream for an assortment of locally made ice cream or grab a coffee at Monogram. If you have more time, be sure to stop by Owl's Nest Books, one of Calgary's fantastic indie bookstores.

Location: Britannia Plaza, Elbow Drive and 49 Avenue SW

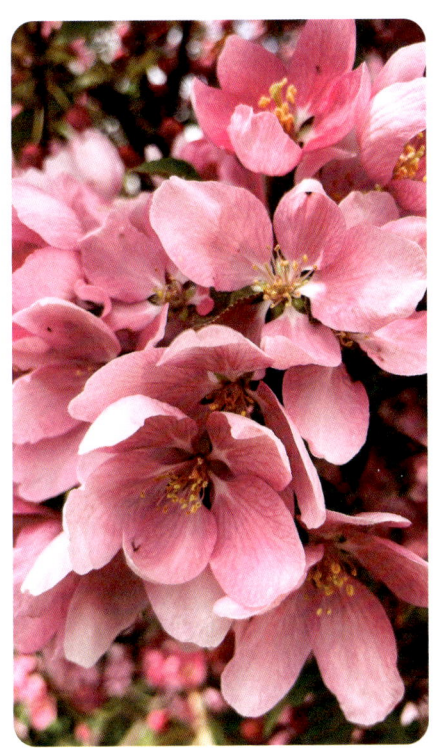

A hidden staircase behind Christ Church takes you off the sidewalk and along shaded pathways. In August these trails are an urban foraging hotspot when the saskatoon berries are deep purple and plump. More dips and climbs lead to a Rocky Mountain viewpoint from the top of the Glencoe stairs in the community of Mount Royal. If the sight of the mountains inspires you, then do a few sets of stairs to train your legs for the mountain hikes that beckon. A long, long time before European and American settlers claimed the land, the Blackfoot people used the base of the Mount Royal hill as a campground before venturing up the Elbow Valley. In 1904 the first homes in Mount Royal were built. The building boom was a result of Canadian Pacific Railway (CPR) development nearby.

Continue to more stairs and stunning downtown views from Evamy Park. Loop through Cliff Bungalow and Elbow Park, back over the Elbow River, before climbing the tucked-away pathway into the community of Britannia or stay low along the river pathway for a flat walk. The Britannia route is a zigzag along the quiet streets of one of Canada's wealthiest neighbourhoods. If you need a coffee, ice cream, or a picnic lunch, Britannia Plaza has it all. Grab your food and head to the escarpment, where you can sit on a bench and watch for birdlife high above or pet a few pooches at ground level. I often see bald eagles soaring low along the Elbow River from this vantage point. A brief walk downhill and then across the Elbow River leads you back to Sandy Beach. Dip your feet in the river, skip some rocks, and relax, or, on a very cold winter day, watch the steam rise from the river – a frigid, yet beautiful, sight.

Sandy Beach - Elbow Park - Britannia

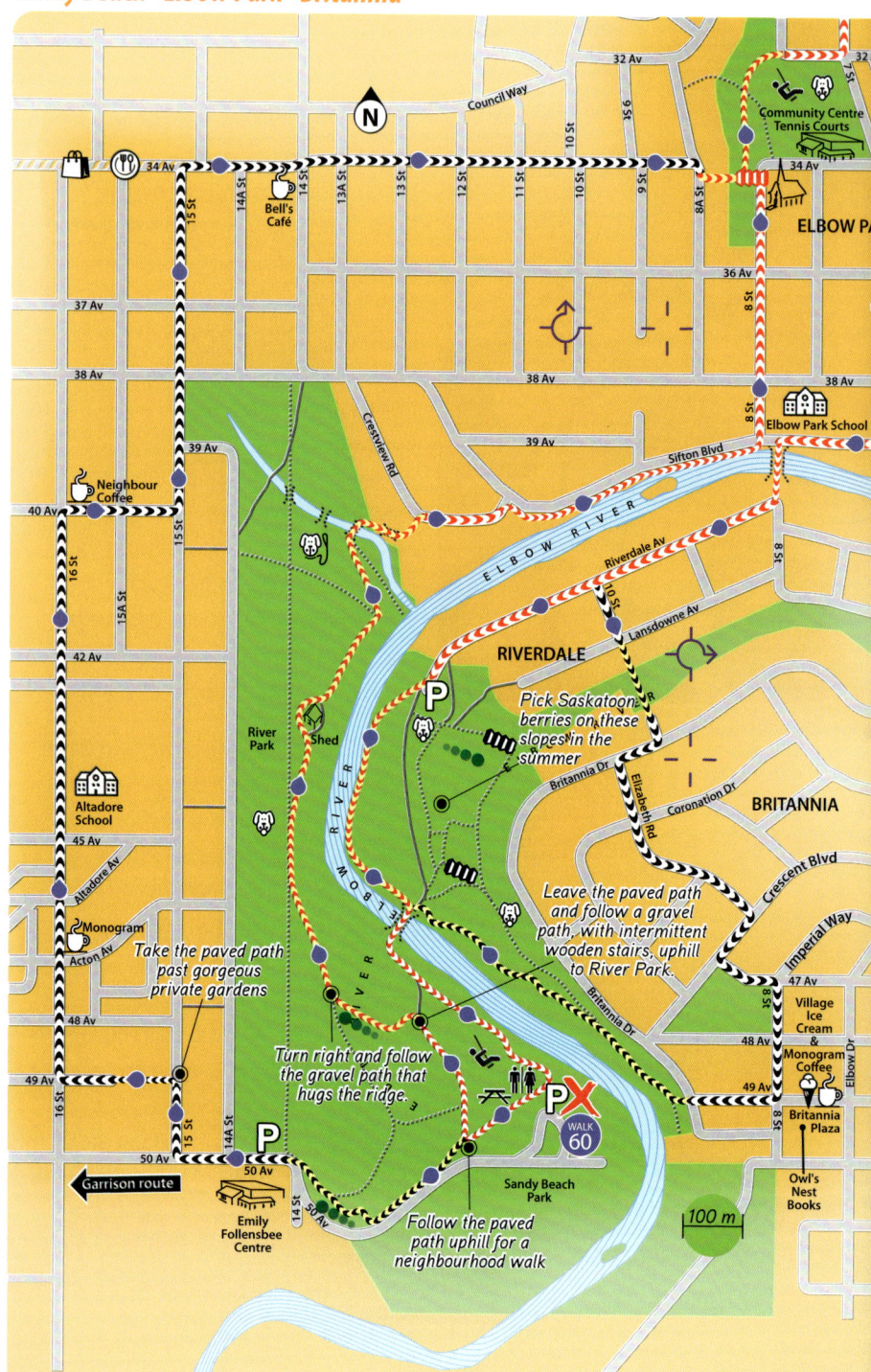

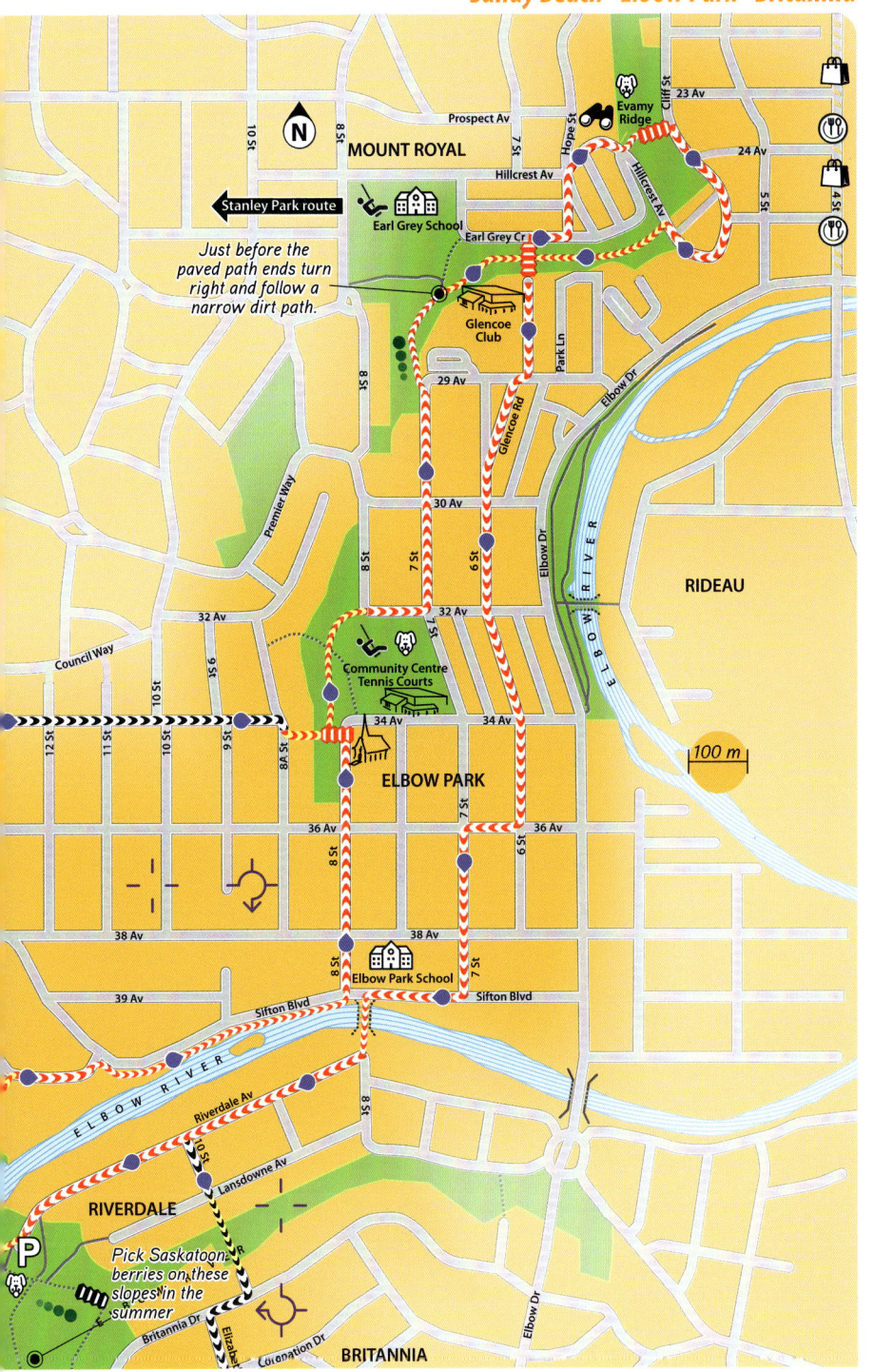

Elbow River to Bow River

Walks 61 and 62

SW

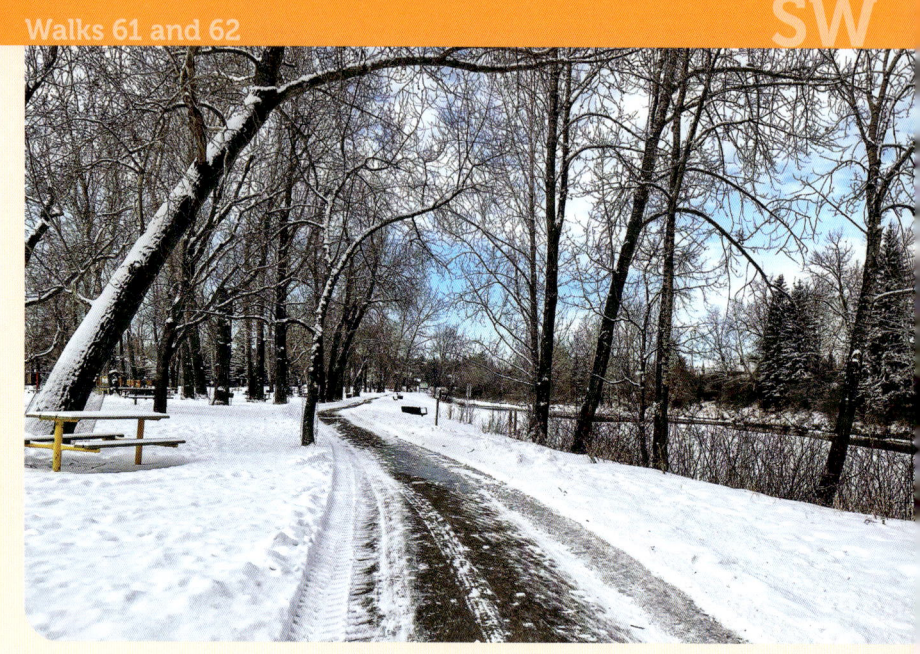

Walks at a Glance:

The Elbow River Pathway from Sandy Beach to the confluence with the Bow River is a wonderful route with many interesting detours. Bring your pups as Walk 61 starts with swimming followed by lots of off leash. Sandy Beach is a popular spot to launch a raft in the summer as the shallow Elbow River makes for the perfect leisurely float.

Connect to to Riverdale Avenue, where you'll enjoy a picturesque stroll past stunning riverside homes before dropping back onto the paved pathway under Elbow Drive. The entire length of the Elbow River Pathway is a wonderful mix of nature and neighbourhoods as you

Details

Categories: LRT, Café, Dog, Nature, Neighbourhood & Parks, People watch & shop, Hilly, Stroller, Historic, Vistas, River, Birds

Start: Walk 61: Sandy Beach Park, 4500 14A Street, SW; Walk 62: 17 Avenue and 9 St SE

LRT: Erlton Station

Facilities: Bathrooms at Sandy Beach Park and Stanley Park (May–October), Sports Centre in Lindsay Park

Distance & Difficulty

Walk 61: Elbow River Loop South: 7.5 km (sidewalks, paved and gravel paths)

Walk 62: Elbow River Loop North: 10 km (hills, sidewalks, paved and gravel paths)

Highlights, Detours & Destinations

Dogs love all the off leashing and swimming around Sandy Beach in River Park and Britannia Slopes. Sandy Beach has an inclusive playground, swimming and picnic sites. Stop by the Stanley Park outdoor pool (summer)

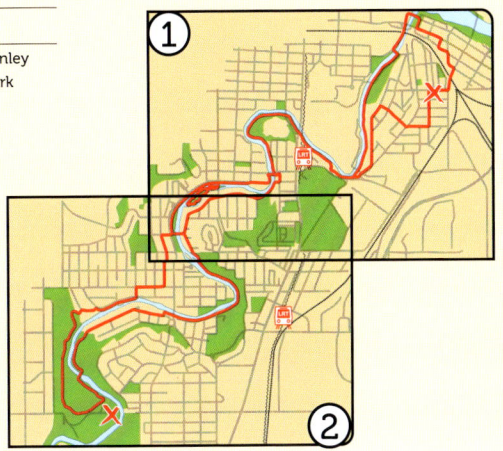

walk by Stanley Park and through Rideau, where a stunning private garden marks the turnoff for Walk 61 and the return loop for Walk 62. Continue along quiet side streets into Roxboro before crossing into Roxboro Park in search of the hidden connector gravel trail at the entrance to Erlton Park, where an optional stair climb leads walkers to phenomenal views. The pathway continues through Erlton, Lindsay Park and under Macleod Trail towards Stampede Park. A set of stairs leads you to the top of Scotsman's Hill where you'll get a bird's-eye view of Stampede Park, the downtown core and the Rocky Mountain peaks beyond or continue

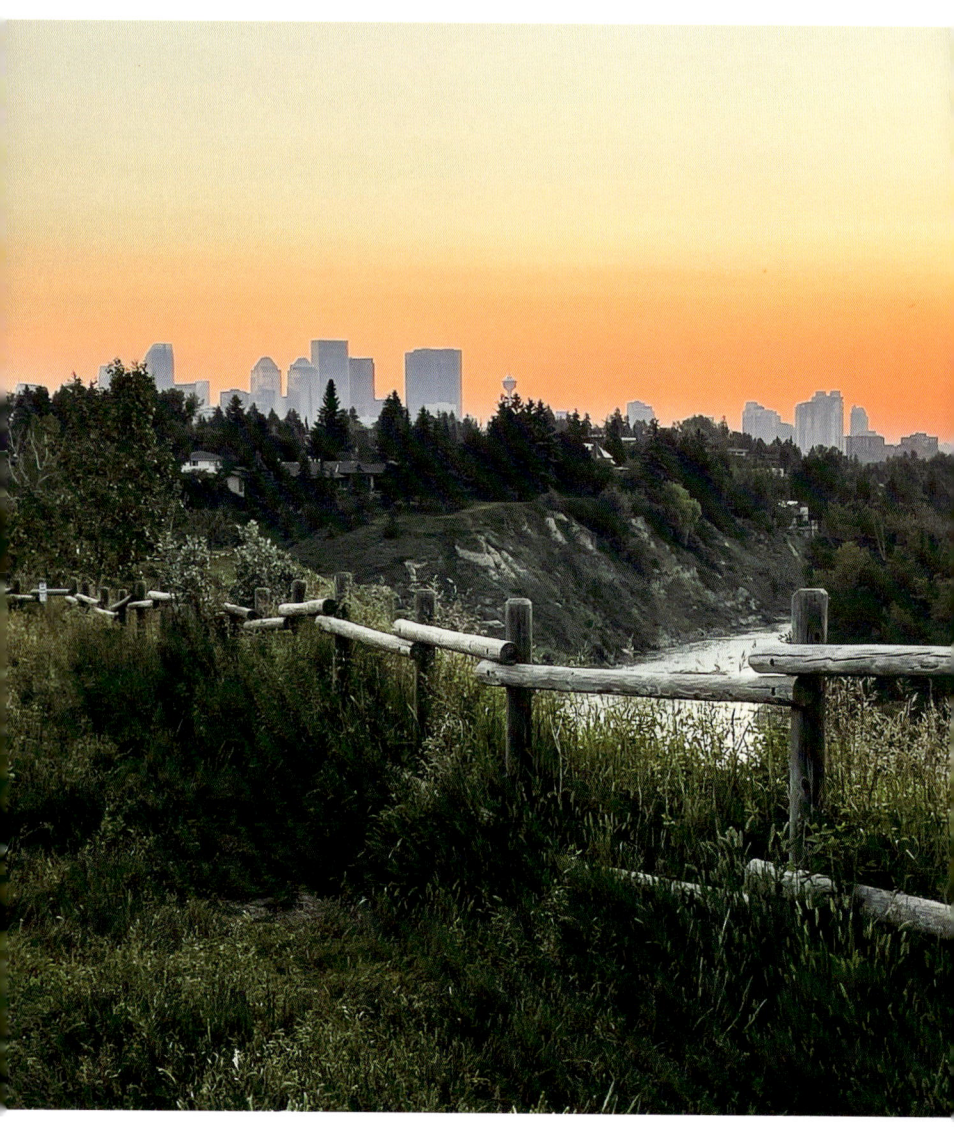

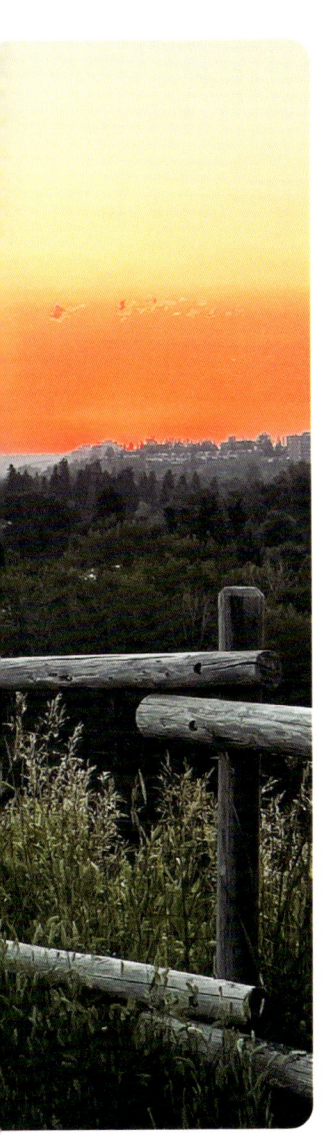

along the paved path to The Confluence Historic Site and Parkland. Explore Ramsay side streets, home to old-fashioned corner stores, historic homes, and buildings from the early 1900s—some renovated and fantastic, some handyman delights. Grab a book from a little-free libraries, watch for folk art and colourful homes and gardens.

The Confluence Historic Site & Parkland

In spring 2024, Fort Calgary changed its name to The Confluence Historic Site & Parkland. This new name encourages a broader narrative to include the many diverse histories of the land. The Confluence Historic Site & Parkland is home to many stories from diverse people. Long before the North-West Mounted Police arrived in 1875, Indigenous peoples have been gathering on this land from time immemorial. The shift from colonization to industrialization also brought a new wave of settlers with different worldviews. While some celebrate this land as the birthplace of Calgary and an icon of national pride, others recount stories of hardship under colonial rule.

This is our layered history, and every story makes it complete. Today, The Confluence serves as a gathering place to share the full history of this land through diverse voices. Like the rivers that meet here, different worldviews and perspectives collide. But as we recognize the truths of our past, we can make sense of our collective identity.

Elbow River to Bow River

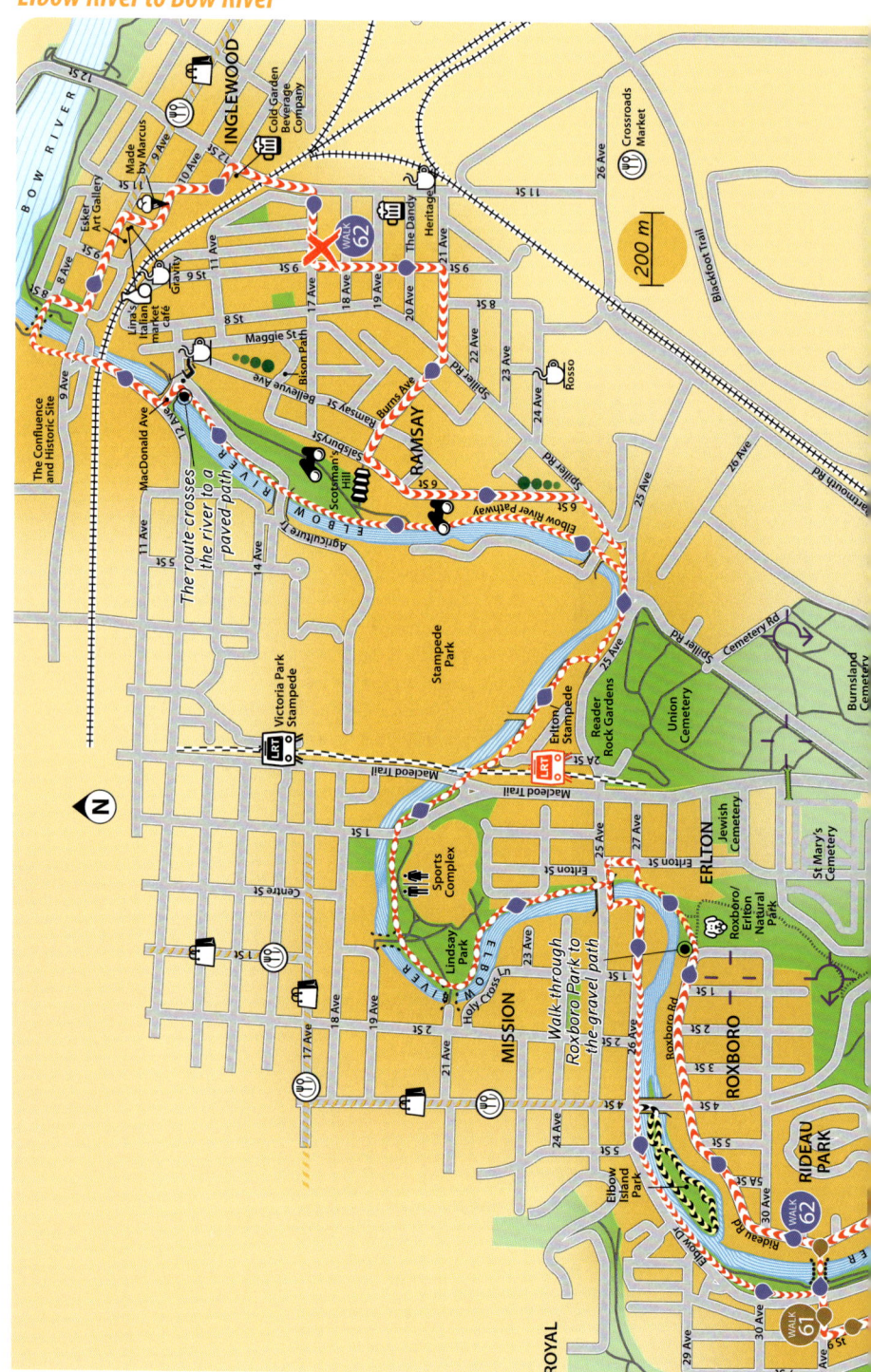

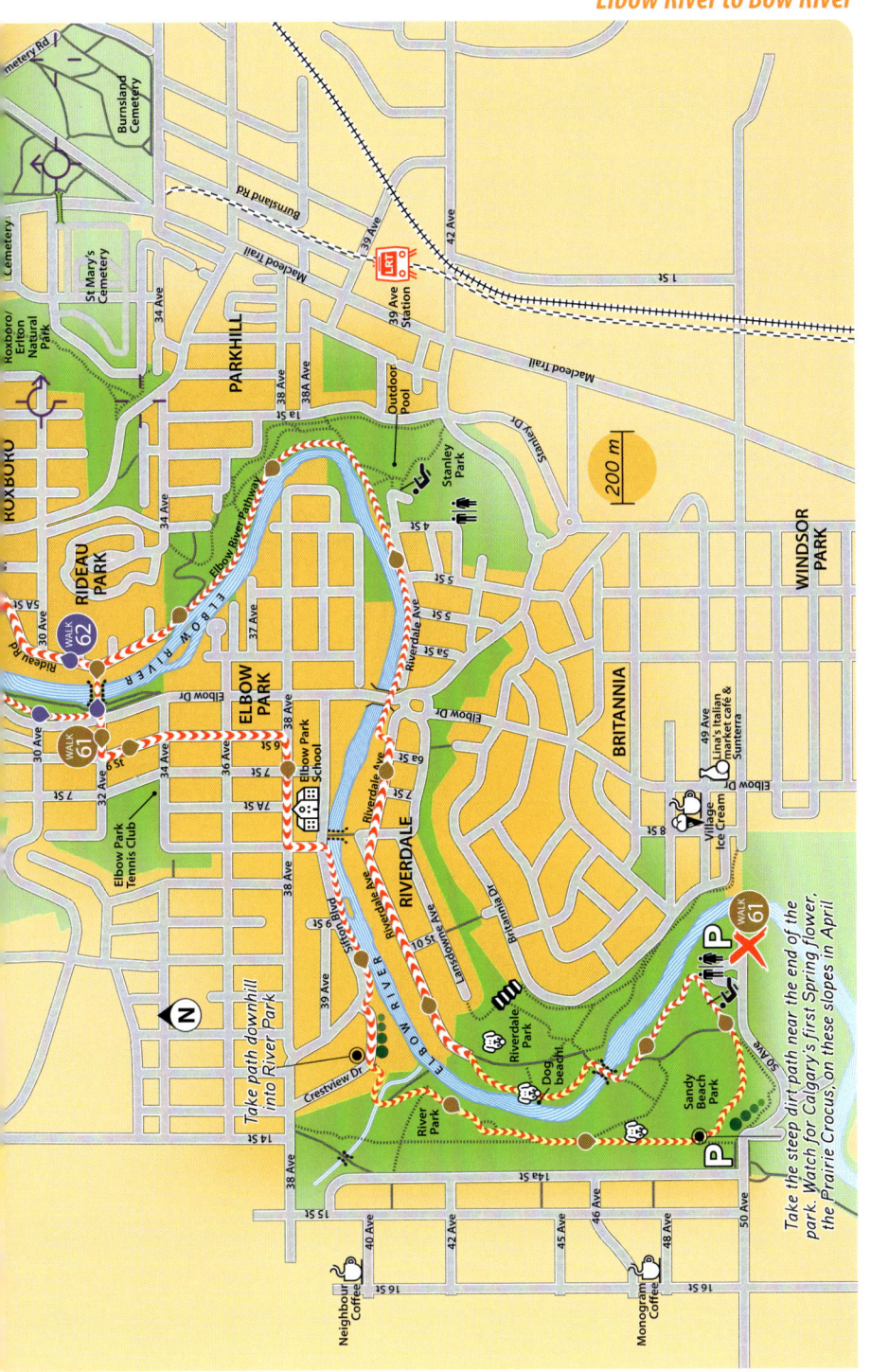

Garrison - Currie - North Glenmore - Altadore - Glenmore Dam

Walks 63 and 64

SW

Walks at a Glance:

Neighbours coming and going, or, in the summer, sitting on porches while their children play in the streets or sell lemonade to passersby, that's Garrison Woods. A new neighbourhood with old roots, these friendly streets were originally part of the Currie Army Barracks.

Built in the 1930s, the community experienced a complete overhaul when the base closed in 1998. The tidy, compact, army houses now share the streets with brick and multi-coloured row houses and sizable single-family homes. The military history is still alive here, with streets named Vimy Ridge and Passchendaele. The Military Museums of Calgary, with tanks and armoured vehicles, also calls this community home.

Details

Categories: Café, Dog, Nature, Neighbourhood & Parks, People watch & shop, Hilly, Stroller, Historic, Vistas, River, Birds

Start: Walk 63: Flanders Park, St Julien Drive and Garrison Boulevard SW; Walk 64: Glenmore Aquatic Centre, 5330 19 Street SW or North Glenmore Park, parking lot D

Facilities: Bathrooms in North Glenmore Park

Distance & Difficulty

Walk 63: Garrison - Currie - Altadore: 7 km (Sidewalks and paved paths)

Walk 64: North Glenmore - Glenmore Park - Glenmore Dam: 7 km (paved paths, sidewalks, stairs and hills)

Highlights, Detours & Destinations

Many cafés, pubs and restaurants along the routes. See sidebar

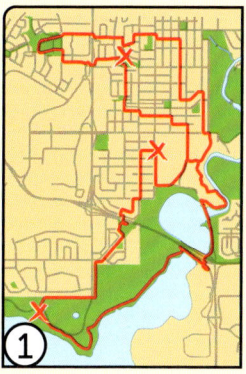

Garrison Woods and Currie - designed to move people on foot, bike, and with public transit - host promenades and cut-through pathways that offer walkers and cyclists efficient and pleasant route options, make walking and cycling easy. With its people-populated porches and free-range kids, the community is a throwback to the days when everyone knew their neighbours and kids made their own fun, meeting in the middle of street and setting up the hockey nets. Listen for "Car!" and "Game on!" as you walk through the area. And Garrison Woods, with its dense housing and abundance of families, is the epicenter of the ultimate Halloween haul. If you live there, you must invest a sizeable portion of your income on mini-chocolate bars and chips come October. Be prepared.

GARRISON - CURRIE - NORTH GLENMORE - ALTADORE - GLENMORE DAM

A short walk away is the Elbow River and the Glenmore Dam. Follow the paved path along the escarpment and descend to the river valley, following a series of haphazard trails below the dam. This off leash area is popular with dog walkers and the treed trail system is a fantastic nature immersion, boosting your chlorophyll quotient. The Elbow River is shallow and perfect for paddling in the hot months so plan a swim post walk to cool off. With many route options, you can meander along the river or through the trees before climbing your way back to the paved path. Soak up the river-valley views while you catch your breath.

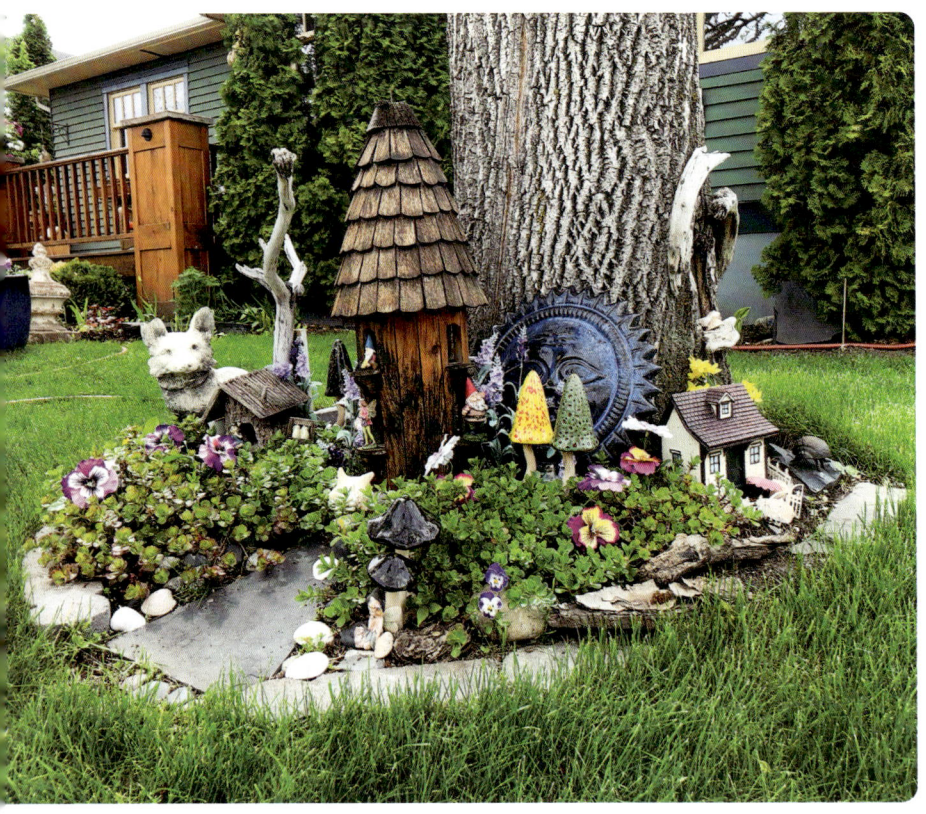

Walk 64 continues up and over Glenmore Trail to connect to the Glenmore Reservoir pathway in North Glenmore Park. Skirt the Earl Grey Golf Club enjoying stunning views across the water. Loop back into the neighbourhood of North Glenmore. Calgary's older neighbourhoods are always growing and changing, like the city itself. Close-knit communities like Garrison Woods, Altadore, and North Glenmore, where neighbours don't just nod in acknowledgement, but become your friends, are the building blocks of a great city.

Need a creative boost, feeling anxious, lacking purpose? Go for a walk.

Creative people walk. The strolling philosopher Friedrich Nietzsche concluded this 125 years ago in Twilight of the Idols, in which he claimed, "All truly great thoughts are conceived by walking." This is my experience, too, and the reason this book exists. I needed to walk to research the routes in the book, true enough. But the reason I created this book is because I need to walk, every day.

A study published in Nature in 2024 found links between physical activity and creative thinking. The study "Habitual physical activity is related to more creative activities and achievements" found that physically active people are more creative, curious, and are less anxious. And creativity helps people find meaning and purpose in life. Another study published early in 2014 in the Journal of Experimental Psychology found links between physical activity and cognitive abilities, specifically, the effect of walking on creativity. The study, "Give Your Ideas Some Legs: The Positive Effect of Walking on Creative Thinking," concluded that when people walk, on a treadmill or in the great outdoors, creative ideas flow. The walkers had better ideas and more of them compared to the sitting group. And the benefits that came from walking continued after the walk was complete, when participants sat down again. A walk also offers some downtime from the constant barrage of information that we all experience today. Moving aimlessly through the streets or pathways, picking your pace, letting your thoughts change with the scenery, and getting into a rhythm: that's the power of a walk. When you put yourself in the position of "observer," you allow your mind to wander and to land where it may, which in turn allows you to gain perspective and solve many a problem.

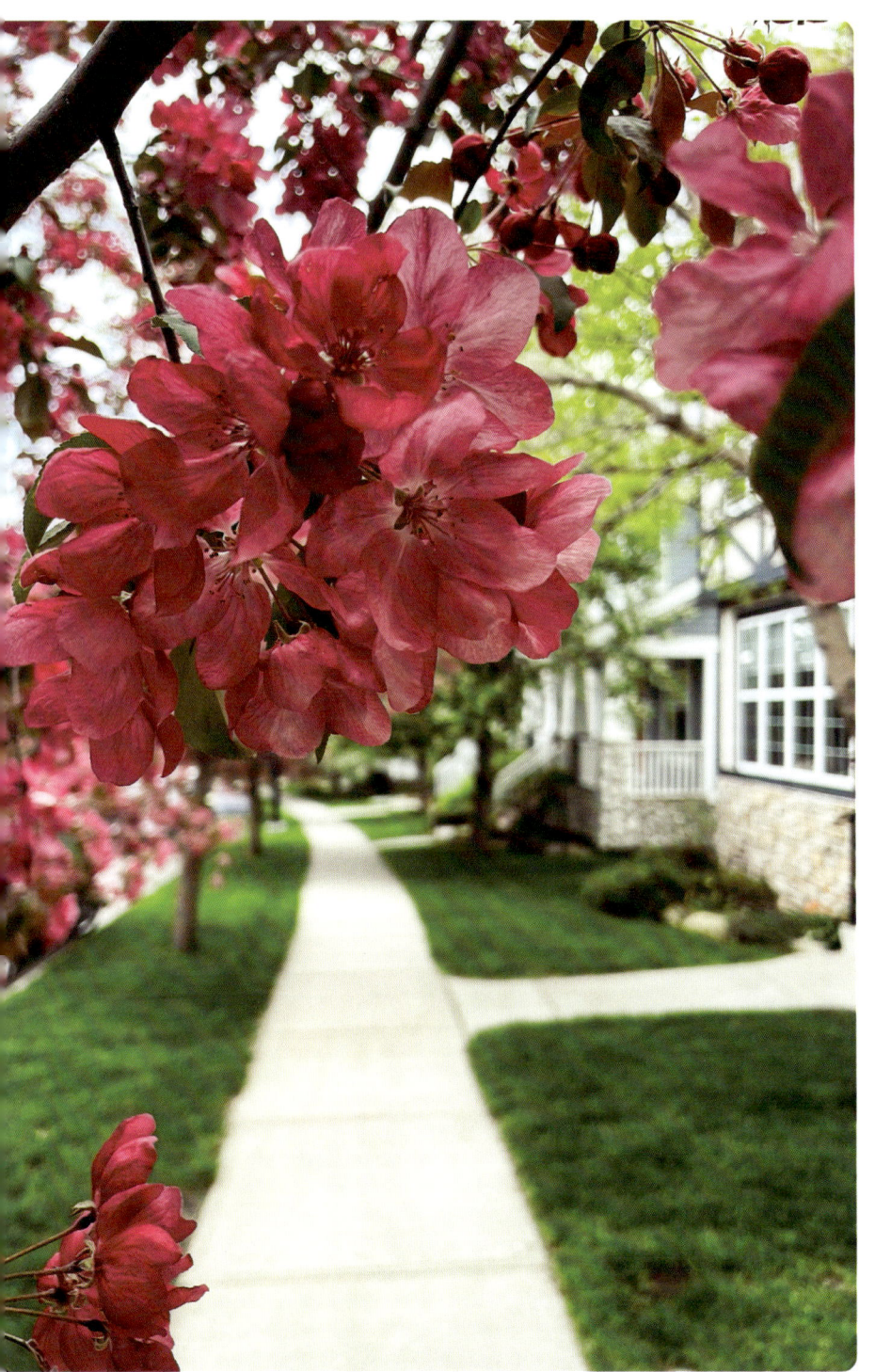

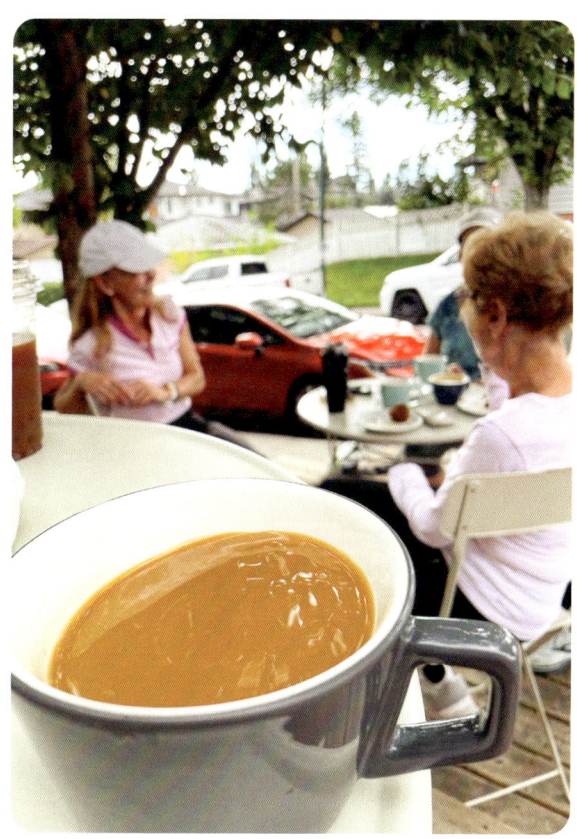

Tasty Pit Stops

Drop by locally owned Sierra Café while walking route 64 through Lakeview. Devoted to coffee, culture and community, this little café makes everything from scratch. Enjoy sandwiches, toasts and expertly made drinks inside or on their big dog friendly patio. Take a short detour to the locally owned Pfanntastic Pannenkoek Haus for some authentic Dutch cooking. Choose from more than 40 varieties of pannenkoeks, a savoury or sweet Dutch Pancake, or you can build your own for unlimited combinations. Walk a little further and grab a lunch or coffee at the Blue Flame Kitchen Café. Their vast and bright 100-metre-long space with vaulted wood ceiling is an architectural wonder and is the perfect place to sit and savour a cappuccino with a good book or to fill a table with your walking friends.

With help from the Calgary Horticultural Society, they harvest herbs, honey, and organic vegetables in ATCO Park's gardens. These homegrown ingredients bring fresh flavours their big breakfasts, rice bowls, soups, sandwiches, baked goods and daily specials. And for those who want a cold drink and a pub meal and a patio, stop by Wild Rose Brewery, Vacay and Veranda at the Stables or The Inn at Officers Garden in Currie.

Location:
Sierra Café: 6439 Crowchild Trail SW
Pfanntastic Pannenkoek Haus: 2439 54 Ave SW
Blue Flame Kitchen Café: The Commons at ATCO Park, 5302 Forand Street SW
Wild Rose Brewery, Vacay and Veranda at the Stables, The Inn at Officers Garden: Currie

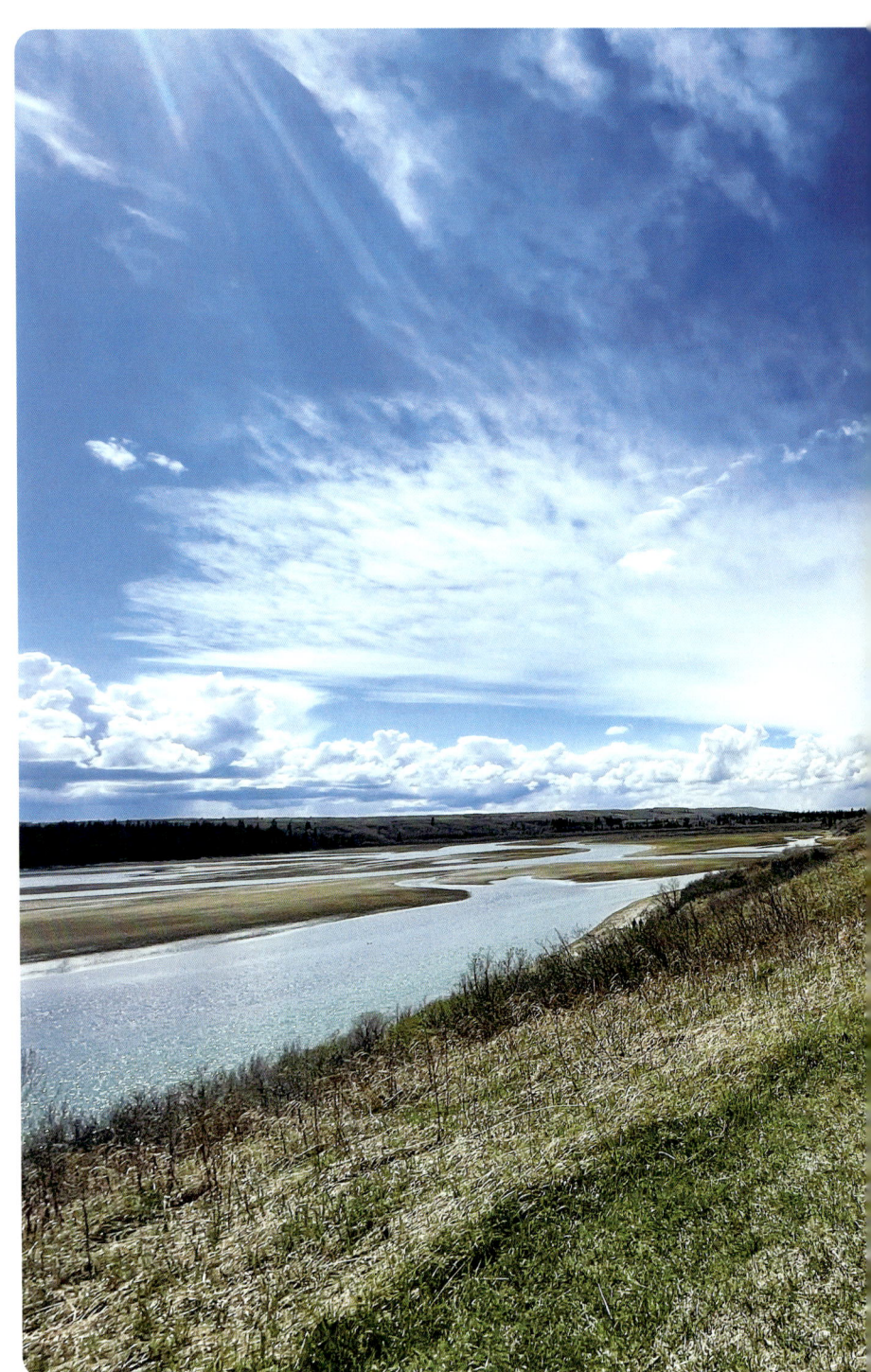

Garrison - Currie - North Glenmore - Altadore - Glenmore Dam

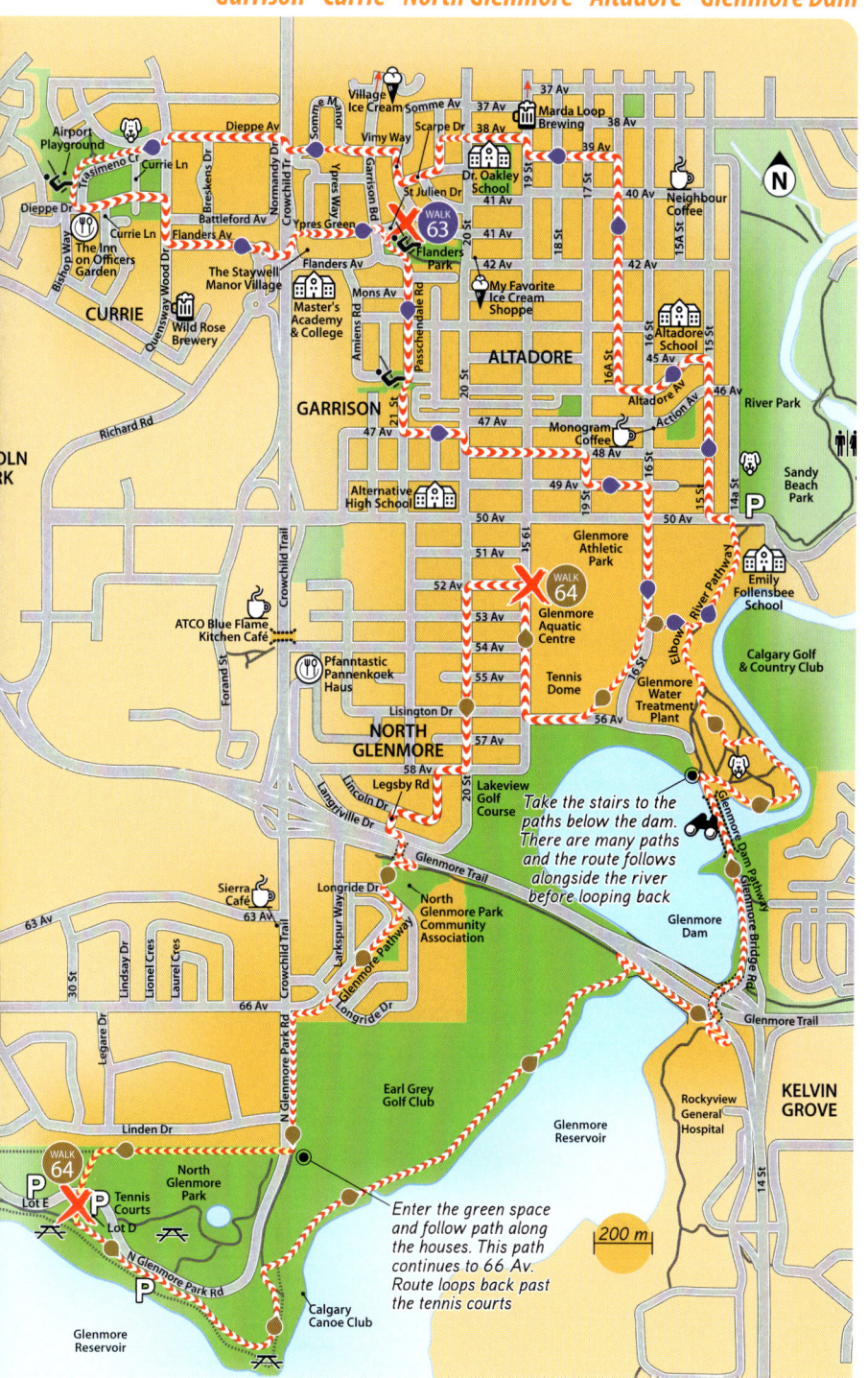

Weaselhead Flats Park & Jackrabbit Trail

Walks 65 and 66

SW

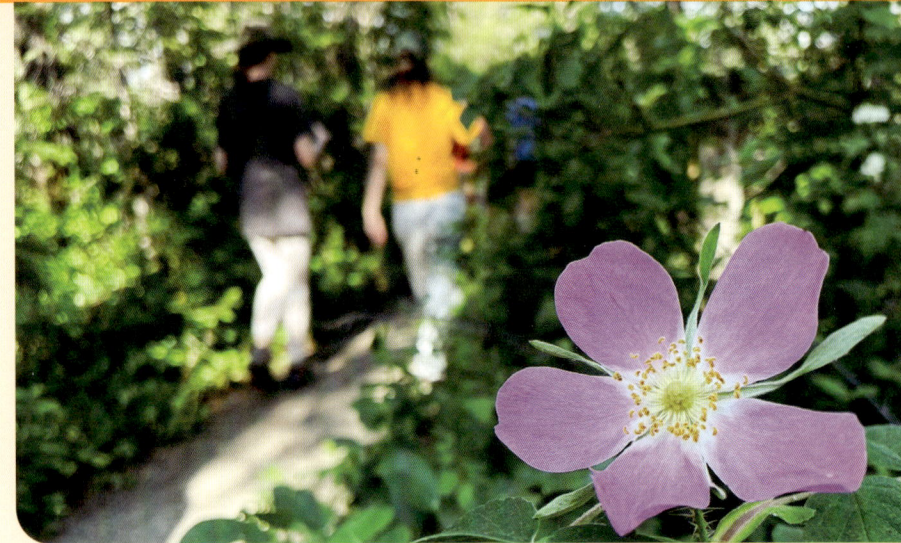

Walks at a Glance:

Wilderness walks with no city noise are urban dwellers' respite, the antidote to constant connectivity. Both featured walks are in the Weaselhead, a park that features some of the greatest biodiversity in Calgary, with over 300 plant species and over 200 species of birds.

Chickadees are your constant companions on the Jackrabbit Trail, my favourite Calgary wilderness walk that dips and climbs through the forest just below the popular Glenmore Pathway. Within minutes of the trailhead, you leave the paved path and begin a shaded walk on a rolling, single-track, dirt trail. All along you enjoy intermittent views of the Glenmore Reservoir.

Walk 65 is a relatively flat walk that starts in North Glenmore Park and follows the paved path along the top of the escarpment, looking west to the Rockies.

Details

Categories: Café, Nature, Hilly, Vistas, River, Birds

Start: Walk 65: North Glenmore Park, Parking lot F or Weaselhead Flats parking lot, 66 Avenue and 37 Street SW; Walk 66: South Glenmore Park, 24 Street and 90 Avenue SW

Facilities: Bathrooms in North and South Glenmore Park

Distance & Difficulty

Walk 65: Weaselhead Flats Park-North Glenmore Park: 9 km or 6.5 km from the Weaselhead parking lot (one hill, paved and gravel paths)

Walk 66: Jackrabbit Trail-South Glenmore Park: 7 km (hilly, paved and gravel paths)

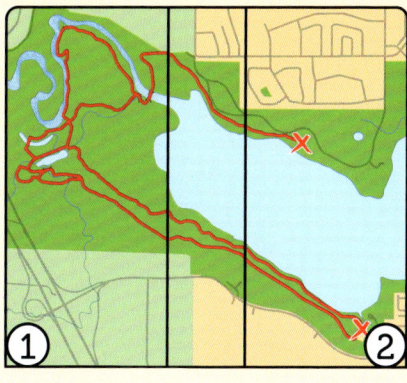

Highlights, Detours & Destinations

No dogs or bikes are allowed on the Jackrabbit and Weaselhead trails, only on the paved regional pathway. Birdlife is abundant on these walks.
Check out www.naturecalgary.com to discover Calgary's best and most unique birding hotspots with maps and bird checklists in English, Spanish, Hindi, French

Following the paved pathway, past the Weaselhead parking lot, descend into tree cover immediately, soaking up the sights and sounds of nature. Enter the Weaselhead trail network, a mix of dirt trails and boardwalks. Keep your map handy since navigating is challenging in this forested area with many paths and no trail signs. Interpretive signs marked on the map in my book will keep you oriented and informed. The route follows the twists and turns of the Elbow River before turning inland on a marshy boardwalk trail over a wetland.

Hit the refresh button on your busy city life with a walk in the Weaselhead's wilderness. A dose of nature calms the mind and engages the senses.

Weaselhead Flats Park & Jackrabbit Trail

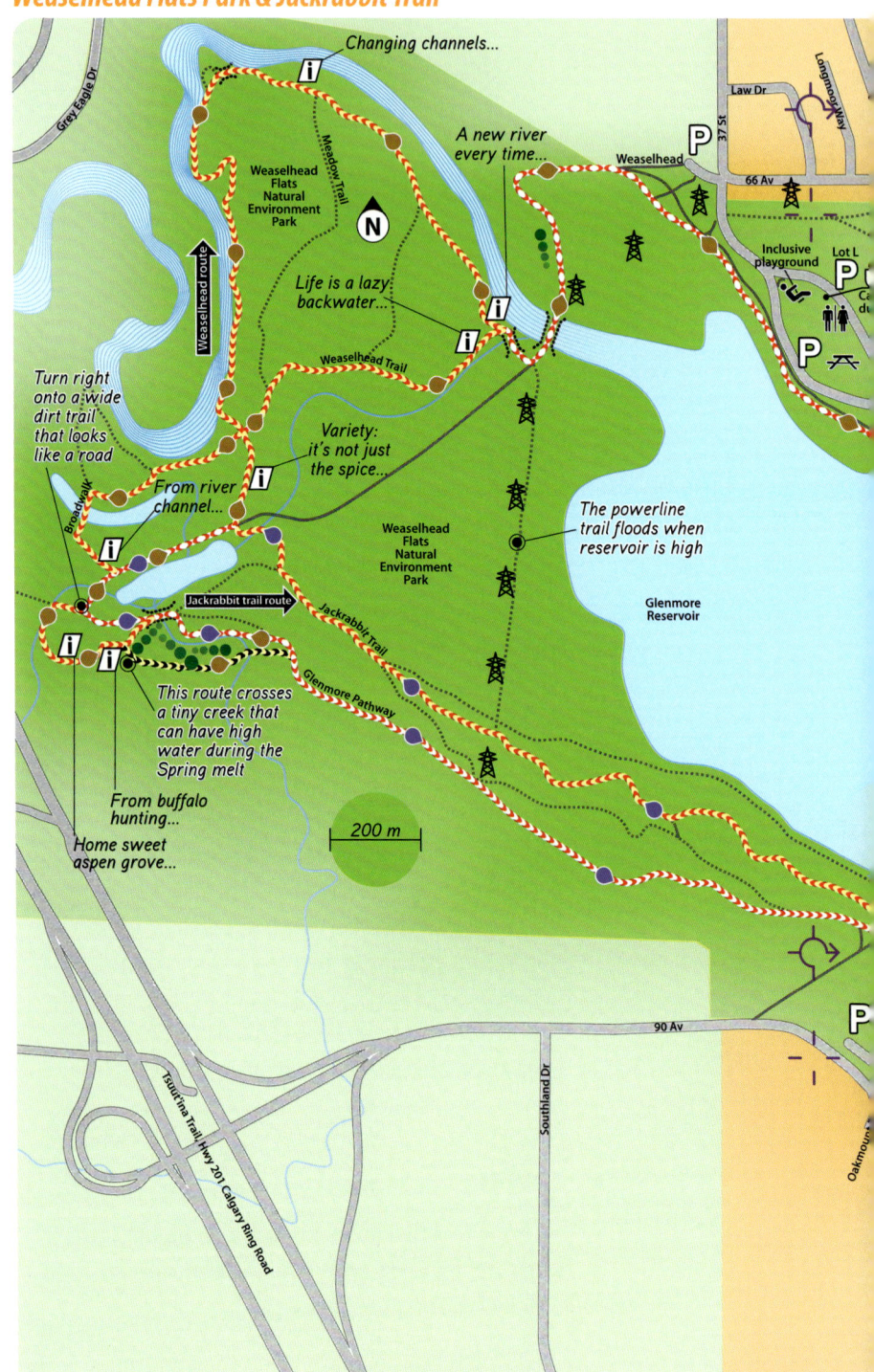

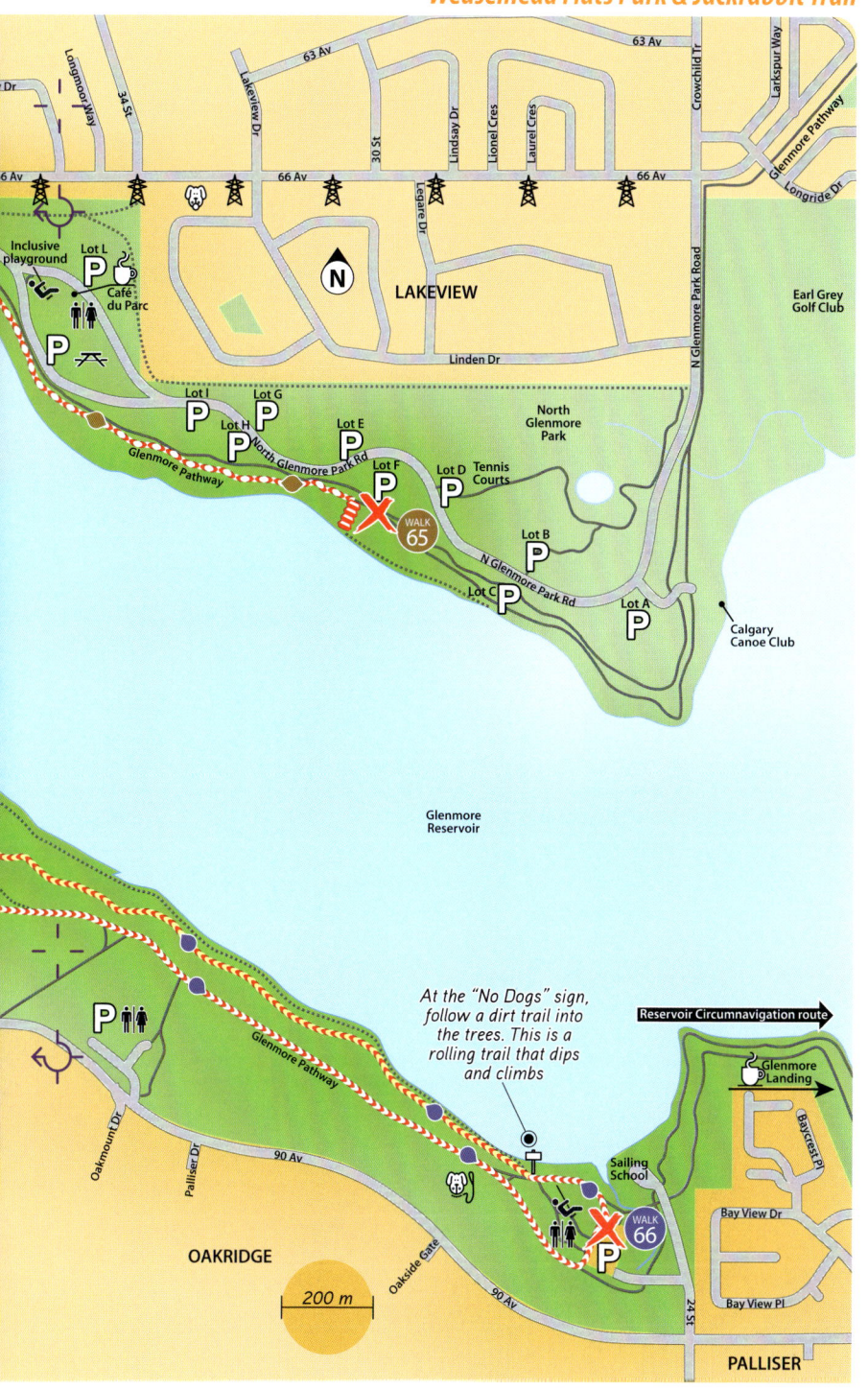

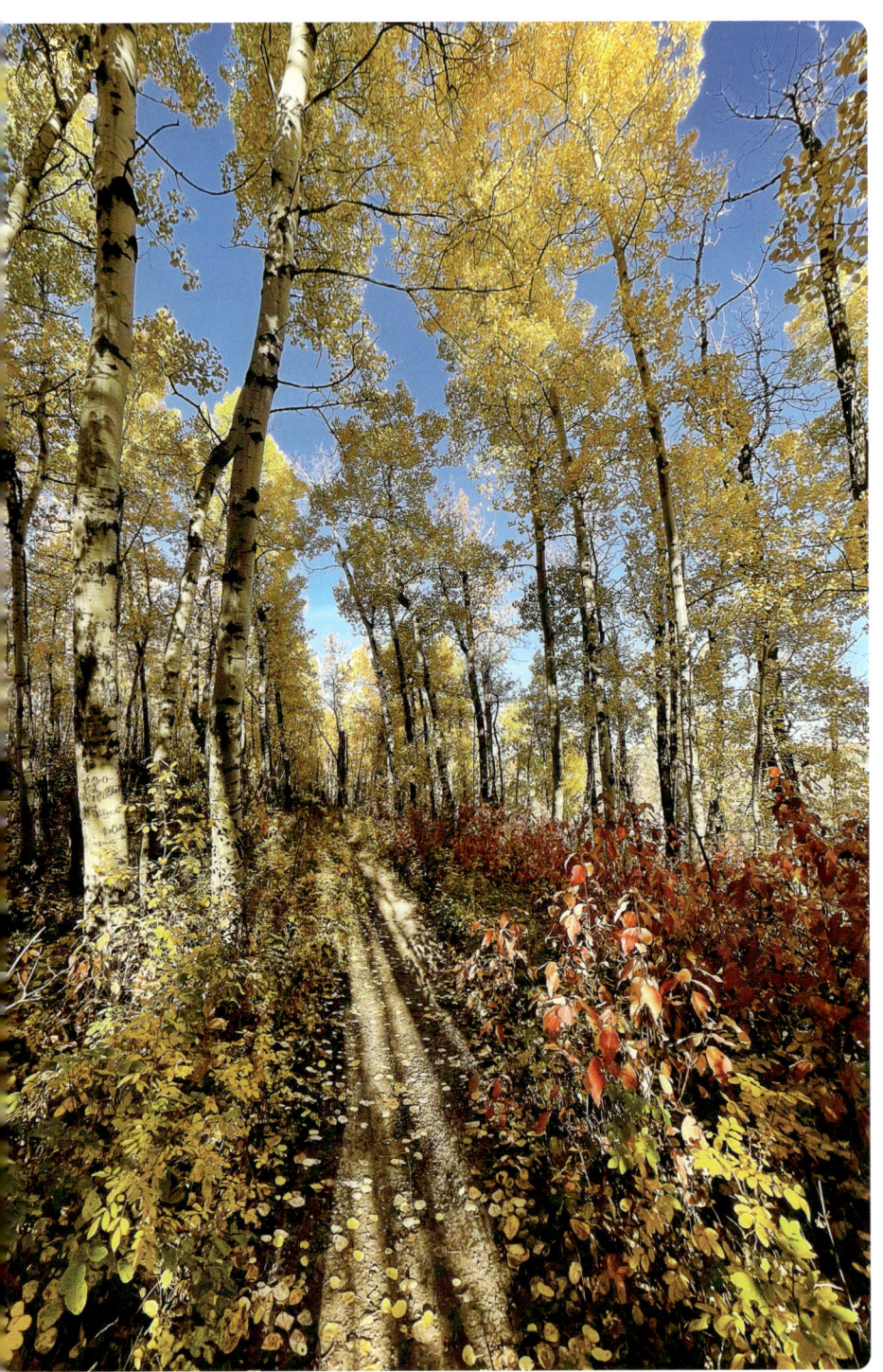

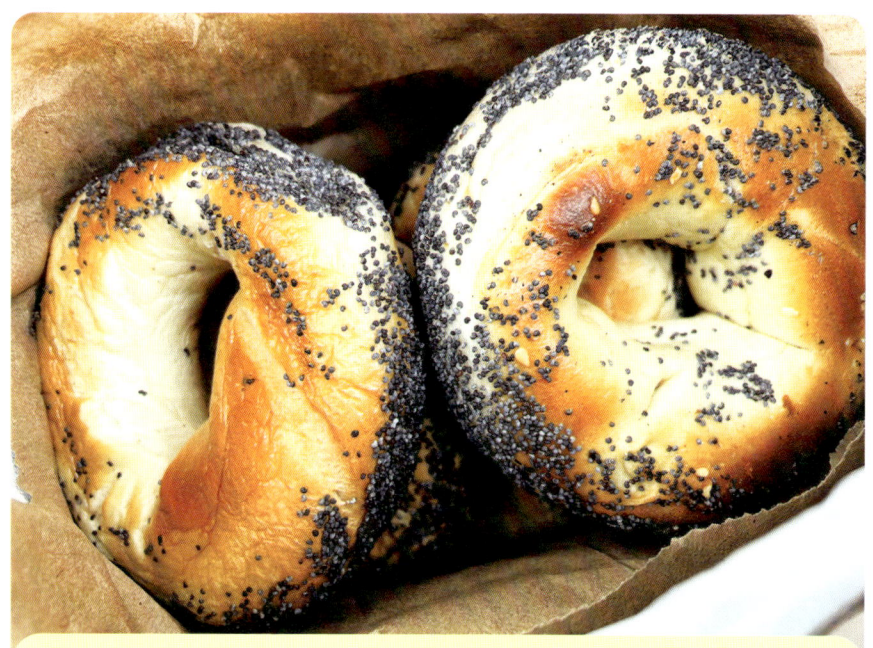

Tasty Pit Stops

On the way to Walk 66 stop by my favourite and the best bagel shop in Calgary, Montreal Bagels. If you hope to buy a dozen or more (cash only!), it is worth calling ahead to have them ready as their bagels sell so fast. At the end Walk 66, continue along the pathway east for another 15 minutes until you arrive at Glenmore Landing or stop on the way to your walk and grab some picnic items. The shopping plaza has many options for food and a grocery store at which you can build picnic lunches. For a nice atmosphere and a good cup of freshly roasted coffee, stop at the Good Earth Café. Another picnic item stop on the south side is the Apple Lady, an independent little shop that brings in BC produce, locally baked goods and breads, seasonal cheesecake jars, prepared salads like quinoa salad with roasted butternut squash and cranberries and many other tasty treats that would be delicious along the walk. And on the north side is the small but mighty Café du Parc in North Glenmore Park right beside the winter skating loop. Selling local Butterblock pastries, ice cream, and all the specialty drinks you can imagine, this little café in a park is fantastic. They also have treats for good dogs.

Location:
Glenmore Landing: 90 Avenue and 14 Street SW
Apple Lady: 3109 Palliser Drive SW, @appleladyyyc
Montreal Bagels: Heritage Drive and Elbow Drive SW
Café du Parc: North Glenmore Park, parking lot L, @cafeparc2023

Glenmore Reservoir - Bel-Aire - Mayfair - Kingsland - Haysboro

Walks 67 and 68

SW

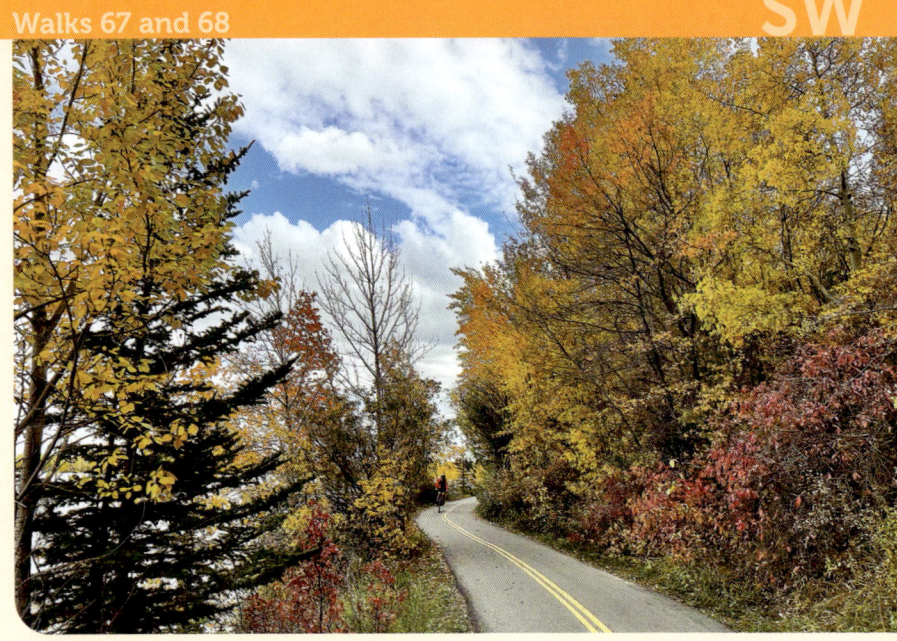

Walks at a Glance:

Views are immediate and constant on Walk 68 as you follow the paved pathway at the top of the bluffs in North Glenmore Park. A popular spot for picnics and family reunions, this people-populated park is a hive of activity in the summer and a peaceful spot in the colder months, when Calgarians hunker down and hibernate.

You can walk the reservoir loop on a straightforward paved path or on the single-track side trails. I provide many off-trail options, popular paths that dip and climb closer to the water. Dogs will be happy to know that much of Walk 67 is off leash party time. Circling the community of Lakeview, this walk is a mix of forested paths, green space walking alongside some sizeable

Details

Categories: Café, Dog, Nature, Neighbourhood & Parks, Hilly, Stroller, Vistas, River, Birds

Start: Walks 67 and 68: Weaselhead parking lot, 66 Avenue and 37 Street SW. Walk 68 alternate: Glenmore Landing

Facilities: Porta Potty at the trailhead. Seasonal and year-round bathrooms in North and South Glenmore Park close to Café du Parc in North Glenmore Park, parking Lot L. Restaurant and public washrooms at Gasoline Alley, Heritage Park

Distance & Difficulty

Walk 67: Lakeview off leash - North Glenmore wetlands: 4 km (gravel and grass paths)

Walk 68: Glenmore Reservoir Circumnavigation: 15 km or 16.5 km for the alternate route to the dam (paved paths, optional gravel paths, hills)

Walk 68: Alternate route to Mayfair & Bel-Aire: 3 km; Kingsland and Haysboro: 5.5 km

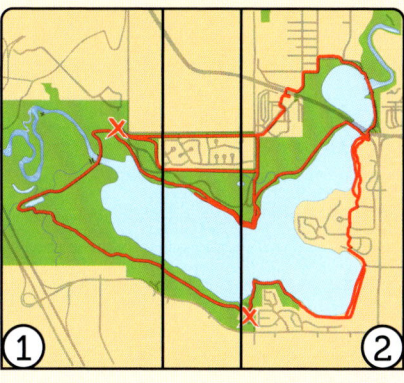

Highlights, Detours & Destinations

For tasty pit stop options see the sidebar in Walk 66. The free skating track in North Glenmore Park is lit up for nighttime fun all winter long. North and South Glenmore Parks have groomed cross country ski trails when snow conditions are good. Birdlife is abundant on Walk 68. Check out www.naturecalgary.com to discover Calgary's best and most unique birding hotspots

---

Lakeview homes, wetlands and off leash running along 66 Avenue. Embark on some urban exploration and explore the pathway network in Lakeview.

After North Glenmore Park, Walk 68 has a choice of routes. Follow the reservoir pathway behind the Earl Grey Golf Club or to take the longer walk into the community of Lakeview over Glenmore Trail, through the neighbourhood of North Glenmore, and over the dam, where impressive downtown and Elbow River views are your reward. The two routes converge at the south end of the Glenmore Trail pedestrian overpass.

Continue along the paved pathway or take the single-track trail at an opening in the fence just below the pedestrian overpass. This narrow pathway leads you along the base of the escarpment overlooking the water. If you stay on the paved path, continue uphill and follow the winding shaded pathway south to a series of benches that perch on the edge of the bluffs. For the explorers out there, walk west of the bench toward to water and find a narrow dirt path that descends through the trees to the shoreline. This off-trail option will add some hills and adventure to your walk.

Once past the Rockyview Hospital, choose between the alternate route through Kingsland and Haysboro or take the paved path descends to the quiet side streets of affluent Eagle Ridge. After a brief side-street walk you return to the pathway and come upon the next attraction en route, Heritage Park Historical Village. A summertime place to visit, it hosts an extensive collection of period buildings and a circa 1890 replica of Calgary's CPR train station. Stop for a snack or continue onward, along the off-trail treed pathway that follows the water or along the paved path all the way to Glenmore Landing: the perfect halfway point at which you can recharge with lunch, a coffee and a muffin. The pathway soon splits, and I suggest taking the lower route, along the paved path closest to the water. Binocular clad birders are also a regular sight here, watching for the varieties of feathered friends that visit the reservoir, many en masse. The Glenmore Yacht Club and South Glenmore Park playground and waterpark soon appear.

For a complete immersion in nature, switch to the Weaselhead route maps, walks 65 and 66. Bordering the Tsuu T'ina First Nation Reserve, the low-lying Weaselhead trails are a network of possibilities, so plan on taking extra time to explore. A hill climb ends the outing and leads you back to fantastic views of the reservoir and the Rockies.

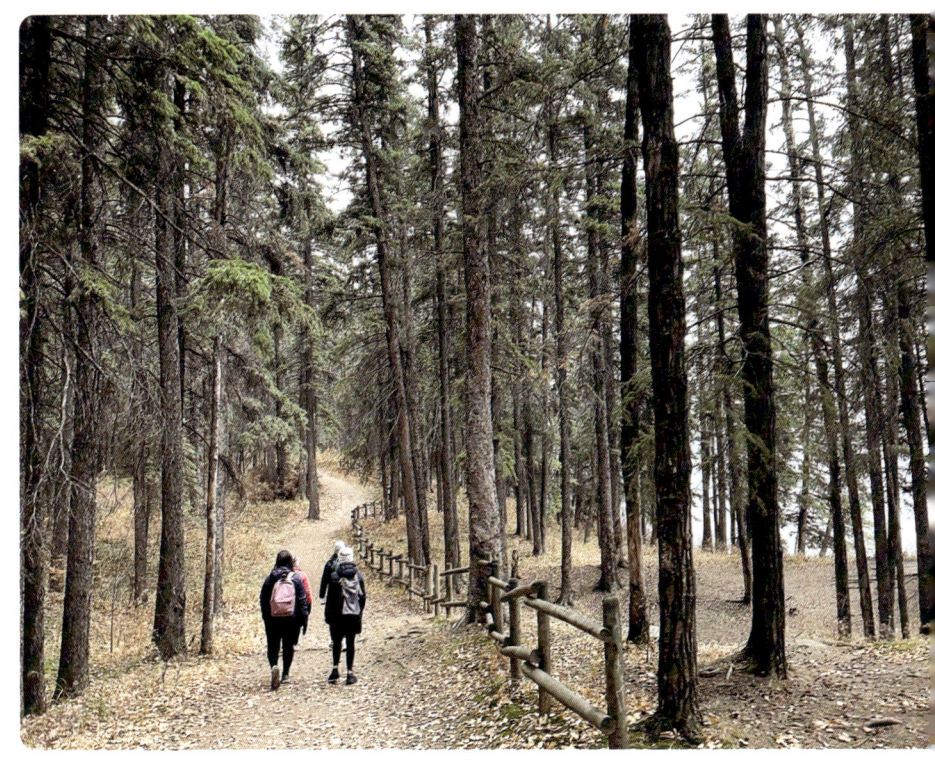

Why is a Walk in the Woods so Good for You?

There is no Wi-Fi in the forest, but trust me, you will find a better connection. Walking in the woods offers a break from distractions. In Japan they call it shinrin-yoku, or "forest bathing." We call it a walk in the woods, and we know that it makes us feel good. Scientists have studied the physical and mental benefits that come from a walk in nature. Many theories suggest various reasons why nature feels good: clean air, lack of noise pollution, and even the fine mist that comes off the trees, that fresh evergreen smell that makes us breathe deeply through our noses. But the most convincing argument for the peace we feel in nature is that the flowers and the birds never aggressively grab our attention. The voluntary attention we pay them is very different from the attention we are forced to pay to a car horn honking, for example. Going for a walk in the park allows your mind to wander, which benefits your brain. Throughout the day, we are required to use voluntary attention repeatedly for cognitive tasks, like responding to texts and e-mail, or remembering our shopping list. Our brain grows tired and inefficient without a break. Going for a walk in the park or a quiet place without distractions gives voluntary attention a break, lets your mind wander, and allows you to be involuntarily engaged by your surroundings. The other benefits of walking in nature are the fresh smells, the clean air, and being surrounded by earthy hues. All of these factors contribute to why a walk in the woods makes you feel good. My hunch, based on anecdotal on-the-trail research, is that the break from distractions plays a pivotal role in making the woodsy walker feel refreshed. Focusing on walking, one foot in front of the other, is therapeutic. Left, right, left, right. And don't forget to put your cell phone on silent.

Glenmore Reservoir Circumnavigation & North Glenmore Park

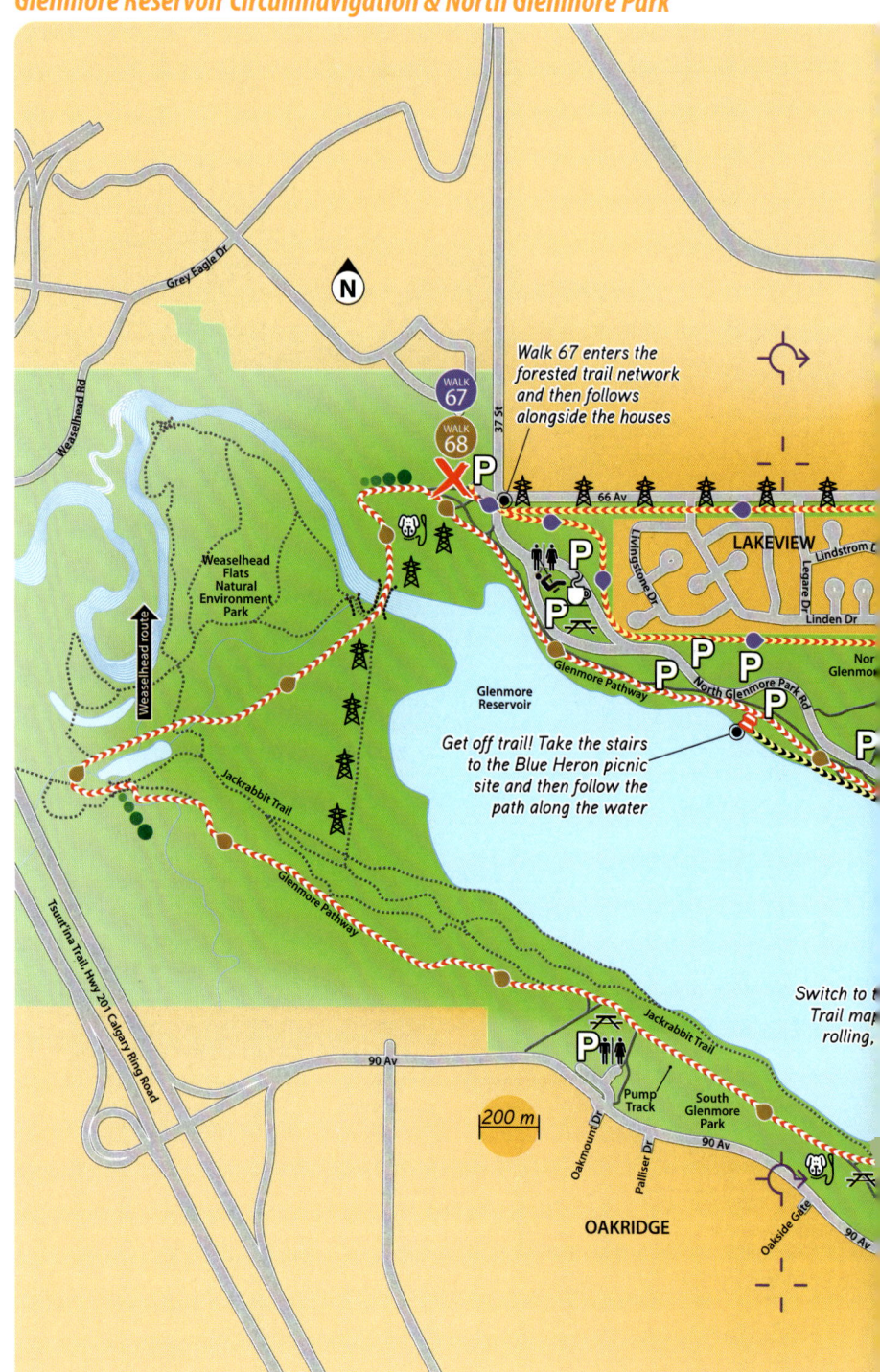

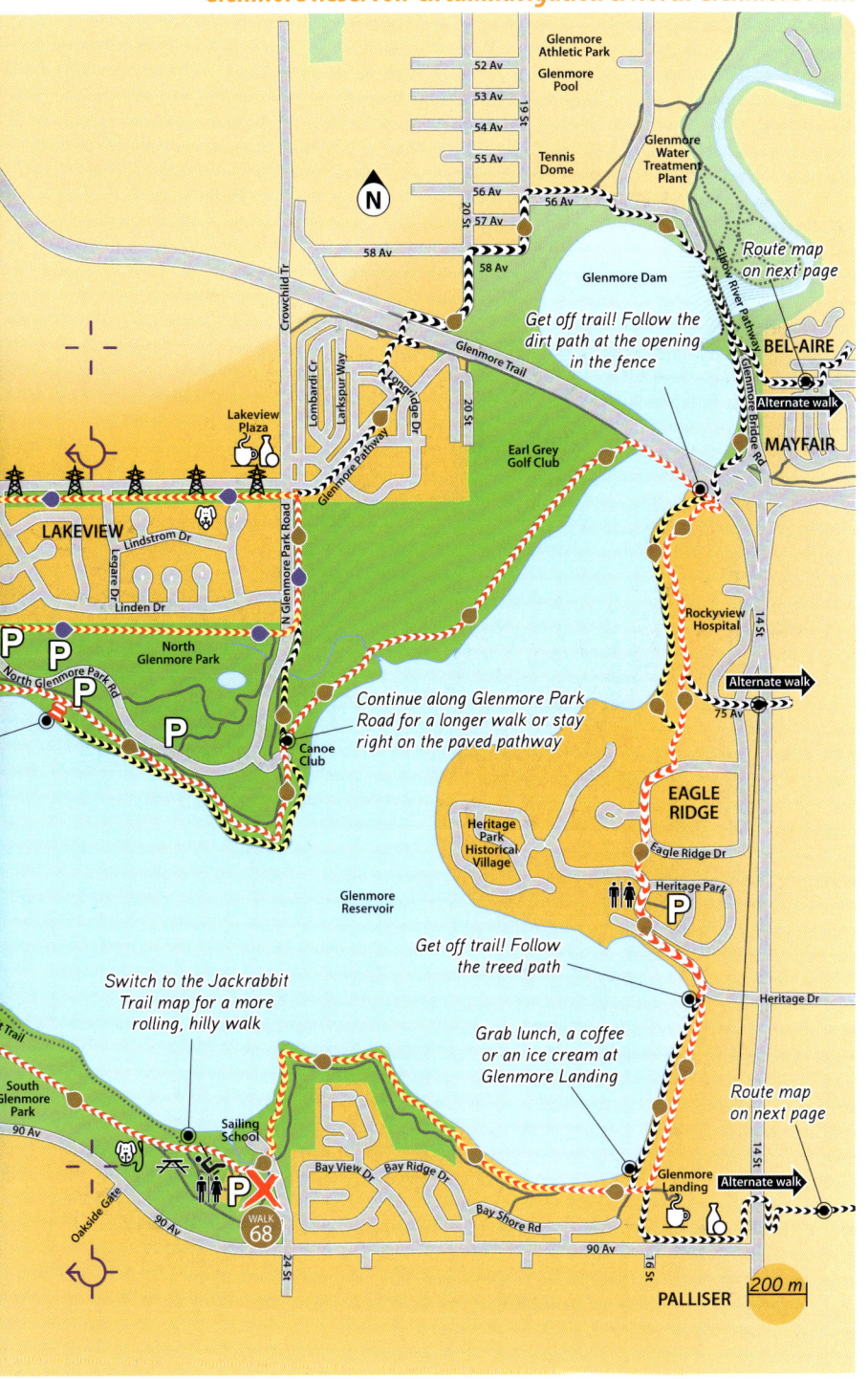

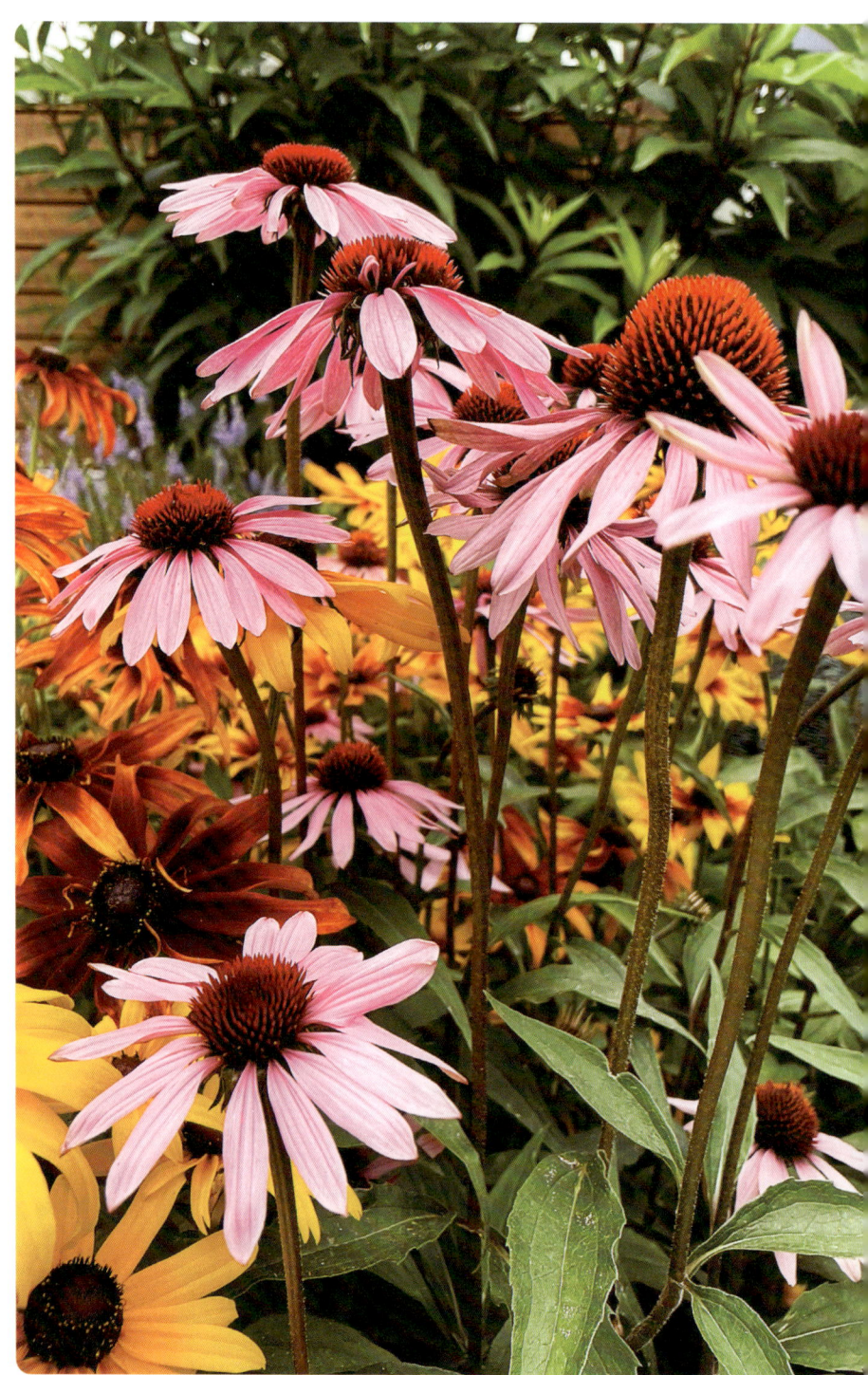

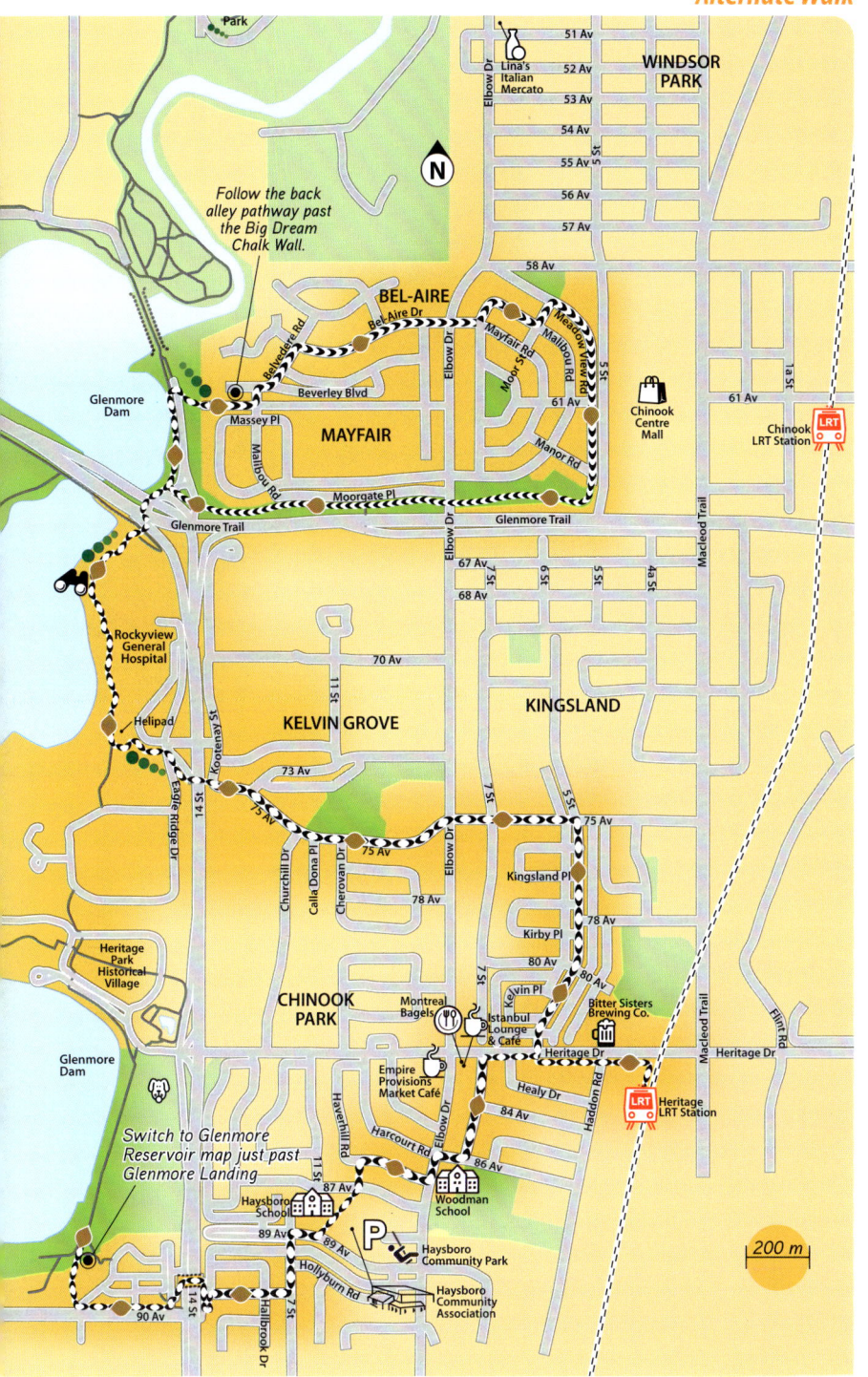

Griffith Woods Park

Walk 69

SW

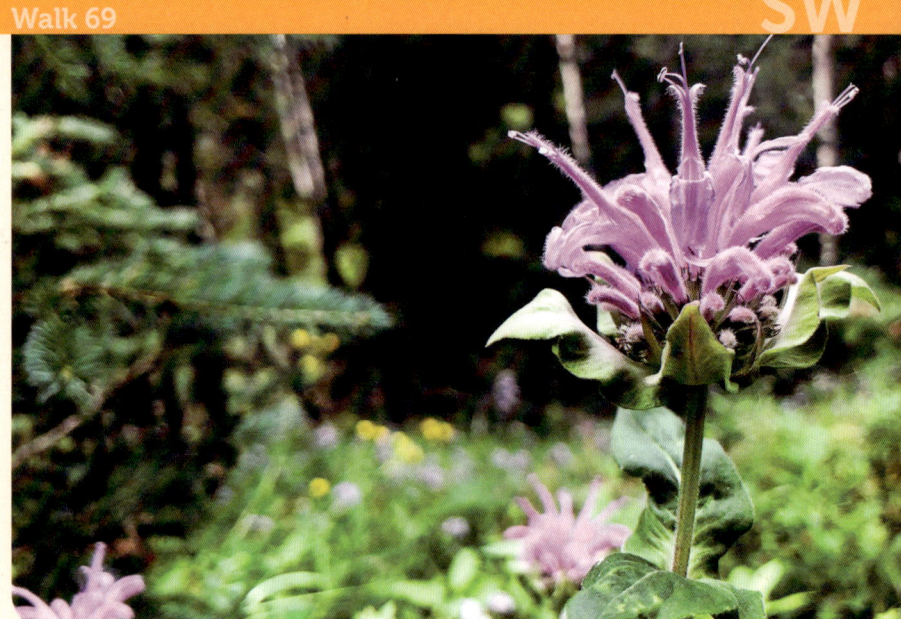

Walk at a Glance:

Peaceful and pleasant, Griffith Woods Park is the perfect spot to slow the pace and collect your thoughts. The mix of paved and gravel pathways weave through a mature, and at times dense, white spruce forest mixed with stands of balsam poplar.

Details

Categories: Dog, Nature, Stroller, River, Birds

Start: Trailhead at the end of Discovery Ridge Link SW.

Facilities: Year-round bathrooms at trailhead

Distance & Difficulty

5 km (Mostly flat on paved and gravel paths)

Highlights, Detours & Destinations

Birdlife is abundant on this walk. Check out www.naturecalgary.com to discover Calgary's best and most unique birding hotspots with maps and bird checklists in English, Spanish, Hindi, French

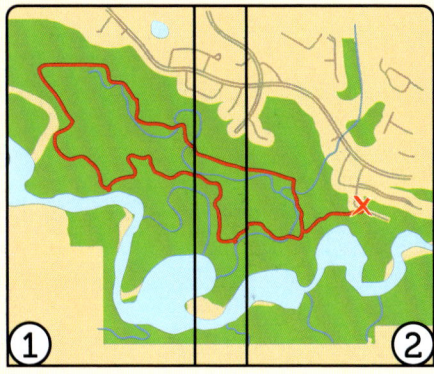

The coniferous forest is home to mule deer, coyotes, porcupines, and the occasional black bear, so keep an eye out. Oxbow wetlands, created when the river changes course, are home to many birds, such as gray jays and red-breasted nuthatches. Tucked away in Discovery Ridge, this suburban park was ranch land from the late 1800s until 2000, when the land was donated to the City of Calgary by Wilbur and Betty Griffith to be set aside as a nature preserve. It is now part of the Rotary/Mattamy Greenway, a 138-km network of parks and pathways that encircles the city and links 55 communities. An oasis of calm, Griffith Woods is a place where you can move slowly and ponder, spend time with family, and enjoy a picnic by the river.

Griffith Woods Park

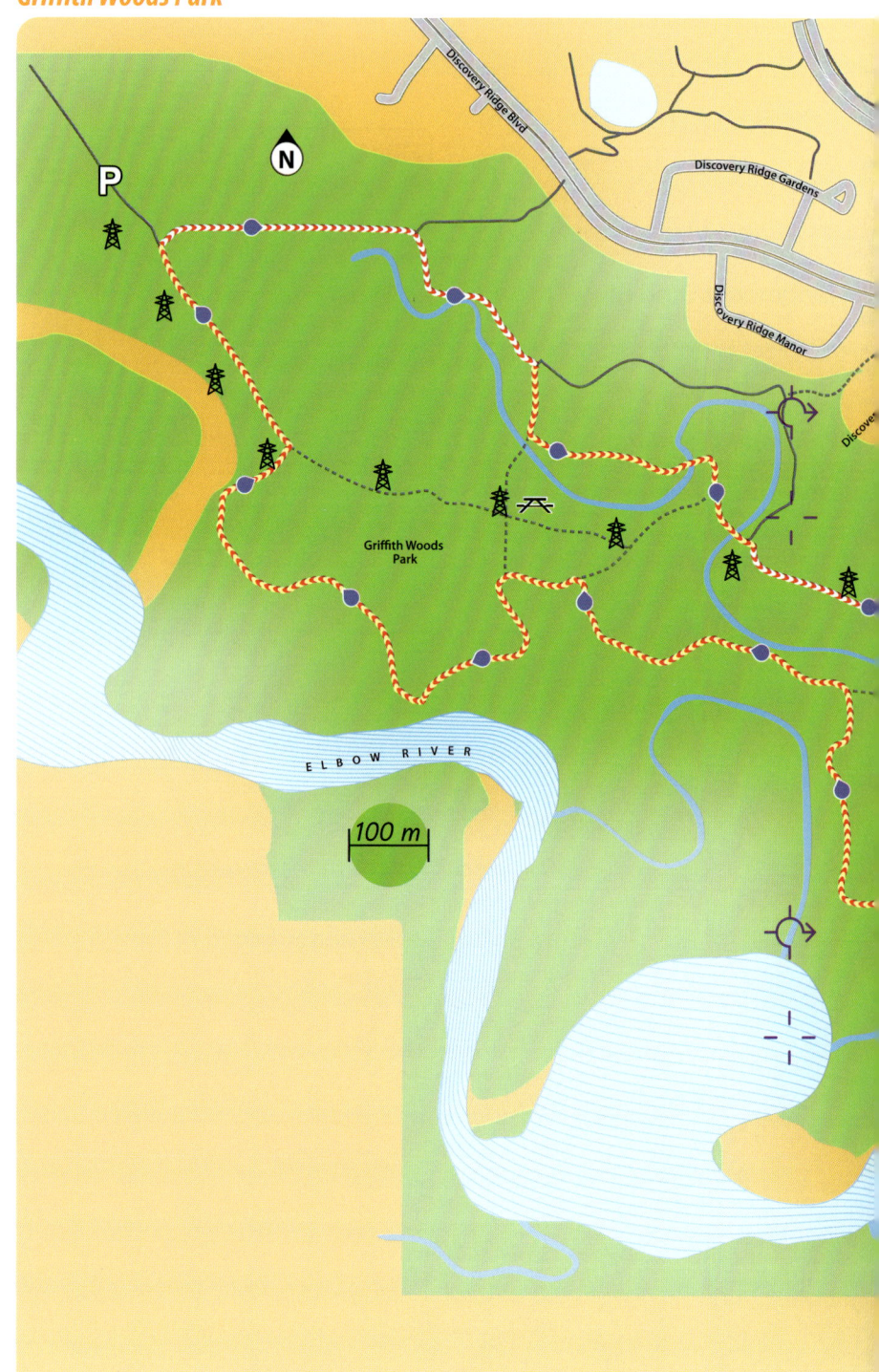

Griffith Woods Park

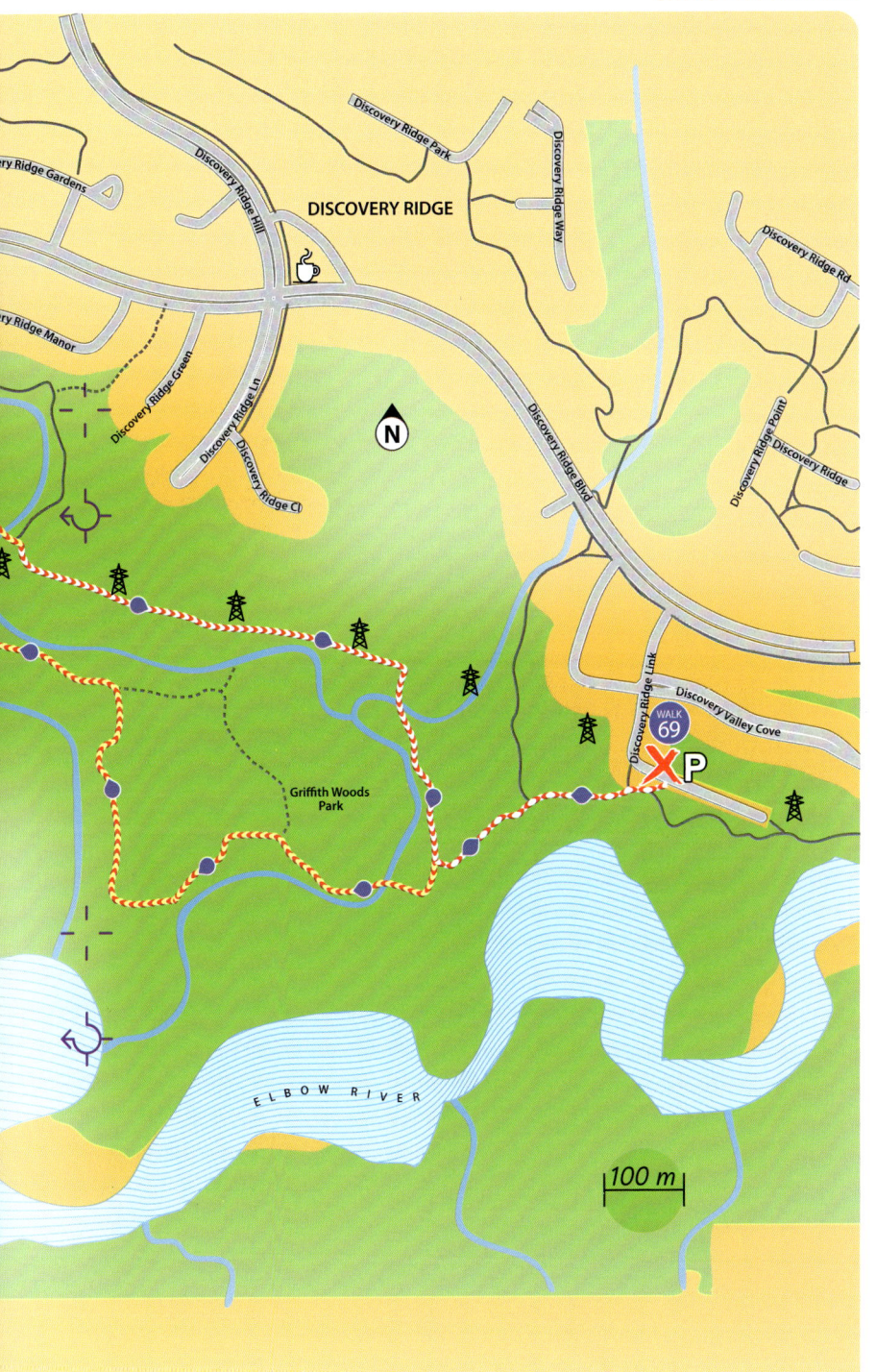

Calgary Road Names: A History

One thing that distinguishes Calgary from other metropolitan areas is how we name our major thoroughfares. The word "trail" is used across our city and pays homage to the old oxcart trail that existed between Calgary and Fort Benton in Montana. Stoney, Blackfoot, Metis, Shaganappi, Sarcee, and Peigan trails are all named in honour of the First People on this continent, although the latter two nations have since changed their names. The Peigan are now known as the Piikani Nation, and the Sarcee are now the Tsuut'ina Nation, but both street names remain. Others, such as Edmonton, Banff, Morley, Beddington, Airport, Spruce Meadows and Bow trails are named after destinations or nearby landmarks. Glenmore Trail is named for a Gaelic word meaning "big valley," thanks to early explorer Sam Livingstone.

Calgary's Ring Road has two names. Stoney Trail was derived from Alberta's Nakoda First Nation. The road's name changes to Tsuut'ina Trail as it crosses Fish Creek into the Tsuut'ina Nation.

Deerfoot Trail, Calgary's fastest freeway, was aptly named after the runner, Api-kai-ees, a Siksika long-distance runner who became a local hero in Calgary's early days. Described as a "human thunderbolt," he more than lived up to the name as he defeated racers from as far away as Europe.

Lieutenant-Colonel James Macleod was the second commissioner of the NWMP and founder of Fort Calgary. Both Fort Macleod and Macleod trails are named in his honour.

Crowchild Trail is named after David Crowchild, Chief of the Tsuut'ina Nation from 1946 to 1953.

Barlow Trail is named for Noel Barlow, a local pilot and ground crewman who had a distinguished career during the Second World War.

The historic Stephen Avenue in Calgary's downtown is named after Sir George Stephen, who was a prominent businessman in Canada and the mastermind behind the Canadian Pacific Railway.

James McKevitt was an early Alberta settler in the Midnapore area and a CPR surveyor. James McKevitt Road in the SW is named after him.

John Laurie Boulevard is named after Dr. John Laurie, who was a prominent educator and political activist in Calgary best known for First Nations advocacy. He became an honorary Stoney Chief in 1948 and was given the name White Cloud.

McKnight Boulevard is named after Flying Officer William Lidstone "Willie" McKnight of the Royal Air Force. He became Canada's fifth-highest scoring ace of the Second World War.

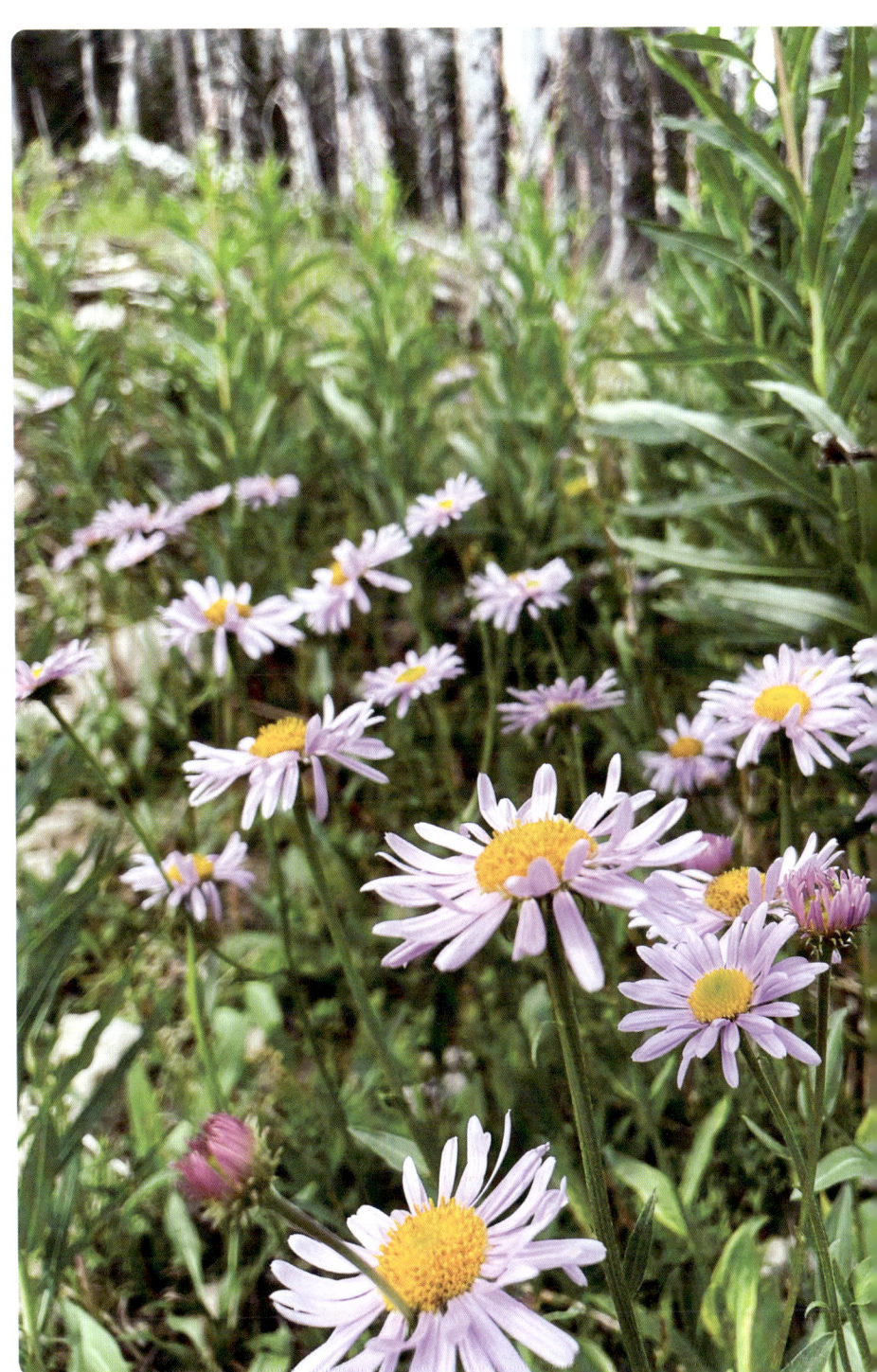

Ann & Sandy Cross Conservation Area, Leighton Art Centre, Brown Lowery Provincial Park

Walks 70-75

SW

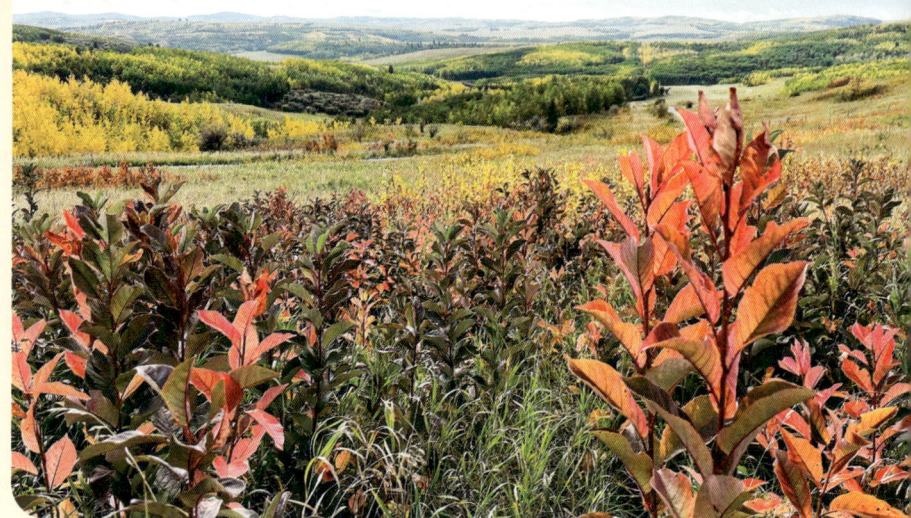

Walks at a Glance:

Prairie paradise walking on the southwest edge of Calgary is the best way to describe the walks or snowshoe days you'll enjoy at the Ann and Sandy Cross Conservation Area and Leighton Art Centre. Consisting of rolling foothills covered in native grasses, aspen forest, and groves of willow, the Cross Conservation Area is a 4,800 acre day-use habitat conservation area and nocturnal preserve.

Unobtrusive trails have been cut into the prairie grasses allowing walkers to navigate the rolling foothills. Aspen forests provide shade and hill climbs get your heart rate up before rewarding you with unobstructed views of the Rocky Mountains.

The Leighton Art Centre sits atop the foothills and hosts breathtaking Rockies views that are a constant as you stroll or picnic on the slopes. Bring your sketchpad and

Details

Categories: Dog (Brown Lowery only), Nature, Hilly, Vistas, River, Birds

Start: Walks 70 -72: Sandy Cross, 160 Street W at Highway 22X There is a per visit fee to park or you can purchase an annual pass.; Walks 73 and 74: Leighton Art Centre, 282027 144 St, Millarville (open Tuesday-Sunday, 10 am – 4 pm); Walk 75: Brown Lowery Provincial Park, Plummers Road

Facilities: Sandy Cross has bathrooms at the start and along the walk. Leighton Art Centre has bathrooms when open. Brown Lowery has bathrooms at the trailhead

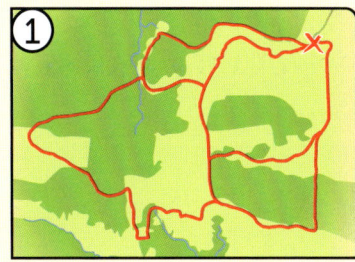
Ann & Sandy Cross Conservation Area

Distance & Difficulty

Walk 70: Paradise Trail: 8.6 km (hills, grass paths)

Walk 71: Fescue Trail: 4.5 km (hills, grass paths)

Walk 72: Aspen Trail: 3 km (few hills, grass paths)

Walk 73: Leighton Art Centre loop: 3 km (some hills, grass paths)

Walk 74: Bird Box Art Walk: 2 km (mostly flat, grass paths)

Walk 75: Brown Lowery Provincial Park: 6.5 km (some hills, gravel paths)

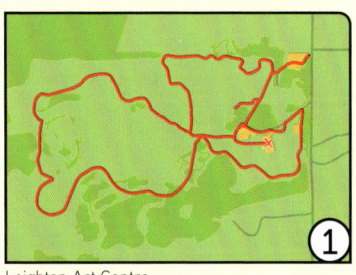
Leighton Art Centre

Highlights, Detours & Destinations

No dogs allowed on Sandy Cross Conservation Area and Leighton Art Centre trails. Pay for parking at Sandy Cross at www.crossconservation.org. Add on a tasty road trip to south or west. See the sidebar below for ideas

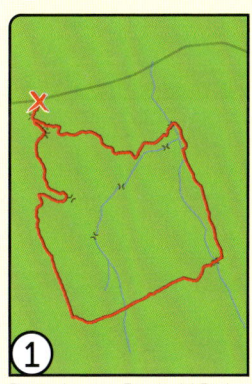
Brown Lowery Provincial Park

Ann & Sandy Cross Conservation Area

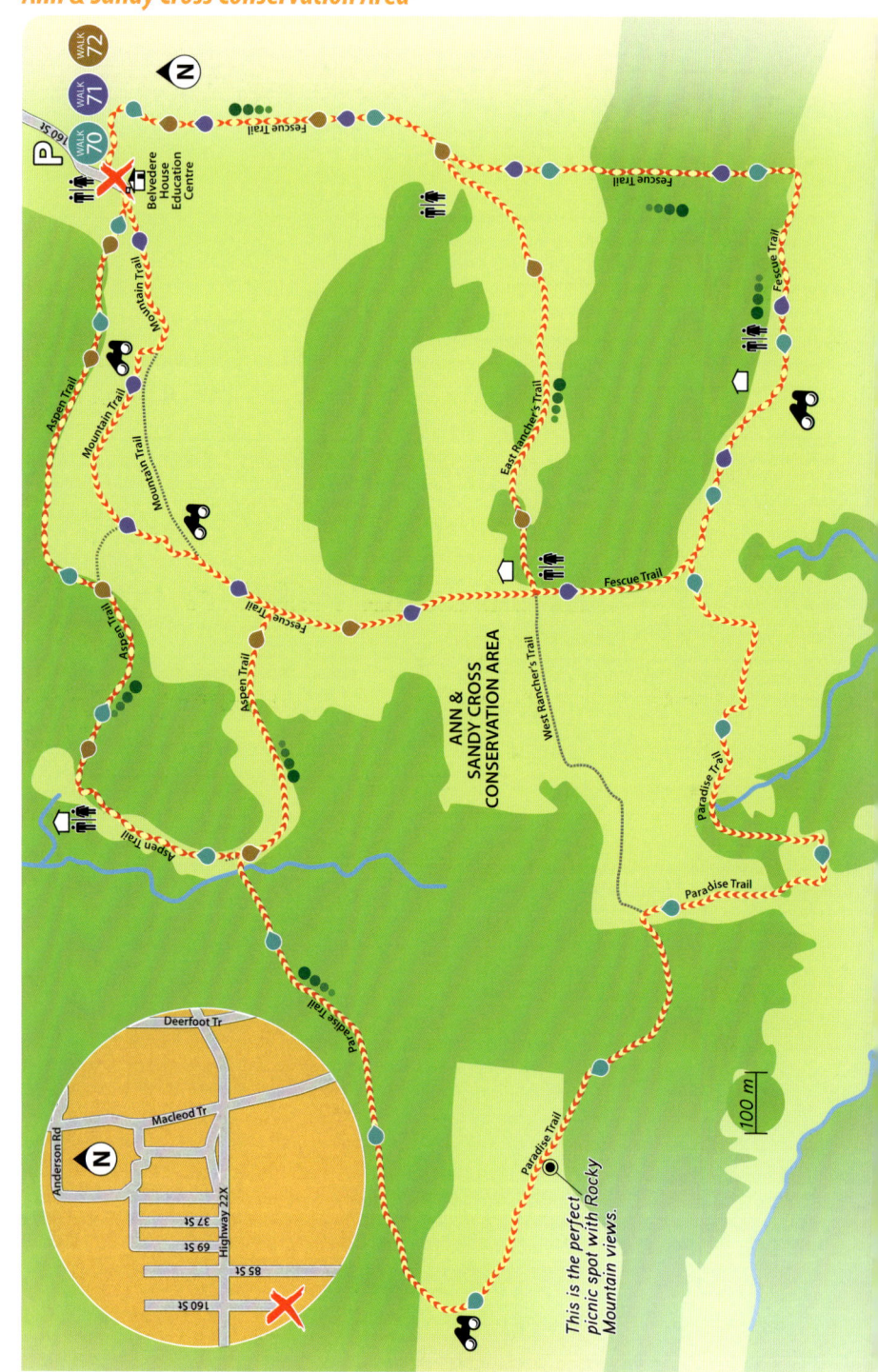

join the artists who create here year-round. A non-profit public art gallery, museum and education centre, plan a visit, to check out the museum or to take a course and get the creative juices flowing.

If you hike or snowshoe in these areas after a fresh snowfall your hidden hiking companions will suddenly become evident. Cougar, deer, moose, herds of elk, beaver, porcupine, red fox, snowshoe hare, and coyote are all regulars to the area and their tracks scatter the landscape during the snowy months. Bring your animal tracks book and have some identification fun with the kids.

Travel 50 km southwest of Calgary to Brown Lowery where walking trails travel through grasslands, mature forests and over small creeks in a rolling foothills landscape that leads to views of the Rocky Mountains and downtown Calgary on a clear day. This small but mighty park offers a complete nature immersion with its variety of wildlife, trees, wildflowers and fungi that live alongside the 12 kilometers of rustic trails. Your potential hiking companions include deer, moose, elk, black bears, lynx, cougar, squirrels, birds and Calgarians. How lucky we are to have these natural gems so close to the city.

Tasty pit stops

There are many tasty and interesting destinations just south of Calgary. Take the back roads for a beautiful ride to the Saskatoon Farm. A U-Pick for saskatoon and sour cherries, summer is when it comes to life with its multiple greenhouses full of plants and flowers, an eclectic old-fashioned street with gift shops, a restaurant with excellent Mexican cuisine (the churros with saskatoon compote and ice cream are delicious) and a seasonal Farmer's Market with local and organic veggies. Okotoks is home to the fabulous family owned French 50 Bakery that specializes in handmade pastries, rustic sourdough, and artisan pizza. Mouth-watering baked goods in a cozy, renovated 110-year-old home, this café makes a wonderful destination for all things delicious. West of Calgary in Diamond Valley is the tiny family-owned Black Sheep Coffee Co. Tasty made in house pastries, sweet and savory, and in house roasted coffee makes for the perfect post walk stop.

Leighton Art Centre

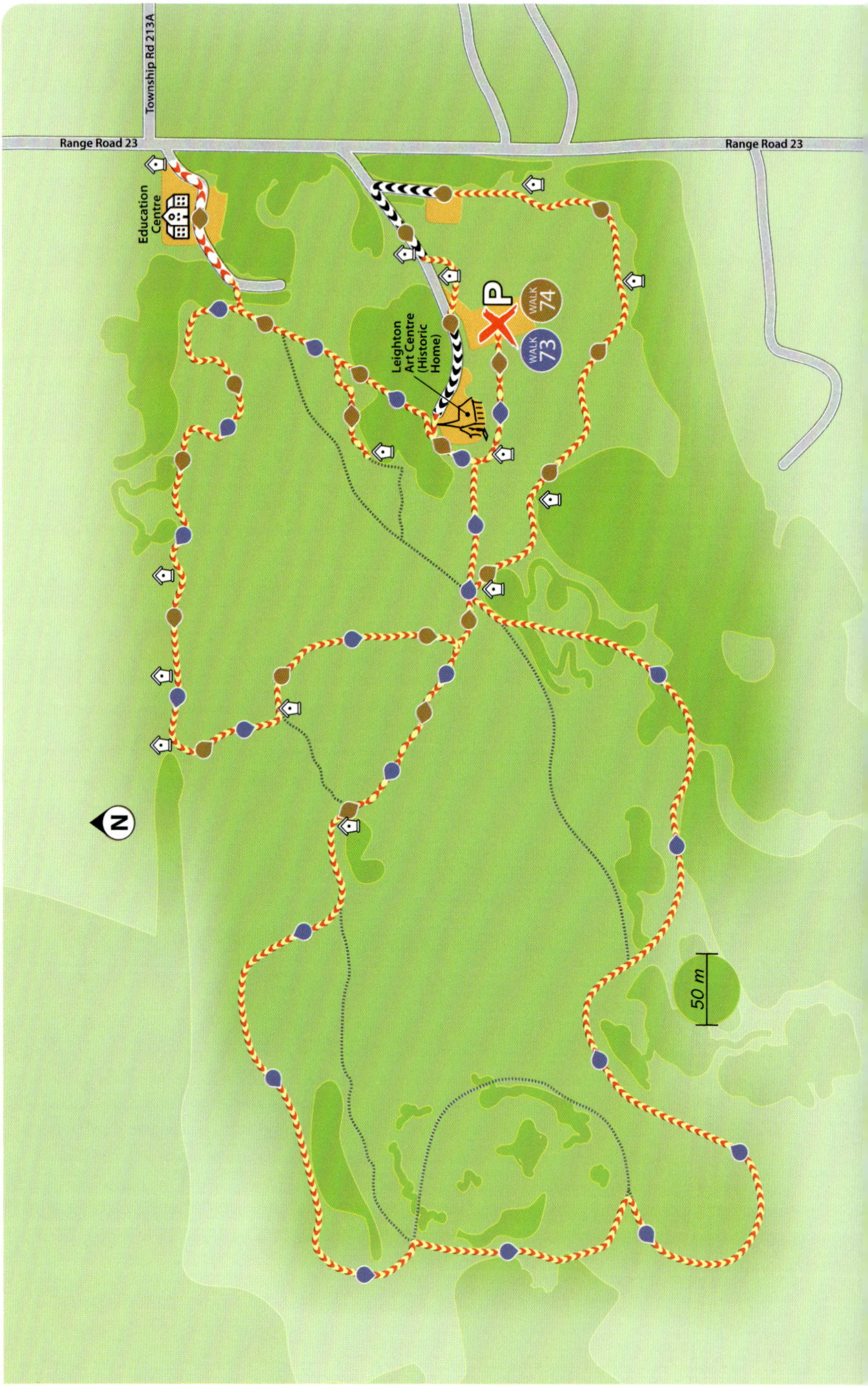

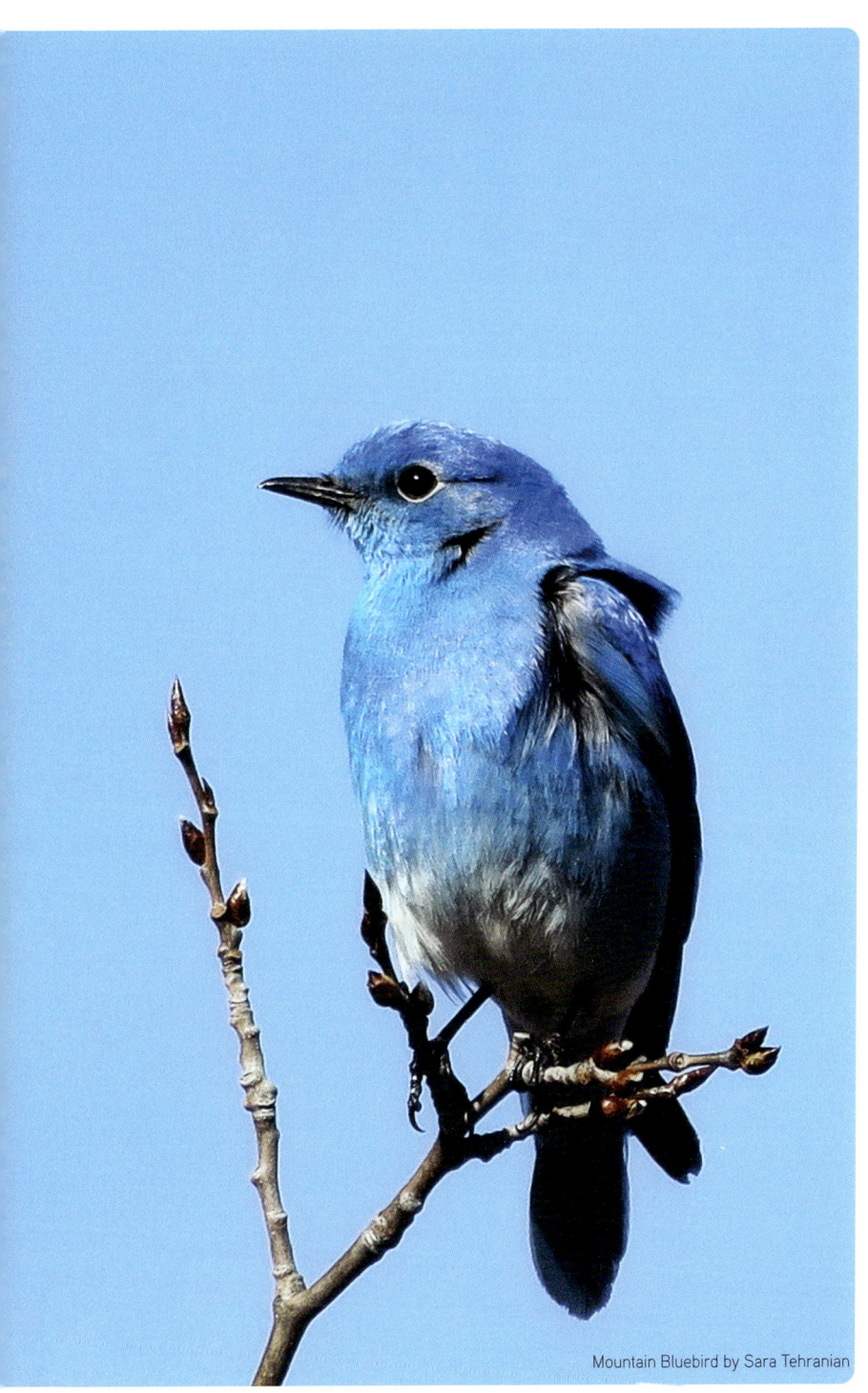

Mountain Bluebird by Sara Tehranian

ANN & SANDY CROSS CONSERVATION AREA, LEIGHTON ART CENTRE, BROWN LOWERY PROVINCIAL PARK

Brown Lowery Provincial Park

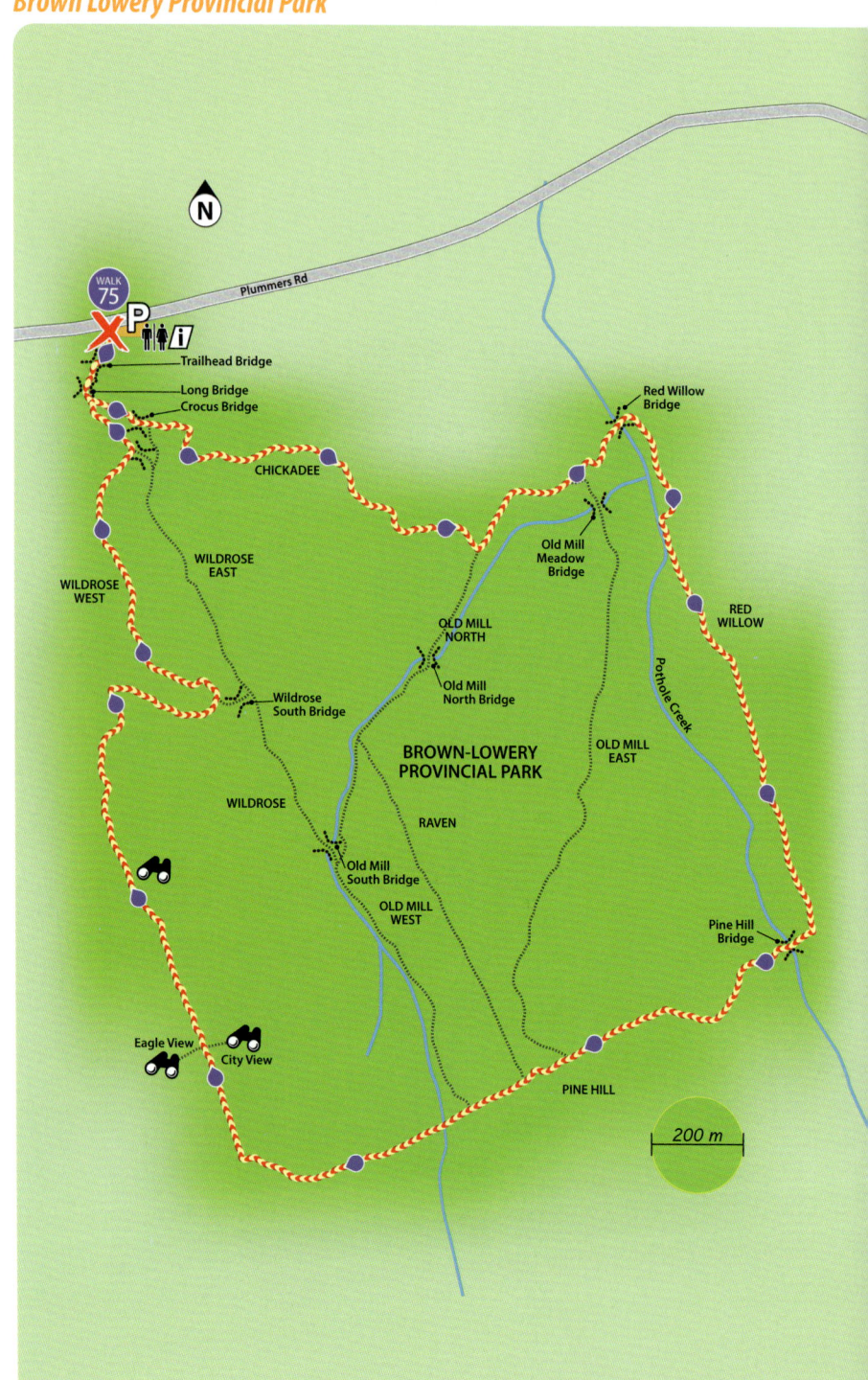

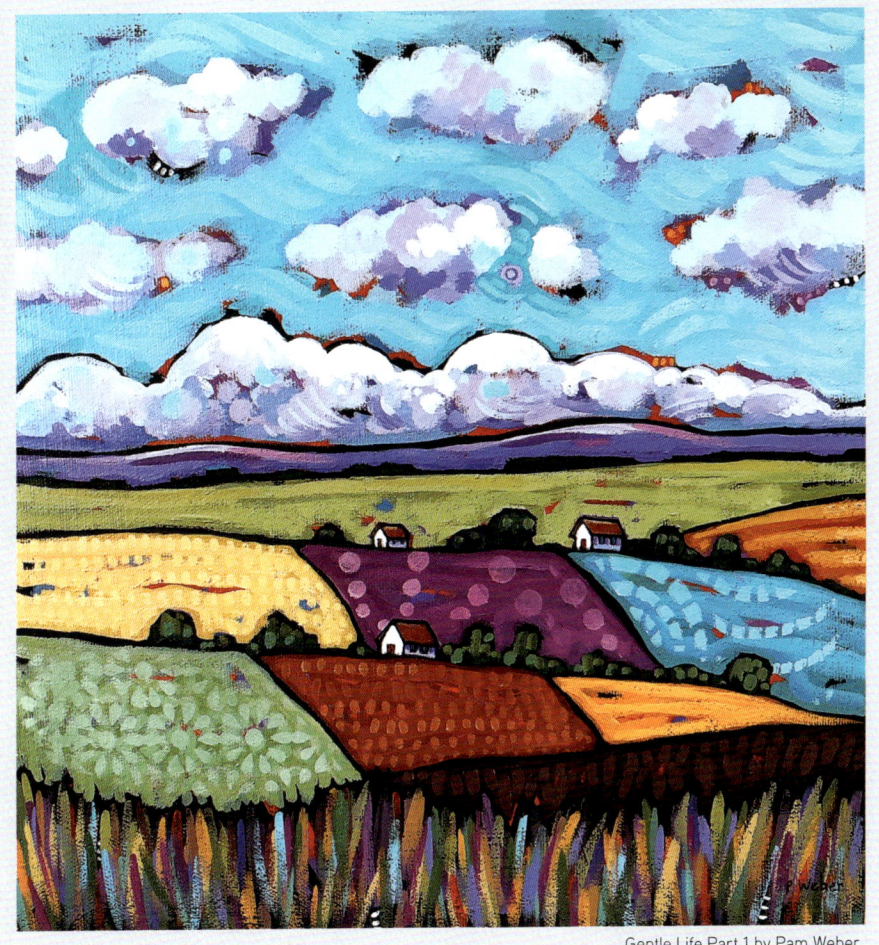

Gentle Life Part 1 by Pam Weber

ANN & SANDY CROSS CONSERVATION AREA,
LEIGHTON ART CENTRE, BROWN LOWERY PROVINCIAL PARK

Fish Creek Provincial Park

Walks 76-81

SW-SE

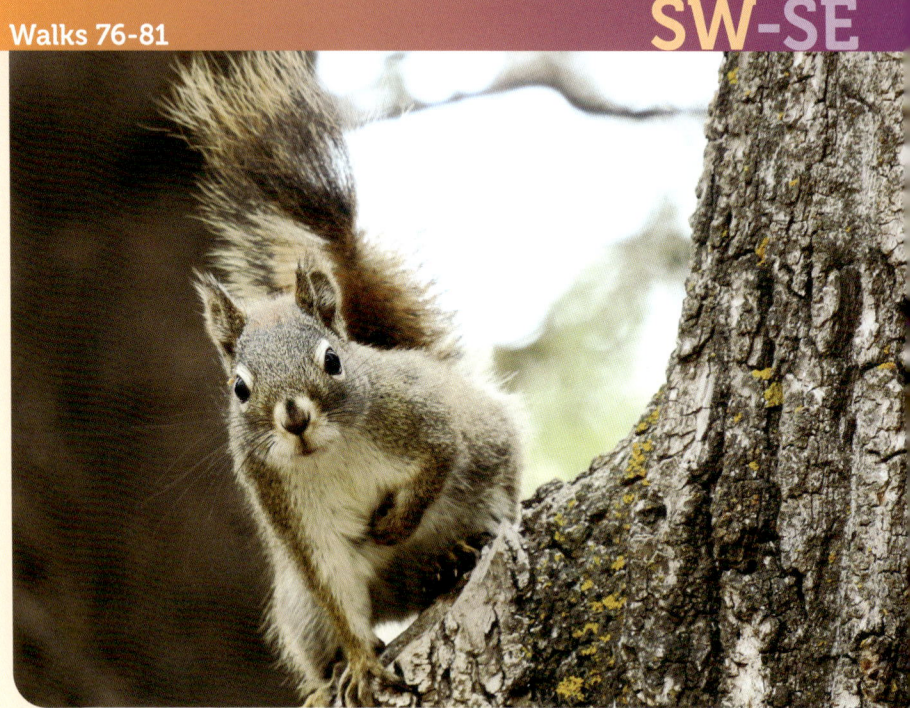

Squrriel by Sara Tehranian

Walks at a Glance:

Vast and peaceful, Fish Creek Provincial Park offers a complete immersion in nature. Stretching 19 km from east to west and encompassing over 13 km^2, it is one of the largest urban parks in North America. More than 100 kilometres of pathways, a mix of shale, paved, and single-track mountain bike trails snake through the park.

Listen for the birdlife in wetlands scattered throughout the park, and spot wildlife as you walk: deer, coyote, snake, frog, and the occasional black bear all call the park home. For those of you inebriated on electronics, going for a walk in Fish Creek will be like hitting the restore button for your mind.

Details

Categories: LRT, Café, Dog, Nature, Neighbourhood & Parks, Hilly, Stroller, Vistas, River, Birds

Start: Walk 76: Votiers Flats, south end of Elbow Drive SW or Shannon Terrace, Woodpath Road SW; Walk 77-79: Bow Valley Ranch, Bow Bottom Trail SE; Walk 79: Mallard Point, Canyon Meadows Drive SE; Walk 80: Rotary Park, 24 Street, SE or Cranridge Heights, SE; Walk 81: Sikome Lake area, Bow Bottom Trail SE or Lafarge Meadows, end of 138 Avenue SE

LRT: Fish Creek Station

Facilities: Bathrooms throughout Fish Creek Park

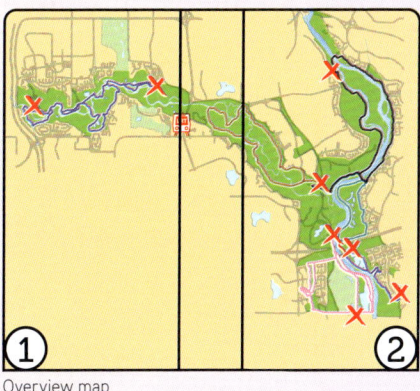

Overview map

Distance & Difficulty

Walk 76: Fish Creek Park West: 12 km or 6 km loop to Bebo Grove (hills, paved and gravel paths)

Walk 77: Fish Creek Park, Bow Valley Ranch: 8 km (hills, paved, gravel and single-track paths)

Walk 78: Fish Creek Park and Dougladale Escarpment: 9.7 km (one hill, paved paths)

Walk 79: Fish Creek Park and Mountain Park Escarpment: 6 km (one hill, paved and grass paths)

Walk 80: Fish Creek Park - Rotary Nature Park - Cranston: 6 km (one hill, paved paths)

Walk 81: Fish Creek Park - Chaparral - Lafarge Meadows: 7 km (Paved paths, optional hill)

Highlights, Detours & Destinations

In a good snow year, cross-country skiing in the west end of the park is wonderful. There are no official ski trails, only skier made tracks. Birdlife is abundant on this walk. Check out www.naturecalgary.com to discover Calgary's best and most unique birding hotspots with maps and bird checklists in English, Spanish, Hindi, French

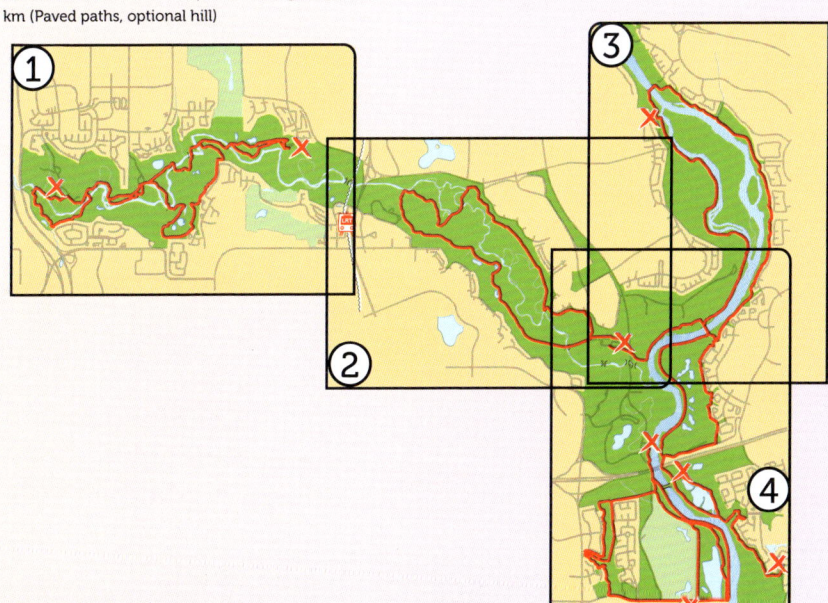

FISH CREEK PROVINCIAL PARK

Fish Creek Provincial Park - Overview

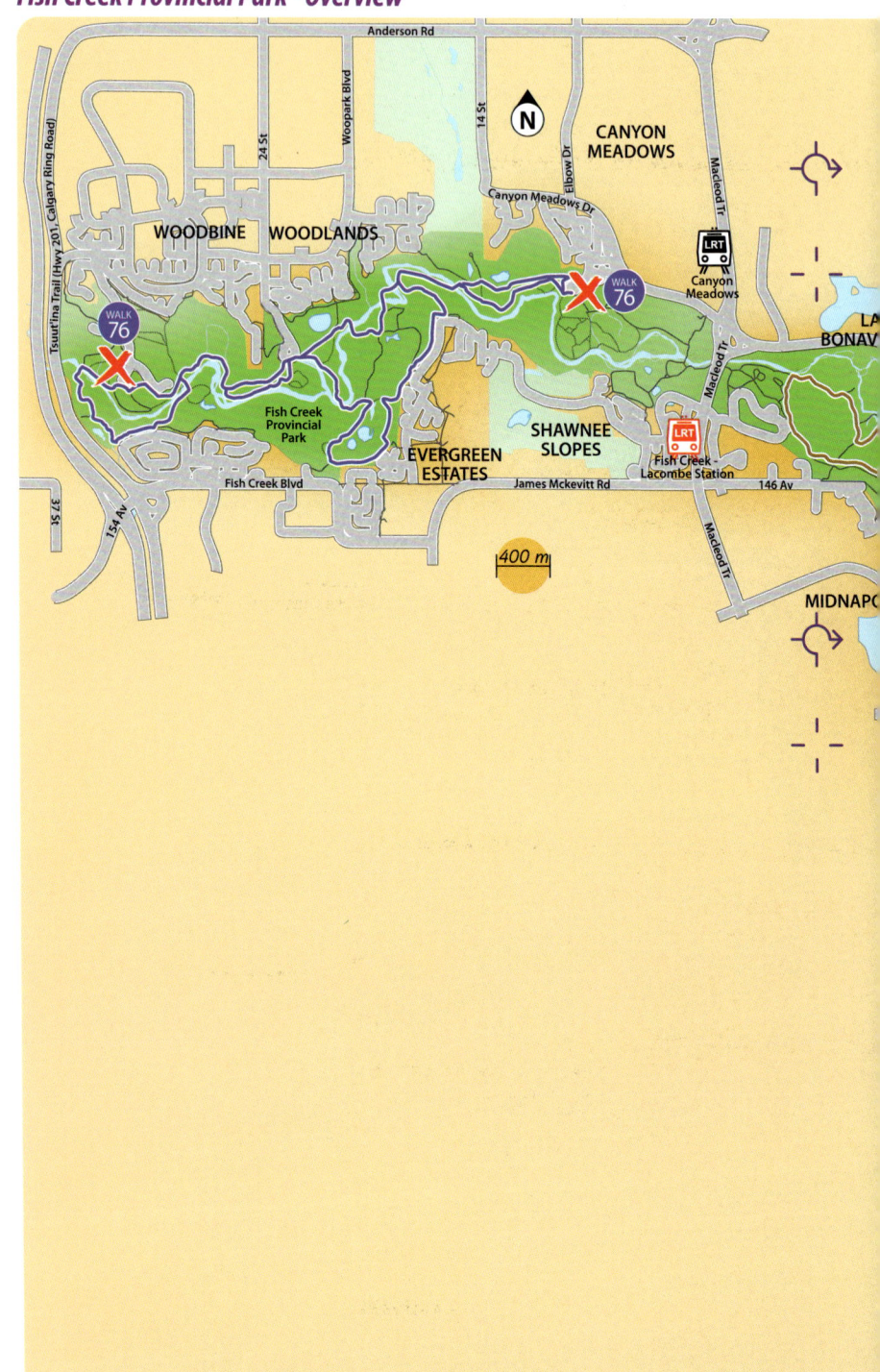

Fish Creek Provincial Park - Overview

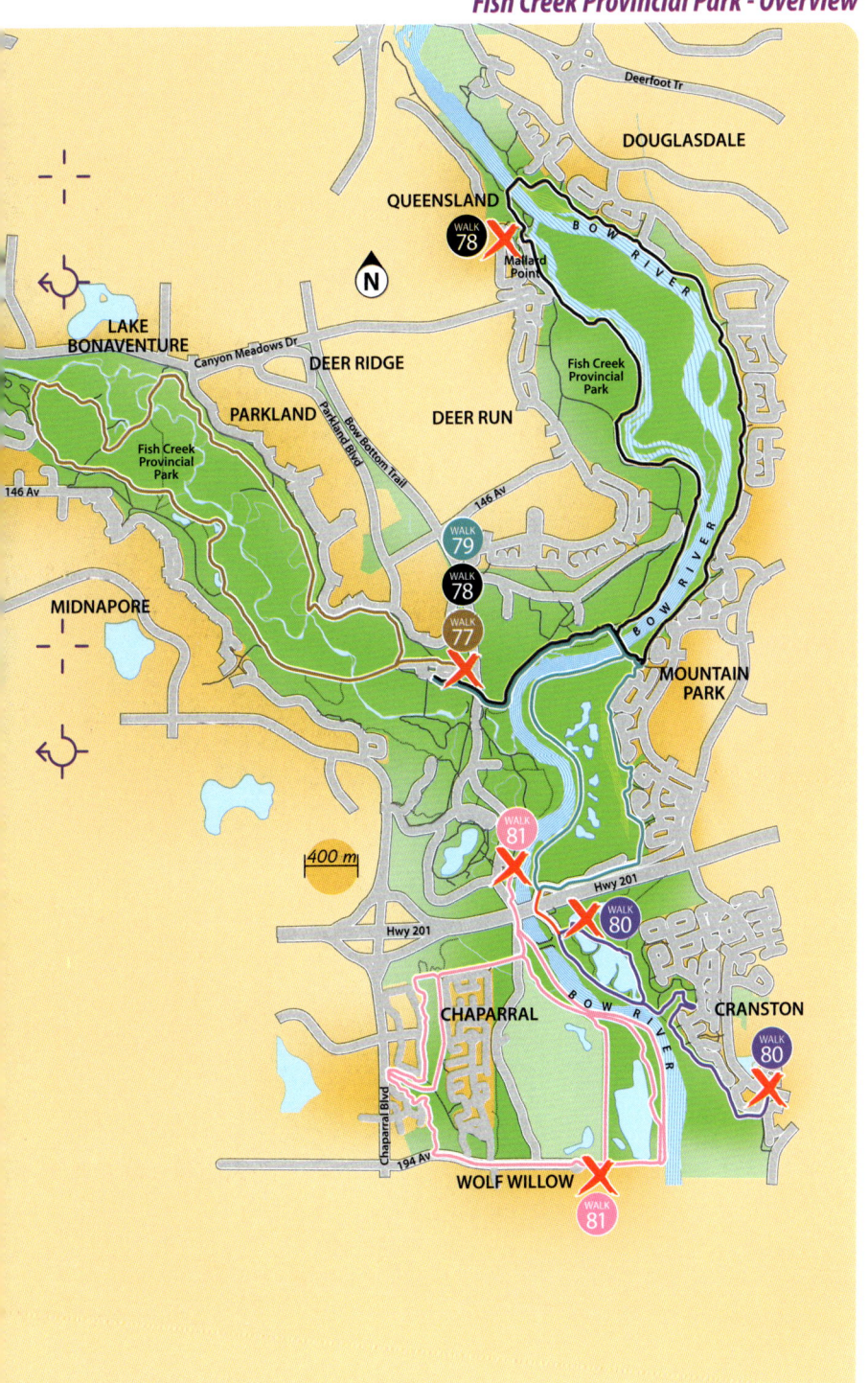

Fish Creek Park West

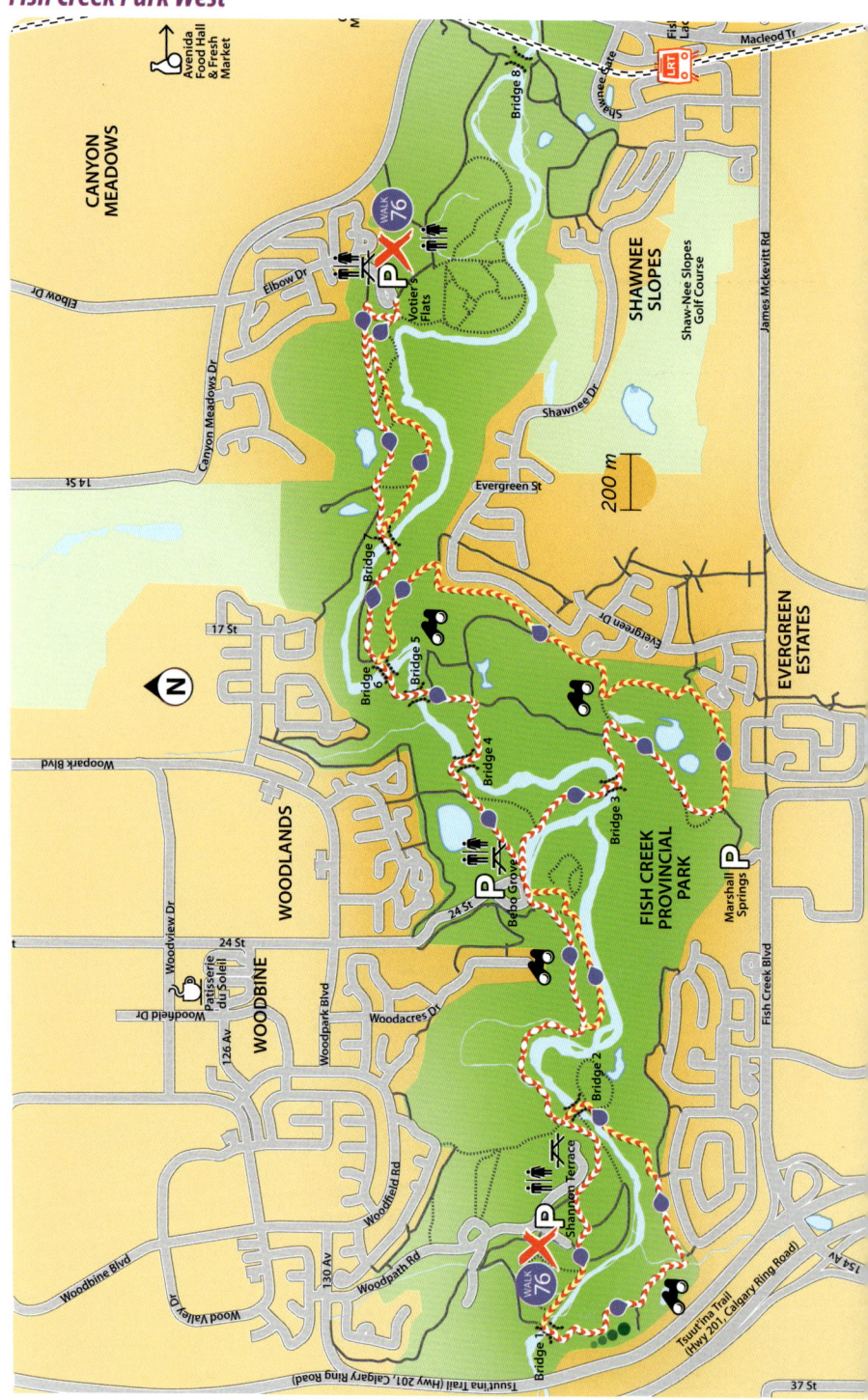

The forested west end is where Walk 76 takes place. It is nicely shaded by a mix of poplar, aspen, and white spruce, is a joy to walk through on a hot summer's day. The sandstone cliffs on the north side of the creek are favourite nesting spots for prairie and peregrine falcons and ravens. The ravens' guttural croak can often be heard high overhead. Bunchberry, purple clematis, kinnikinnick (bearberry), buffaloberry, and red-osier dogwood are just some of the native flowers and shrubs that surround you in the far west end of the park. Just past Shannon Terrace, climb to the community of Everglades and continue on paved paths past significant homes that back onto the park. Descend back into the park and follow the creek trails, listening for the call of wetland birdlife. Past the wetlands, a climb leads to mountain views and a good chance of seeing mule deer in the open grassy areas. As you walk the forested trails, keep your eyes high for a chance sighting of a great horned owl atop the poplars.

Continue east and the terrain changes to grassland with some riparian forest along the creek. Wildflowers are abundant here in the warm months, May through

Pelicans on the Bow River

The American white pelican arrives in Alberta in late April. From the Douglasdale and Mountain Park escarpments, it is easy to identify these birds, one of the world's largest, because of their distinctive, long, flattened bills and brightly coloured, yellow-orange pouches used for feeding. They fill their pouches with young, warm-water fish such as perch, stickleback, northern pike, and lake whitefish. Pelicans also take salamanders, frogs, and a variety of aquatic invertebrates when they are abundant. Pelicans are often seen feeding in the same area as double-crested cormorants. When cormorants dive, they flush fish to the surface, making easy pickings for the pelicans. A group of pelicans may mob and rob the cormorants of their fish finds, too. This aggressive behaviour is necessary for the pelicans to reach their daily consumption goal: 2 kg of food. Young pelicans are fed regurgitated food by their parents. As soon as young chicks can lift their heads, they begin begging by making loud croaking sounds while flapping their wings and weaving their heads back and forth. They bite the base of their parents' bills and pouches to signal that they are hungry. As the chicks get older, they boldly reach into their parents' throats for food, sometimes even farther to extract the gizzard's half-digested contents. The mobbing, persistent harassment by the young, leads the adults to cough up and fly away fast. By late September, the birds head south to the Gulf of Mexico where they winter alongside all the human Canadian snowbirds.

Fish Creek Park, Bow Valley Ranch

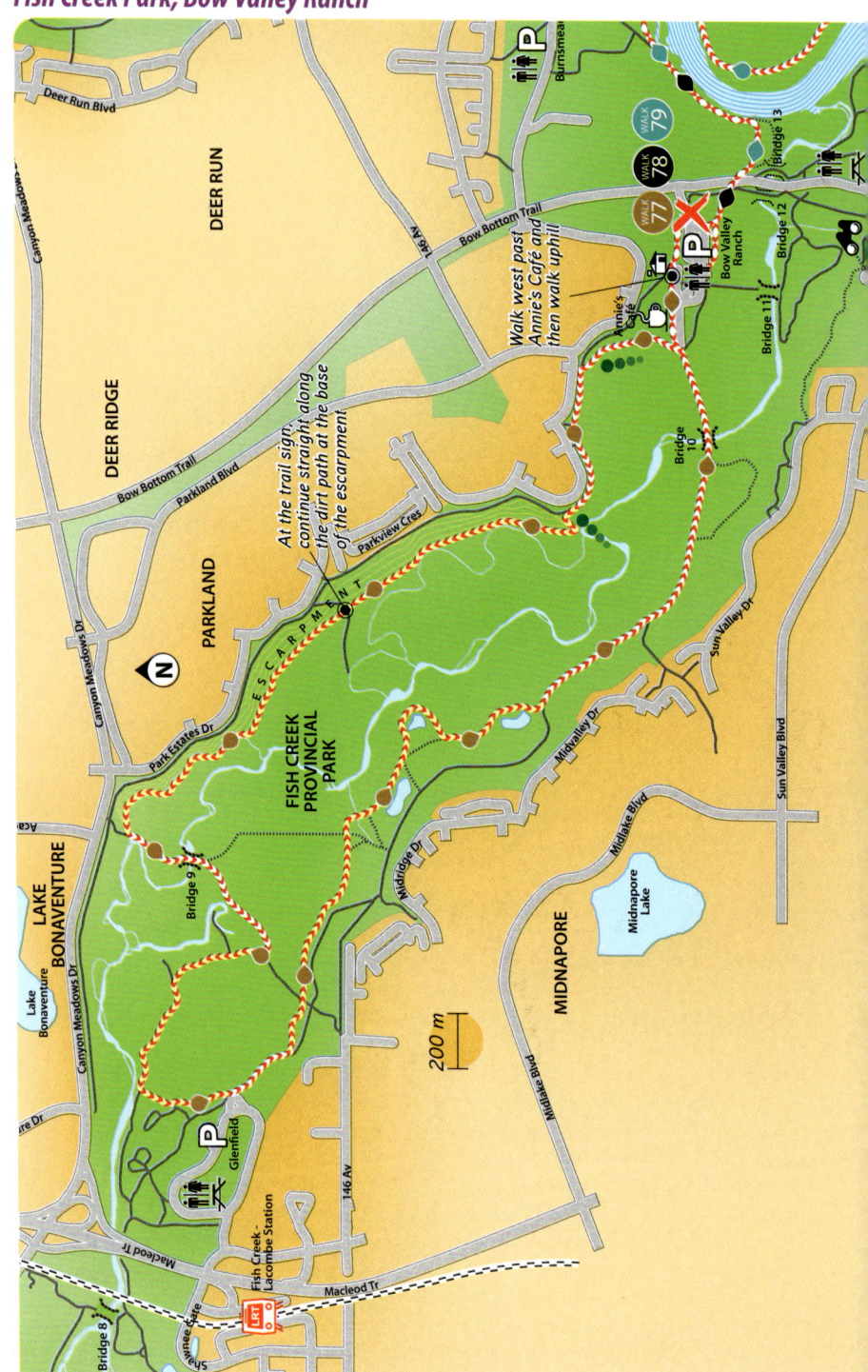

September. Walk 77 leads you past the Artisan Gardens and Annie's café at Bow Valley Ranch. Climb to the community of Parkland and follow the escarpment trail. Soak up the expansive views of the park below and the Rockies beyond before descending back into the park and continuing along the valley bottom.

Pelicans visit the Bow River in the spring and summer, so keep your eyes on the river as you climb the escarpment trail to the community of Douglasdale and Mountain Park on Walks 78 and 79. Both walks have stunning Rockies and downtown Calgary views from the escarpment.

The History of Fish Creek Park

As you walk through the park, you can ponder the changes to the landscape that has happened here over time. Glaciers covered Fish Creek Provincial Park in 13,000 BCE. The glaciers retreated over time, and humans are believed to have first settled in small numbers in the Fish Creek Valley around 6500 BCE. More than 80 archeological sites have been identified throughout the park. The University of Calgary archeological team has uncovered evidence of early buffalo hunts, Indigenous weaponry, campsites, cooking utensils, and other ancient artifacts. At least four locations in the park have been identified as buffalo jumps and kill sites used by hunters between 2500 BCE and 1700 CE. The oldest identifiable artifact found in the park to date is a broken atlatl head, dated around 2500 BCE.

In 1873, John and Adelaide Glenn became the first European settlers in the Fish Creek valley. They set up a small trading post and farm in 1874. The Blackfoot Confederacy signed Treaty No. 7 in 1877. The First Peoples were paid cash and given reserves totaling close to one million acres. In return, they gave up large tracts of land. The federal government purchased places like that of the Glenns as instructional farms. In 1879, Glenn sold his farm to the Dominion Government, and it became Indian Supply Farm #24. The idea was to assist the Blackfoot to adjust to their new way of life. William Roper Hull and John Hull bought Fish Creek Supply Farm in 1892. Experts in the cattle industry, the Hulls had found ranching success through irrigation and hay-stacking efficiencies, using techniques that were copied across Canada. William Roper Hull sold his meat operations and the Bow Valley Ranch to Patrick Burns in 1902. He then moved to Calgary, a two-hour ride away at that time. Starting with nothing, Patrick Burns came to dominate the western Canadian meatpacking and dairy products industries. To Burns, the Bow Valley Ranch was an integral but small part of his empire. Burns bought out all the nearby ranches and farms. He came to own all the land between the Bow Valley Ranch and his packing plant in the southeast part of Calgary on Blackfoot Trail. The Bow Valley Ranch remained in the Burns family until the provincial government bought it in 1972 and opened it as a park in 1975. We are lucky to have such a vast park, one of the largest urban parks in North America, in the heart of the city.

Fish Creek Park and Douglasdale

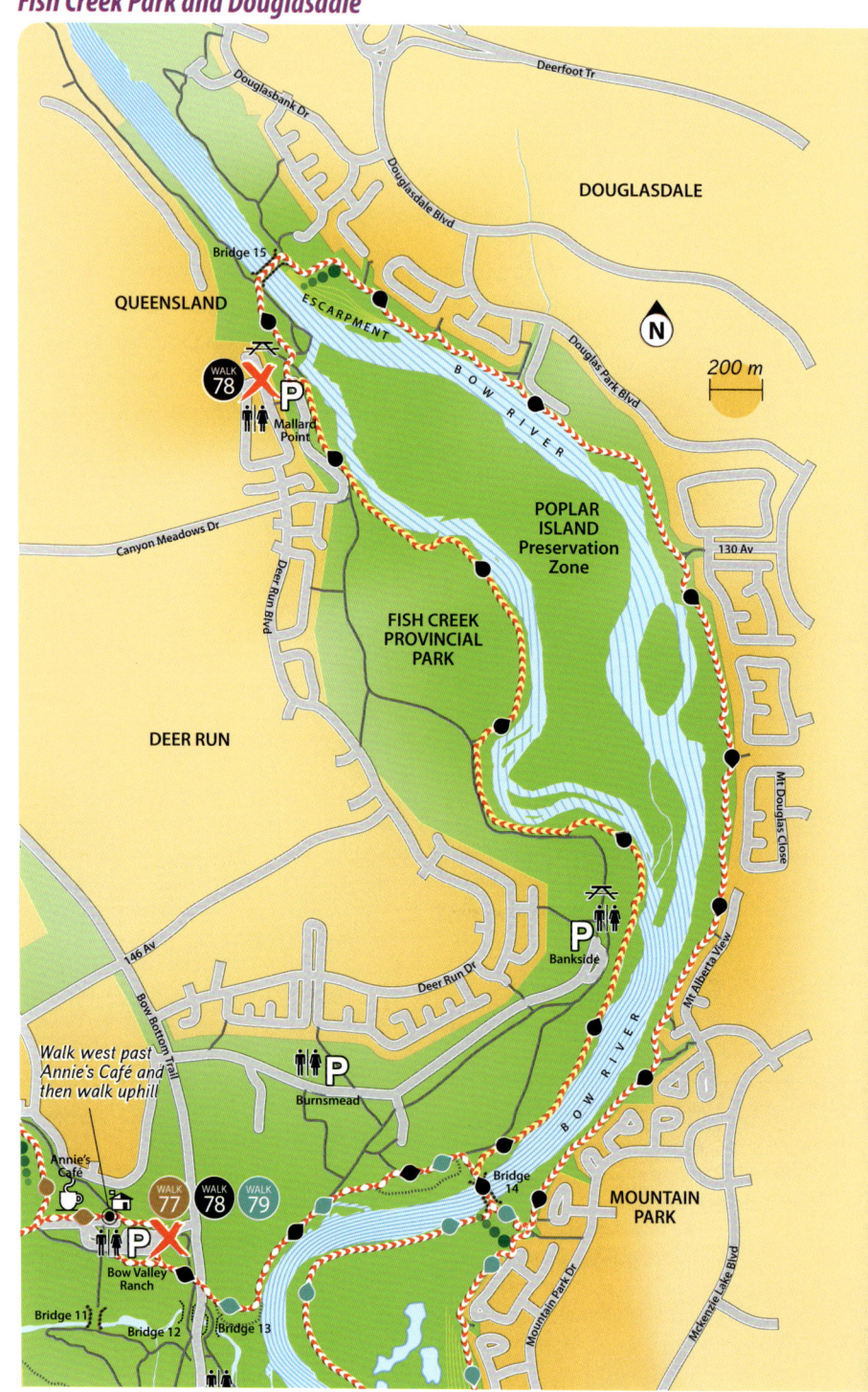

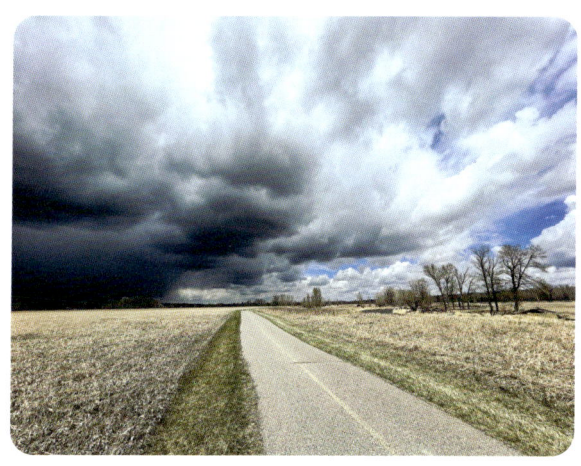

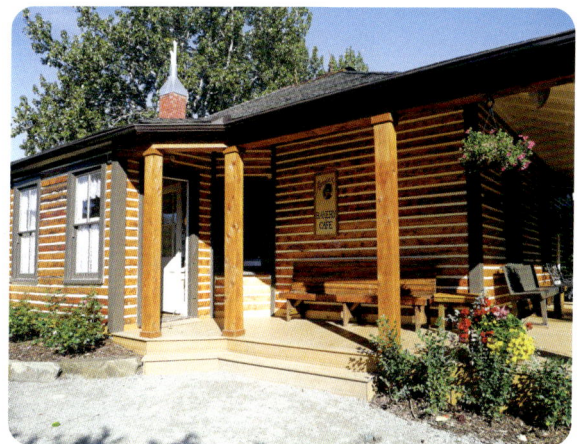

Tasty Pit Stops

Plan to fuel up with made-from-scratch pastries, a big breakfast, or lunch at Patisserie du Soleil in Woodbine. Popular with the locals, this family-run bakery café has a patio for summertime outdoor eating. Swing by the Avenida Market to grab picnic supplies. Choose from the flavours of Mexico, the Caribbean, Bangkok, and El Salvador, to name a few. Annie's Café at Bow Valley Ranch was once part of the Patrick Burns ranching and meat packing empire. Once the foreman's house, this cozy café is named after Annie Bannister, the foreman's wife. Muffins, scones, and cookies tempt post-walk taste buds. Sit on Annie's deck with a lemonade and watch the world go by. Family run Christie's Café in Wolf Willow is the perfect pit stop on Walk 81. Chat with Christie herself as you order up a drink and grab some house made cookies, squares, cinnamon buns, soups or sandwiches. Detour from the Douglasdale escarpment to Lina's for a tasty Italian treat. Follow the pathway alongside 130th Avenue to reach this supermarket café that serves up big breakfasts, lunches, and so many types of pizza, pasta, and paninis. Take it to go or grab a table, Lina's is top-notch deliciousness.

Fish Creek Park, Mountain Park, Rotary Nature Park, Chaparral

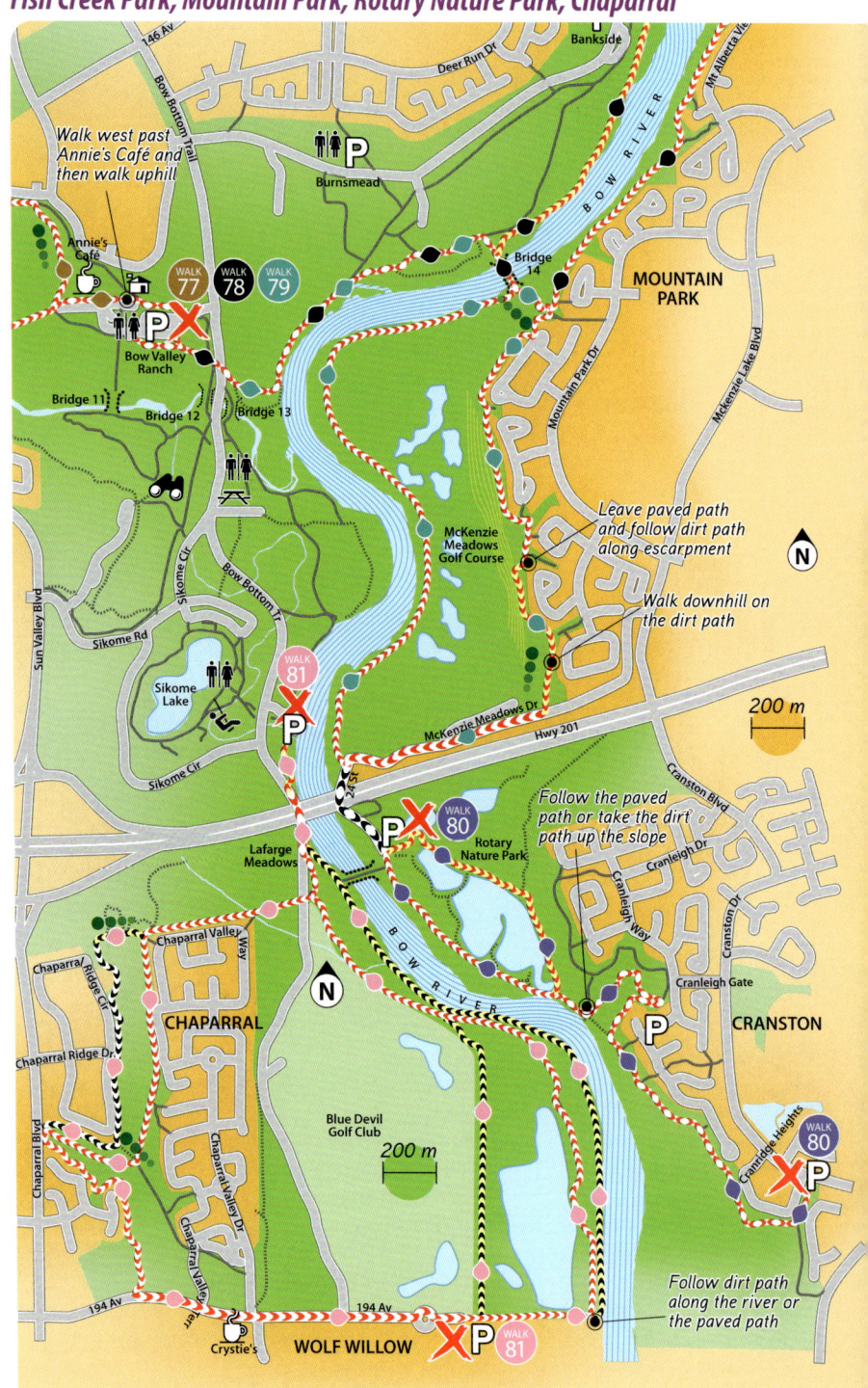

Walk 80 explores Cranston and the Rotary Nature Park wetlands. At one time a gravel pit, the area was reclaimed into its natural state and now hosts 40 acres of wetlands that attract waterfowl and upland birds, making this park the perfect sanctuary for birdwatching. Walk 81 travels through the Lafarge Meadows to big views from Chaparral on the west side of the Bow River.

Enjoy the randomness of nature, the chance sightings of wildlife and disconnect from the city's fast pace. Restore and recharge with a complete wilderness experience in the heart of the city.

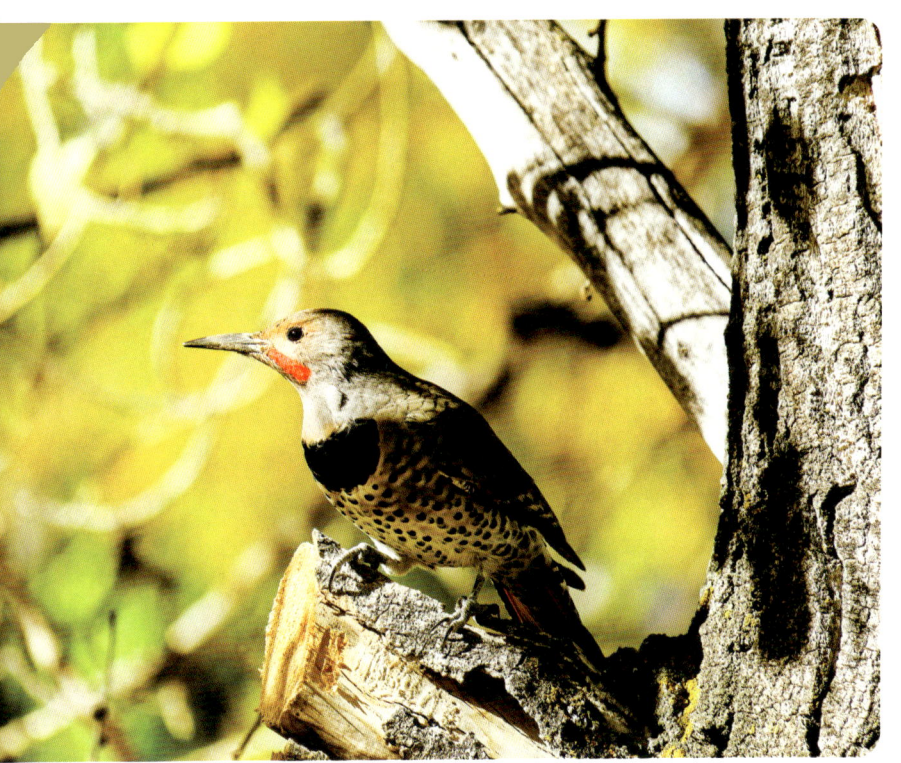

Northern Flicker by Sara Tehranian

Legacy Environmental Reserve

Walk 82   SE

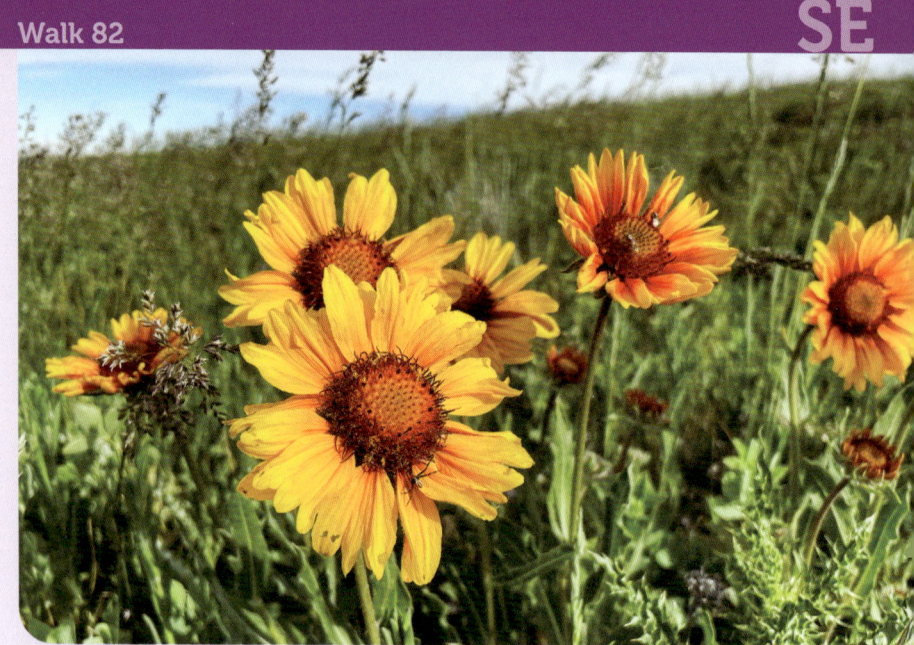

Walk at a Glance:

Wild ravine walkabouts that skirt neighbourhoods are a wonderful surprise. Beginning on paved paths, soak up big views of the Legacy Environmental Reserve, the 300 acre wilderness that follows West Creek. The walk soon follows a forested path and descends to the creek.

Dogs love the big open of these ravines and both kids and dogs will have fun following treed trails that dip and climb. Meander along the creek before climbing back to the top of the escarpment to explore the slopes.

This is the perfect spot for a picnic lunch and to watch the sky for ravens soaring overhead. Ravens are mountain and northern-forest birds, so it is unique for

Details

Categories: Dog, Nature, Hilly, Vistas, River, Birds

Start: near All Saints High School, Legacy Village Way SE

Facilities: Grocery store and other services nearby

Distance & Difficulty

6.5 km (hills, sidewalks, paved paths and single-track trails)

Detours, Destinations & Suggestions

West Creek is narrow and small however the current can be strong in the spring and the water levels can be high enough to soak your feet, well into the fall

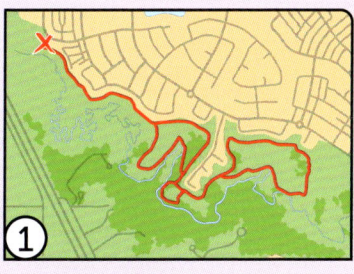

them to nest in the parkland and prairies. Members of the corvid family, scientists continue to be astounded by just how clever these avian Einsteins prove to be. Cliffs are their favourite nesting spots and just north of Legacy in the west end of Fish Creek Park there are the perfect corvid cliff condos. Distinguishing between ravens or crows can be challenging. Ravens are usually larger and with heavier bills than crows have, and they soar overhead while crows flap their wings steadily as they fly. Smart scavengers, ravens will eat anything. They talk to each other with "rawks" and "tocks," but it is the guttural "croak" made by the raven that gives it away. Ravens have full-blown cognitive skills and before reaching full maturity. Problem-solving crows perform similarly to

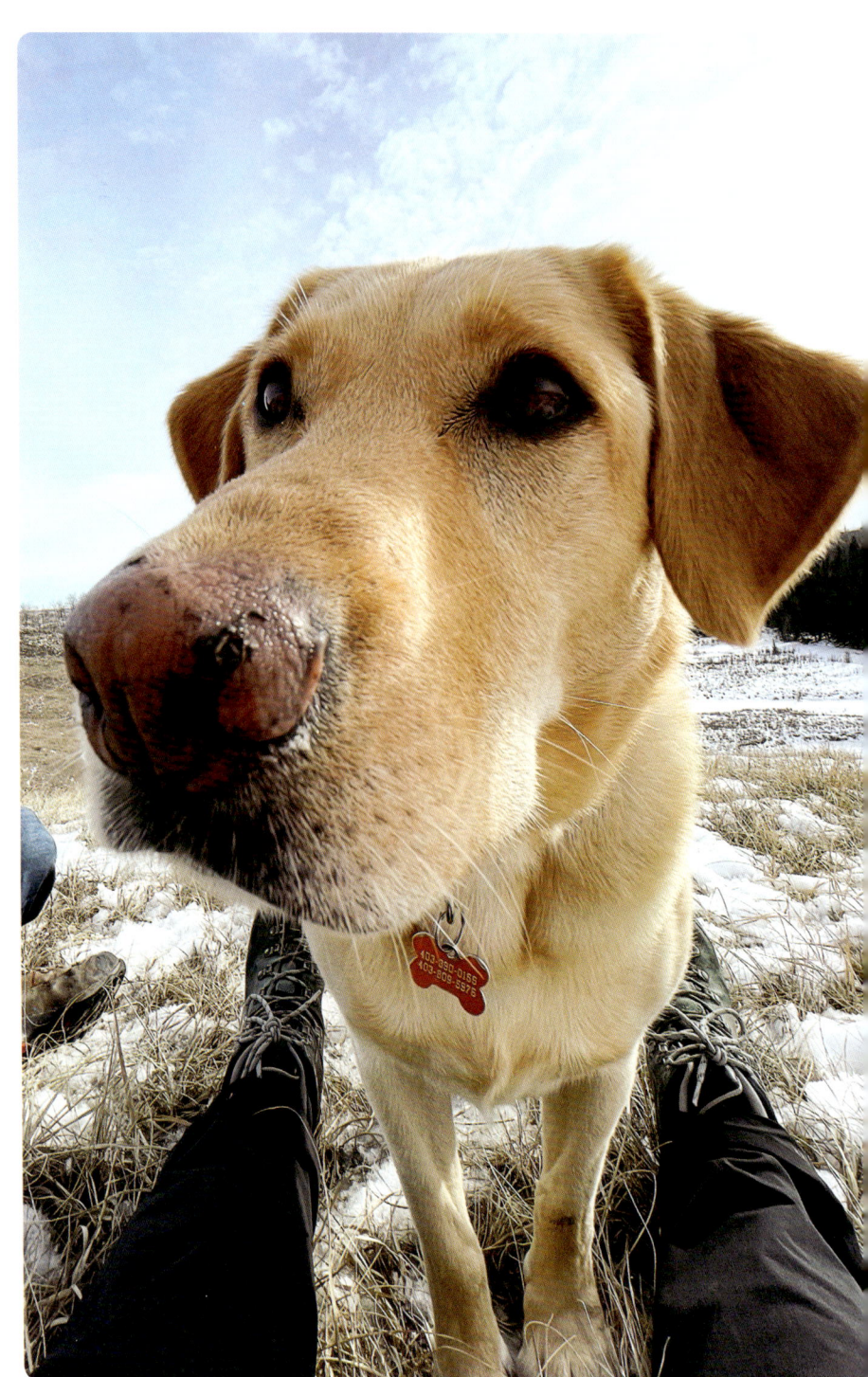

children under seven years of age. They plan, have great memories and they use tools. They also hold grudges so don't tick them off as they will tell their friends what you look like, and you will be dive bombed for years.

Walk the slopes, do some hill training or simply descend to the creek and enjoy the calm. Keep an eye out for deer and then spot the deer differences. Mule deer have large ears rimmed with black and tails that are white with a black tip. They travel in small bands of does, yearlings, and fawns; the bucks travel alone. White-tailed deer have brown tails. When alarmed they lift their tails to expose the white underside and a white rump patch. They wave this furry flag to warn their friends of possible danger. Being quite solitary and shy, white-tailed does are usually alone or with their offspring from that year.

Climb out of the valley and enjoy the dips and climbs on the return route or stick the paved path for an easy stroll.

Pole It for Stability!

Avoid knee injuries and get an upper body workout by hiking with two poles on hilly walks. Two poles are better than one because four points of contact make you more stable than three. It is important to adjust pole length to suit the terrain. When hanging onto the handle, your forearm should be parallel to the ground. That means you must shorten the pole on the climb and lengthen it on descent. As you press the poles down and away behind you, you'll feel your abdominal, back, and arm muscles getting a workout. Poles not only increase your calorie burn and offer downhill stability, but they also significantly reduce the lower-body impact of hiking. Your knees will thank you.

Legacy Environmental Reserve

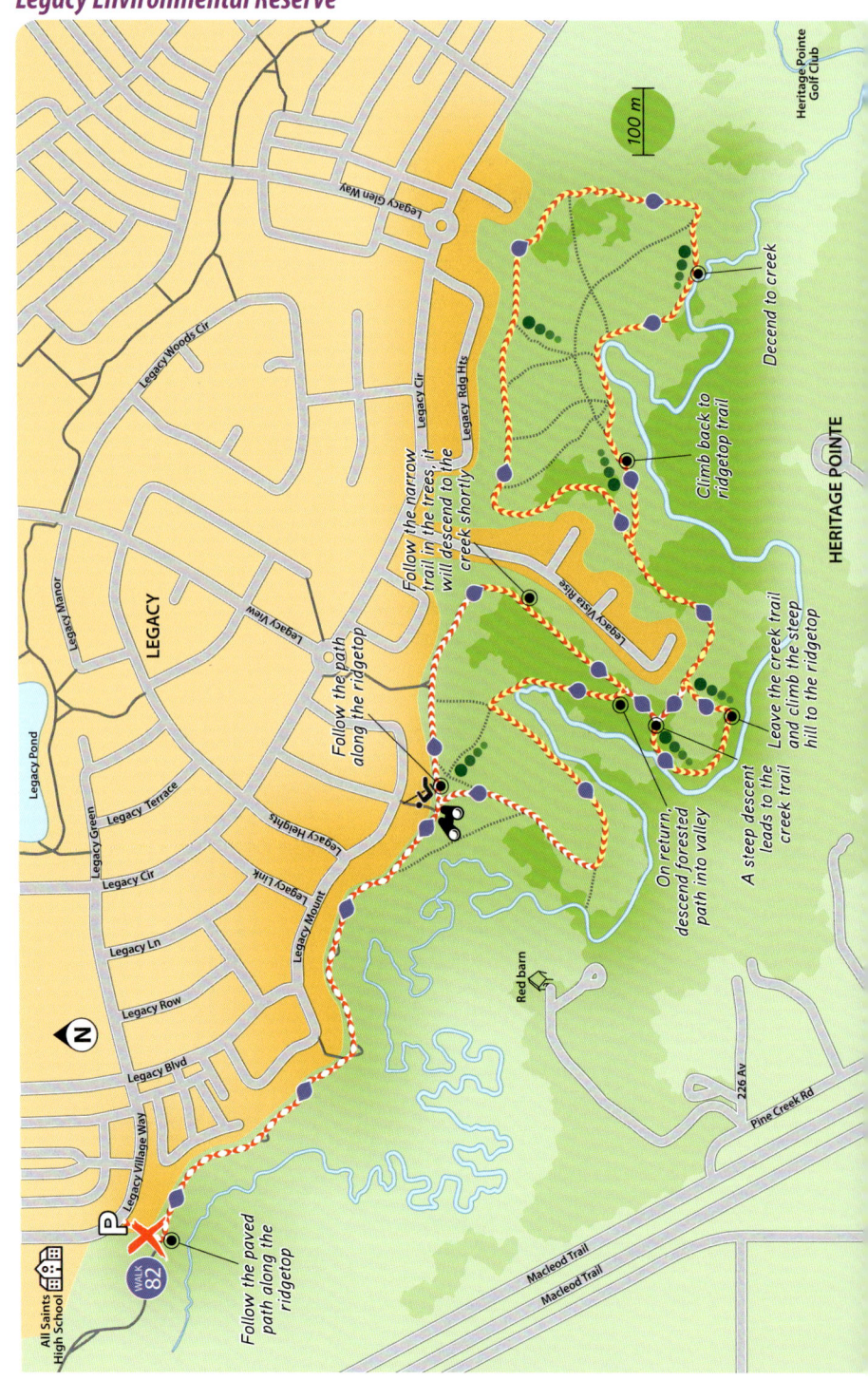

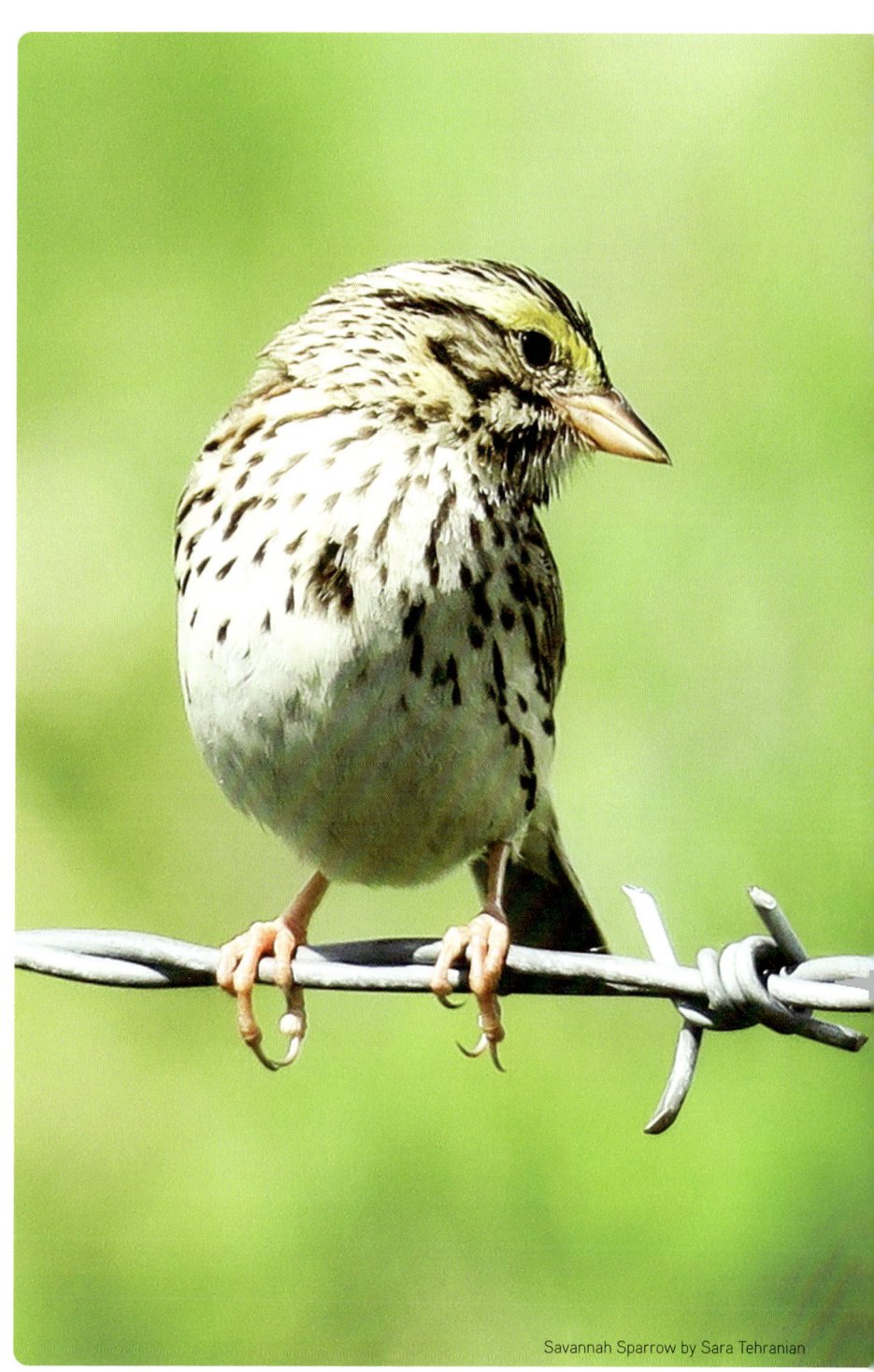
Savannah Sparrow by Sara Tehranian

Sue Higgins, Carburn, and Beaverdam Flats Parks, Lynnwood, Ogden

Walks 83 and 84

SE

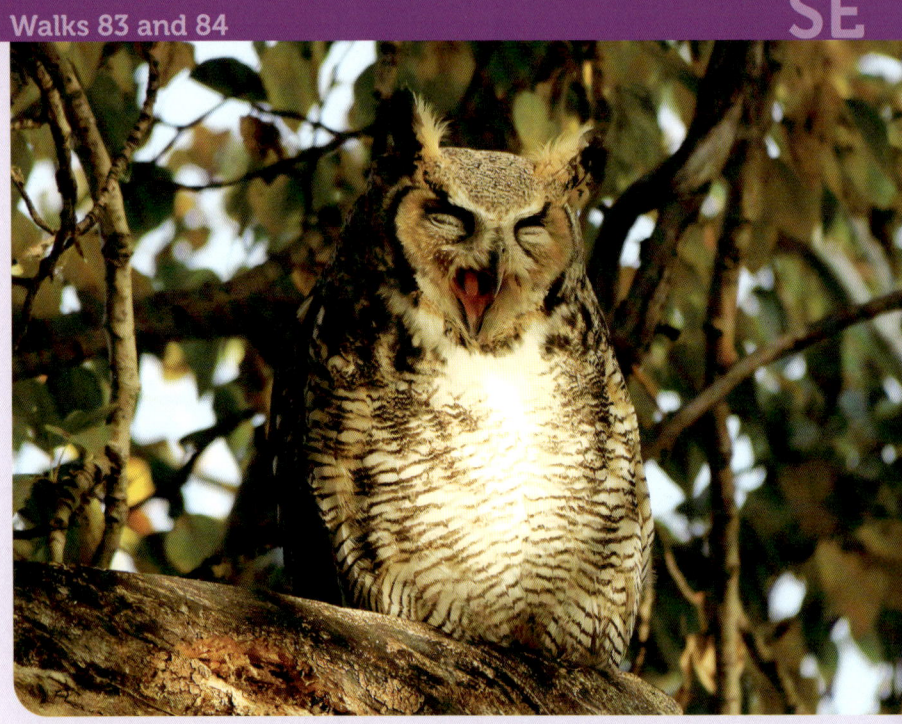

Great Horned Owl by Sara Tehranian

Walks at a Glance:

Families looking for a post-dinner stroll to relax, or to allow the kids to burn off some energy, will enjoy a visit to Carburn Park. This trek is perfect for all ages with its water features, wildlife, and mostly paved pathways. And when the trees are full, this extensive suburban green space becomes a refreshing nature getaway.

Balsam poplars offer shade while shrubs like saskatoon, choke cherry, American silverberry, and Canada buffaloberry provide textures and colours along the trail. Pelicans, double-breasted cormorants, and bald eagles all frequent this area, and many deer call the park home.

Details

Categories: Café, Dog, Nature, Neighbourhood & Parks, Hilly, Stroller, Historic, Vistas, River, Birds

Start: Walk 83: Carburn Park, 67 Riverview Drive SE or Sue Higgins, end of Southland Drive SE; Walk 84: Millican Ogden Community Association, 2110 69 Avenue SE

LRT: Future Green Line Station

Facilities: Bathrooms at Sue Higgins and Carburn Park

Distance & Difficulty

Walk 83: Sue Higgins, Carburn, and Beaverdam Flats Parks: Carburn Park start: 8.5 km; Sue Higgins Park start: 10.5 km (paved and gravel paths, hills)

Walk 84: Ogden- Lynnwood loop: 7.5 km (paved paths, sidewalks, and stairs)

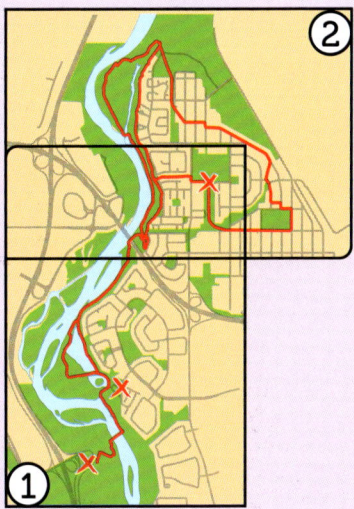

Highlights, Detours & Destinations

There is a skating loop and firepits on the lake at Carburn Park in the winter. Birdlife is abundant on these walks. Check out www.naturecalgary.com to discover Calgary's best and most unique birding hotspots with maps and bird checklists in English, Spanish, Hindi, French

Walk 83 follows the paved Bow River Pathway from Sue Higgins Park through Carburn Park, under Glenmore Trail, and up the escarpment to Lynnwood and views of the Rocky Mountains, the downtown core, and industrial Calgary. The southeast of many cities tends to be where industry thrives, and Calgary is no different. In fact, just north of Beaverdam Flats Park along the Bow River Pathway lies Old Refinery Park, a former Imperial Oil Refinery location that has been reclaimed for use as a park. The two walks meet at this point. Walk 83 descends along a narrow pathway through prairie

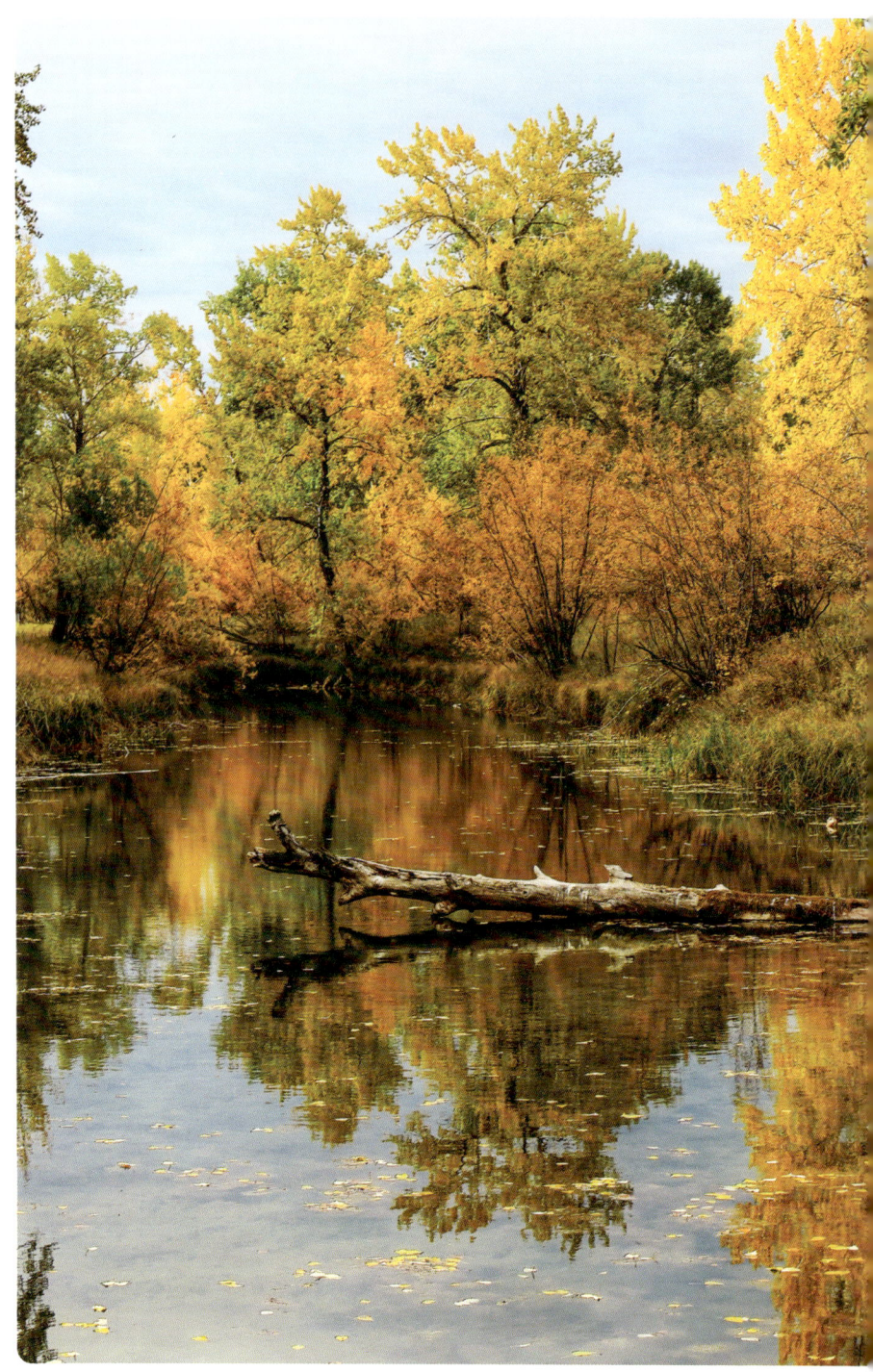

Carburn Park by Sara Tehranian

grasses to Beaverdam Flats Park while Walk 84 stays high and explores the neighbourhoods of Lynnwood and Millican Ogden, one of Calgary's oldest communities. Named after the former Vice President of the Canadian Pacific Railway, it is arguable Calgary would not exist had it not been for the CPR, the Ogden Locomotive Shops, and the founding of the town of Ogden.

End your walk in Ogden or if you have just got your walking pace and want to keep going, follow the Bow River Pathway all the way to Fish Creek Park to the south or go north to Inglewood and beyond.

Workaholic Beavers

In Carburn and Beaverdam Flats Parks you'll see beaver dams in the streams and many fallen trees along the stream banks. And if the trail you want to walk on is covered by water, you might want to blame a beaver. Beavers use the trees to build dams; they eat the bark, leaves, and twigs. Beavers are bit driven. For instance, they are attracted to the sound of running water. Play the sound of running water on a speaker close to a beaver and watch the building frenzy that erupts as she covers the speaker until the sound is muted. Do beavers ever stop building? They do in the short term, like in the winter, but not in the long term. Their food eventually runs out and they must dismantle the dam, move on, and start from scratch.

Sue Higgins, Carburn, and Beaverdam Flats Parks, Lynnwood, Ogden

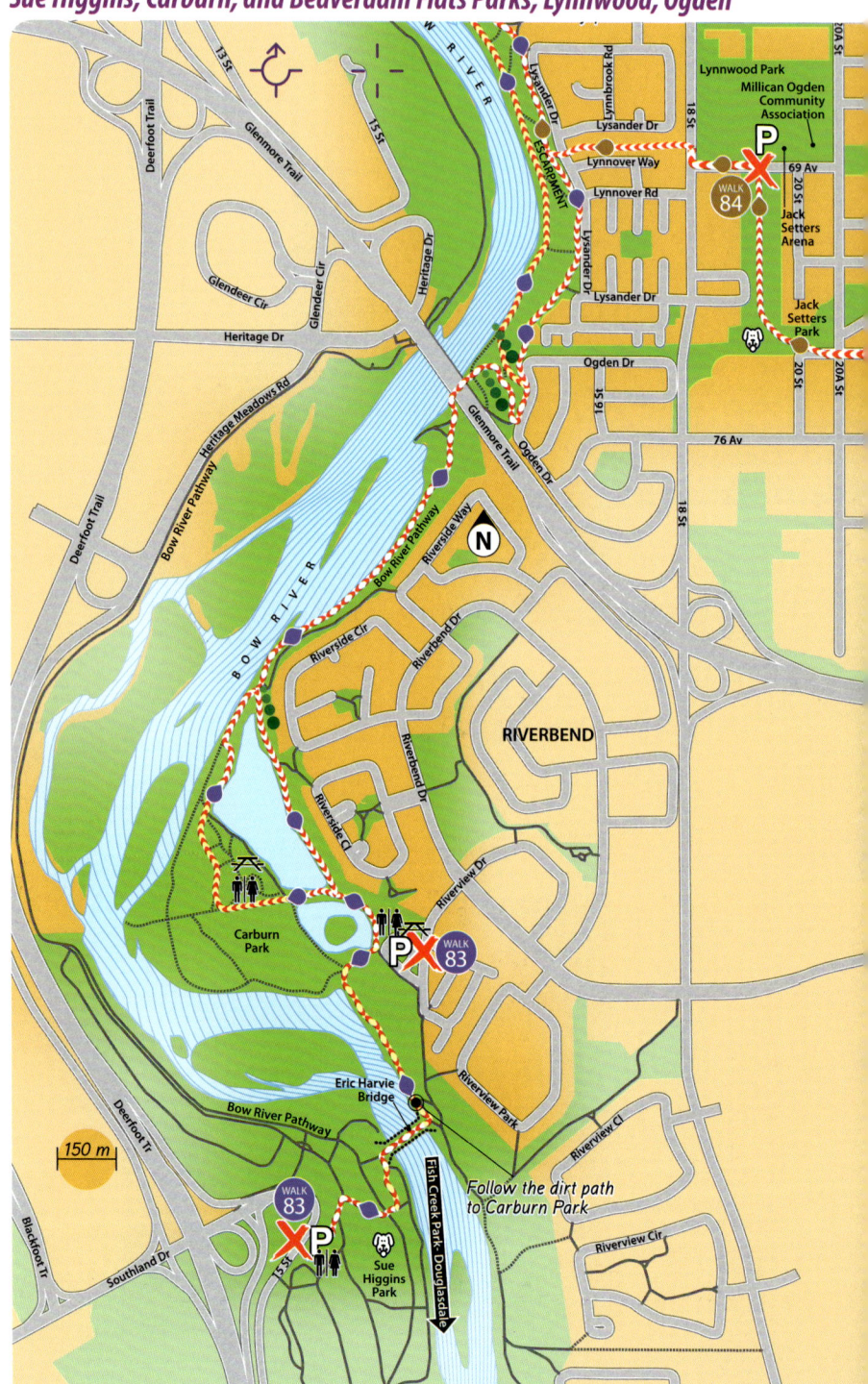

Sue Higgins, Carburn, and Beaverdam Flats Parks, Lynnwood, Ogden

Tasty Pit Stops

Brian's Café is a new addition to Ogden. Situated beside George Moss Park in the Mustard Seed, Brian's Café has a goal of becoming a community hub where people from all walks of life can come together and enjoy great coffee, delicious pastries, and meaningful connections. The Italian Centre is one of my favourite Calgary shopping and eating experiences. Like stepping into Italy, the produce, meats and cheeses are not only varied and fantastic but so reasonably priced. You'll find BC produce when in season, parmesan by the kilogram (priced at wholesale for 1 kg!) and products from around the globe. The café hosts a pup friendly patio and a popular indoor area where you can enjoy pizzas, sandwiches and so many decadent desserts. And the cappuccino is authentically Italian! Such a pleasant place to browse and then enjoy a pastry with friends.

Location:
Brian's Café: 74 Avenue and 23 Street SE (open weekdays, 7 am – noon)
The Italian Centre: 9919 Fairmount Dr SE Calgary, AB

The Italian Centre

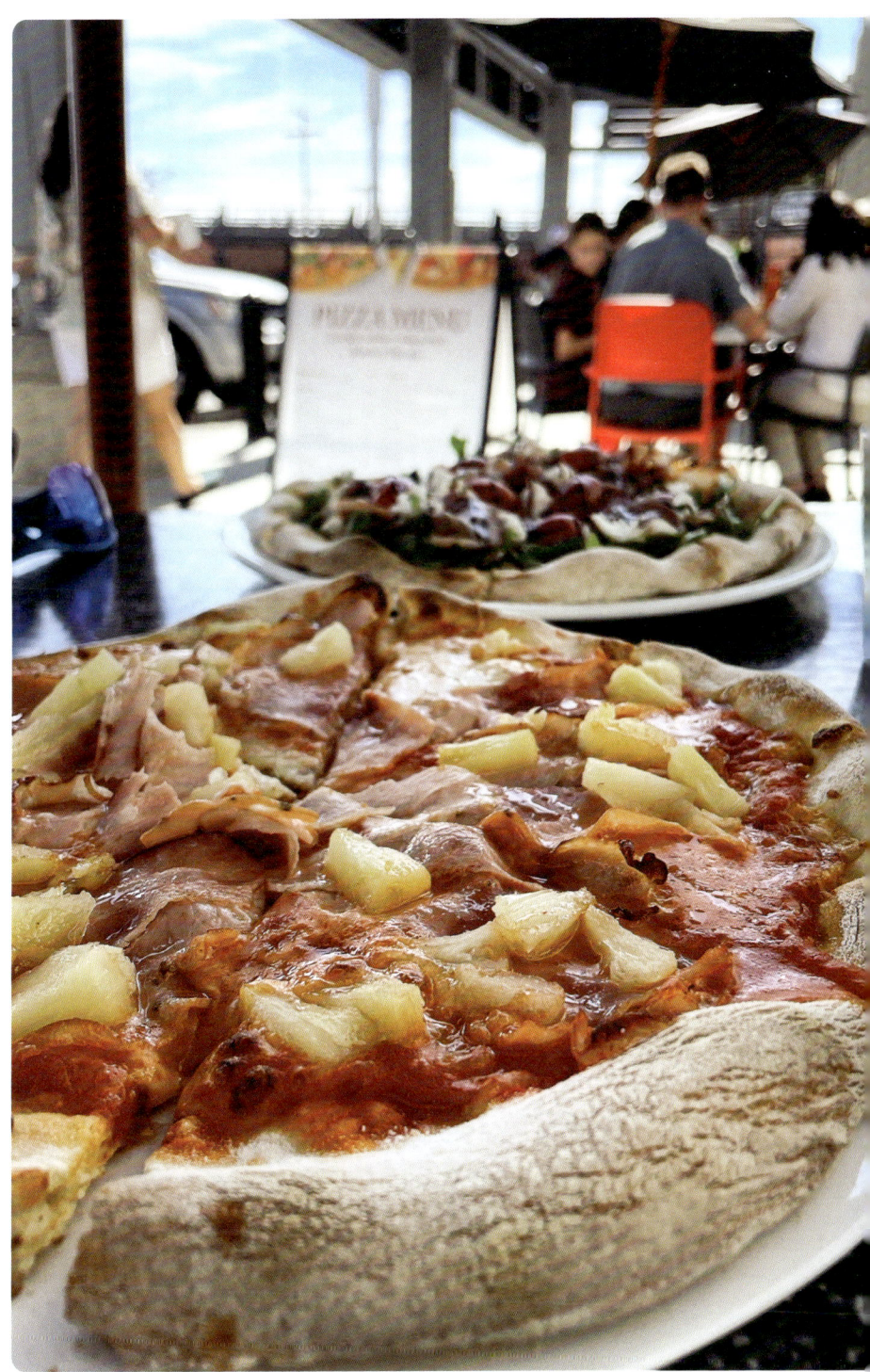

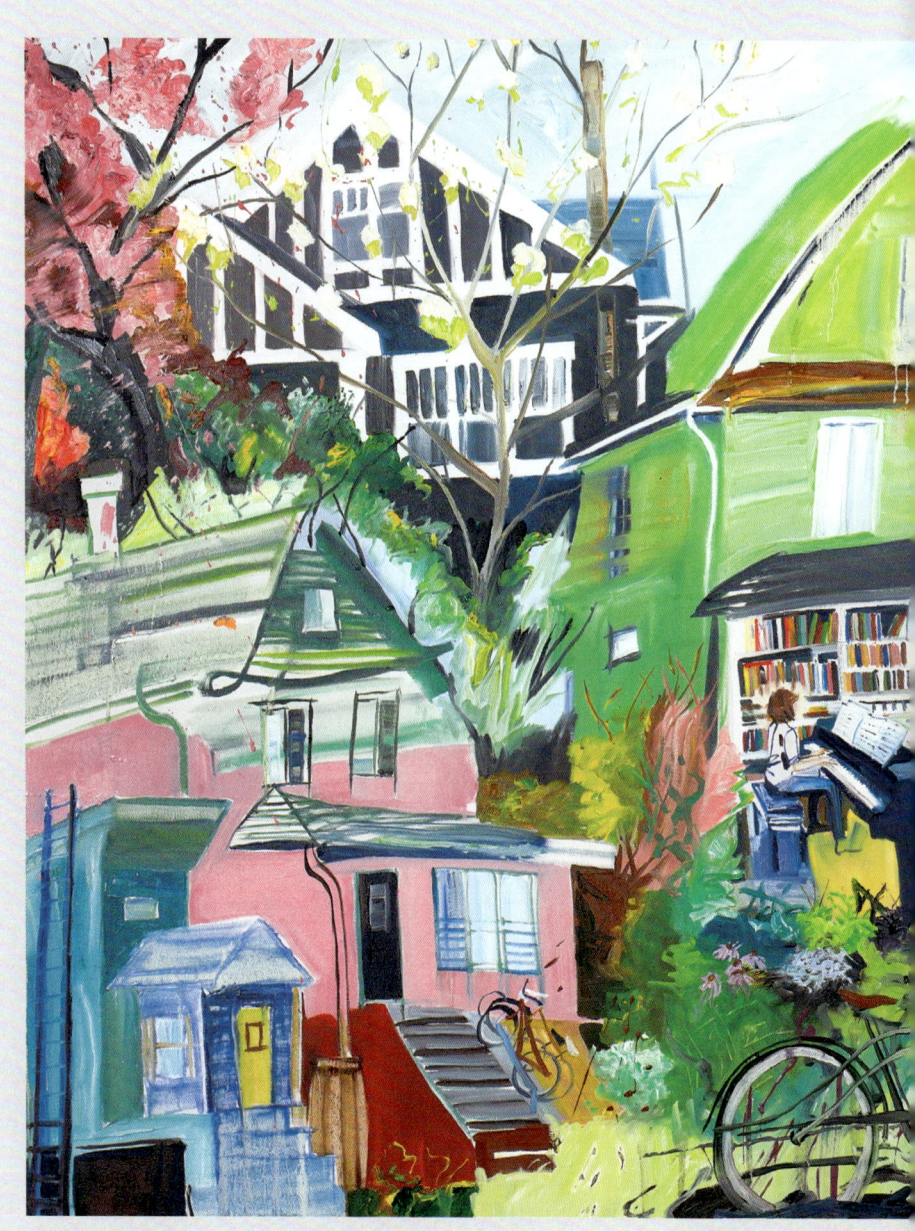

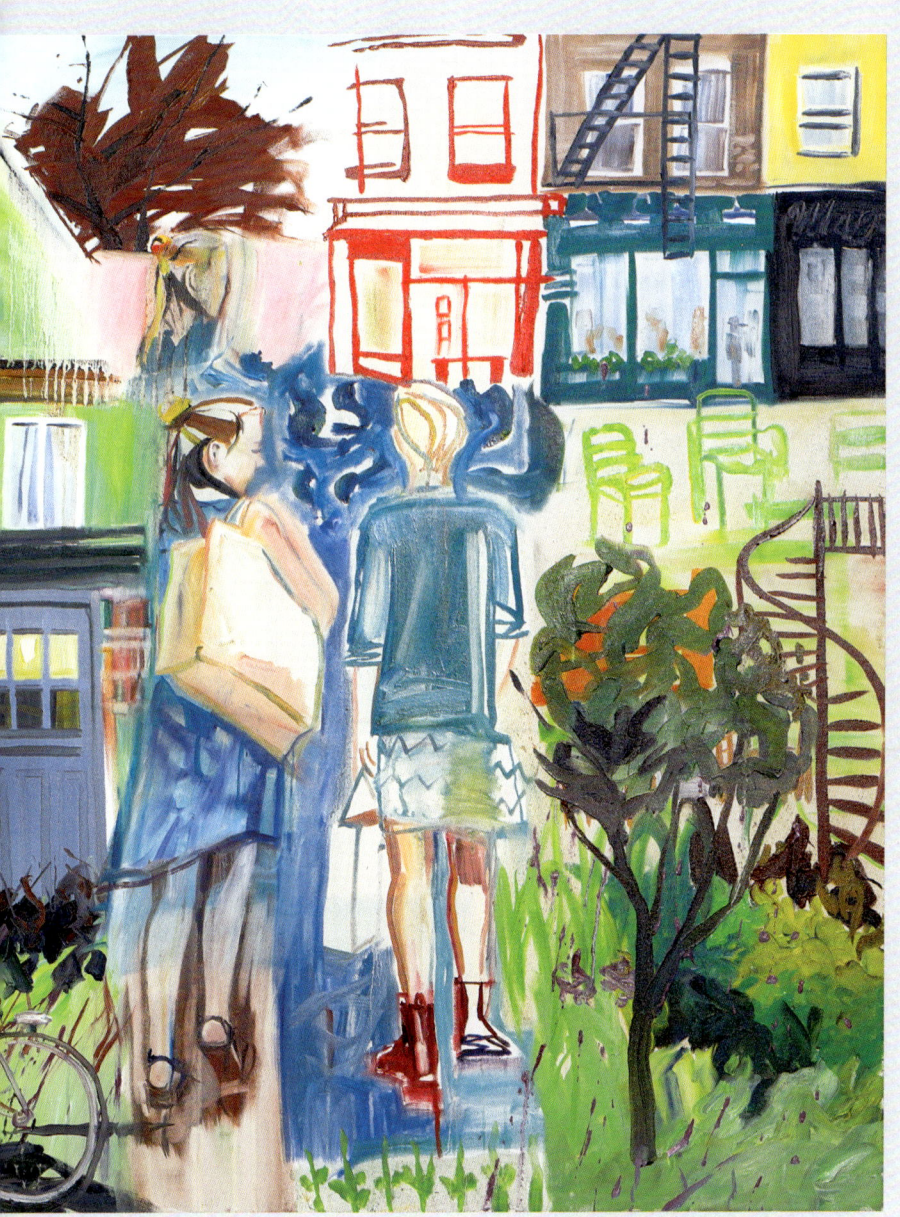

Urban Garden Interlude, Urban Garden Series by Jill Thomson

Elliston Park, International Avenue, Forest Lawn, Southview, Dover, Irrigation Canal Pathway

Walks 85-89

SE

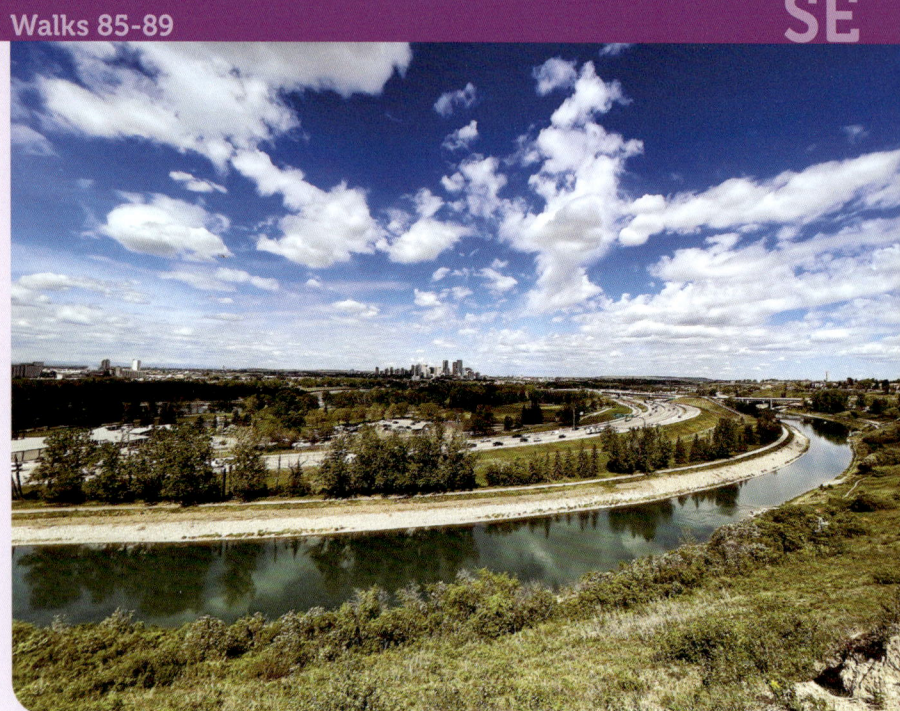

Walks at a Glance:

Impressive Rocky Mountain, Bow River and downtown views are highlights in all these southeast walkabouts. Walk 85 and 86 begins on the paved path overlooking the canal. Drop down to the canal path on Walk 85 or connect to neighbourhoods of Southview and Dover on Walk 86.

Named after Mary Dover, a historic alderman and environmentalist, the community was developed in 1970. Dover has a unique kid friendly design where front yards flow into shared tree-canopied green space and the back lanes serve as the streets. Combine these two routes for a longer 7 km walk.

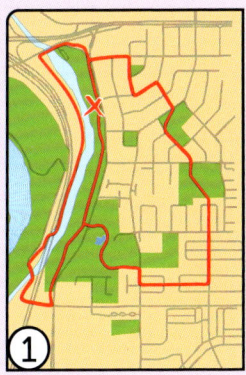
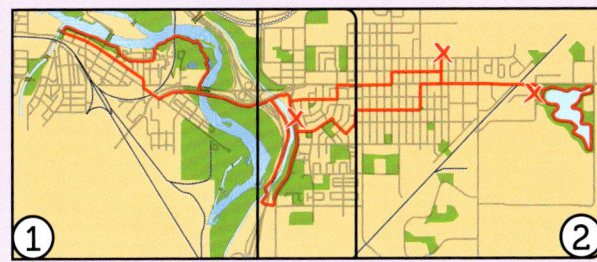

Southview, Dover, Irrigation Canal Pathway

Elliston Park, International Avenue, Forest Lawn, Inglewood

Details

Categories: LRT, Café, Dog, Nature, Neighbourhood & Parks, People watch & shop, Hilly, Stroller, Historic, Vistas, River, Birds

Start: Walks 85, 86, 89: 26th Street and 22nd Avenue, SE.
Walk 87: Elliston Park: 17th Avenue and 60th Street SE.
Walk 88: Forest Lawn Library, 4808 8 Avenue SE

LRT: Max Bell or Zoo Stations

Facilities: Walk 87: Elliston Park has seasonal bathrooms, open mid-May to mid-October. Walk 88: Bathrooms at Forest Lawn Library. Walks 85-89: There are many shops and restaurants along 17th Avenue SE.

Distance & Difficulty

Walk 85: Southview - Irrigation Canal: 3 km (sidewalks, paved and single-track paths, one hill)

Walk 86: Southview- Dover: 4 km (Sidewalks, paved paths)

Walk 87: Elliston Park: 3.5 km

Walk 88: Forest Lawn- International Avenue- Southview: 7 km

Walk 89: Southview - Inglewood: 8 km

Detours, Destinations & Suggestions

Valleyview Park in Southview is a great spot with kids. Enjoy the pond, playground and spray park in the summer. Elliston Park is a birding hotspot. Check out www.naturecalgary.for maps and bird checklists in English, Spanish, Hindi, French. Globalfest, an international fireworks festival, takes over Elliston Park during the last half of August. www.globalfest.ca

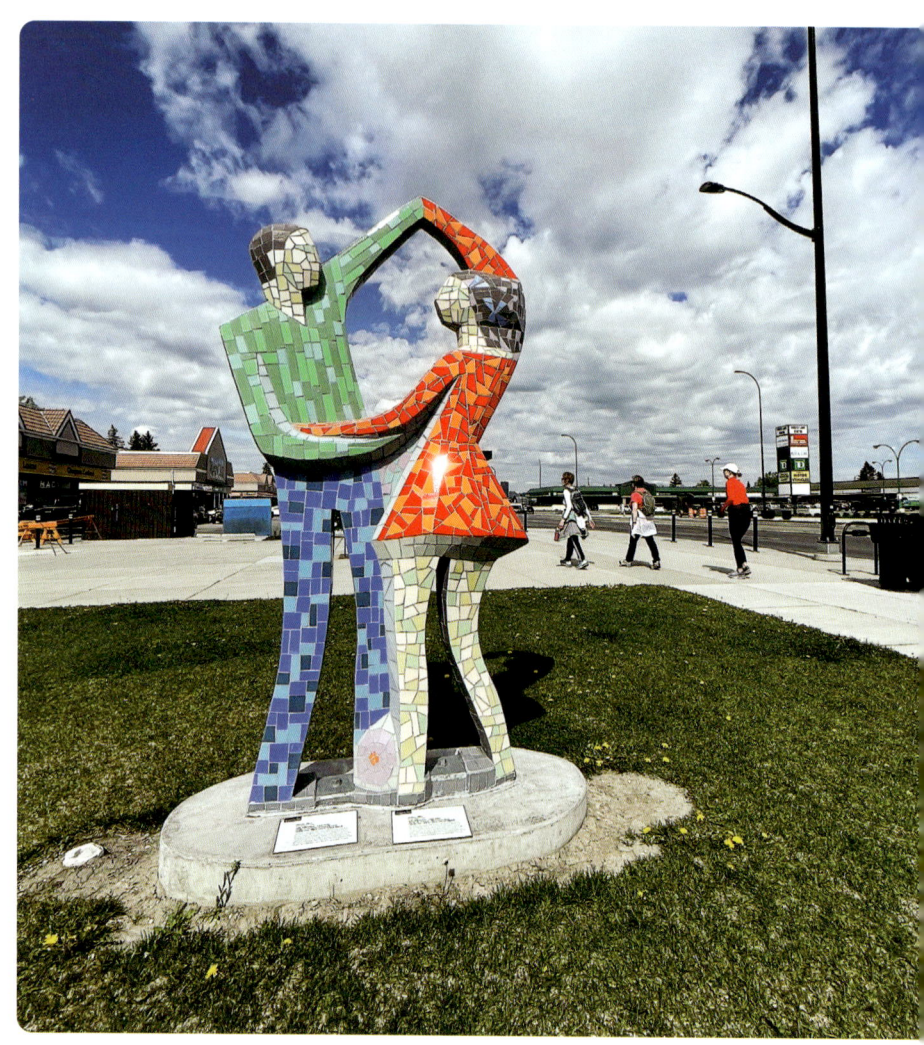

Walk 87 explores Elliston Park, a small park that is a birding hotspot where 175 species of birds have been spotted. This route allows visitors to stretch their legs after a nice meal or a shopping spree along International Avenue. Rolling hills surround Elliston's lake, and trees and shrubs have been planted on hillsides. The route circumnavigates the lake, and there are lots of dirt path detours for those who like to explore.

Connect to Walk 88 by walking west along 17 Avenue into Forest Lawn. Follow a mix of paved paths and side streets while walking towards International Avenue, Calgary's most diverse shopping and eating area. Grab some picnic supplies and walk to the escarpment to soak up big views while enjoying your snacks or connect to Walk 89 and keep walking. You'll pass by Journey to Freedom Park, a monument to honour the Vietnamese Boat People who lost their lives escaping Vietnam after it fell to the communists in 1975. Just after the monument, the path leads over Deerfoot Trail and into Inglewood. Travel down 9 Avenue if you need a coffee or some shopping at local shops or stick the route through the neighbourhood to enjoy the homes and gardens. Inglewood's flood plain soil and slighter warmer weather means the flowers start earlier and last longer. Loop back along the Bow River Pathway and check out the Harvie passage white water park on the river before connecting back to your starting point.

Southview, Dover, Irrigation Canal Pathway

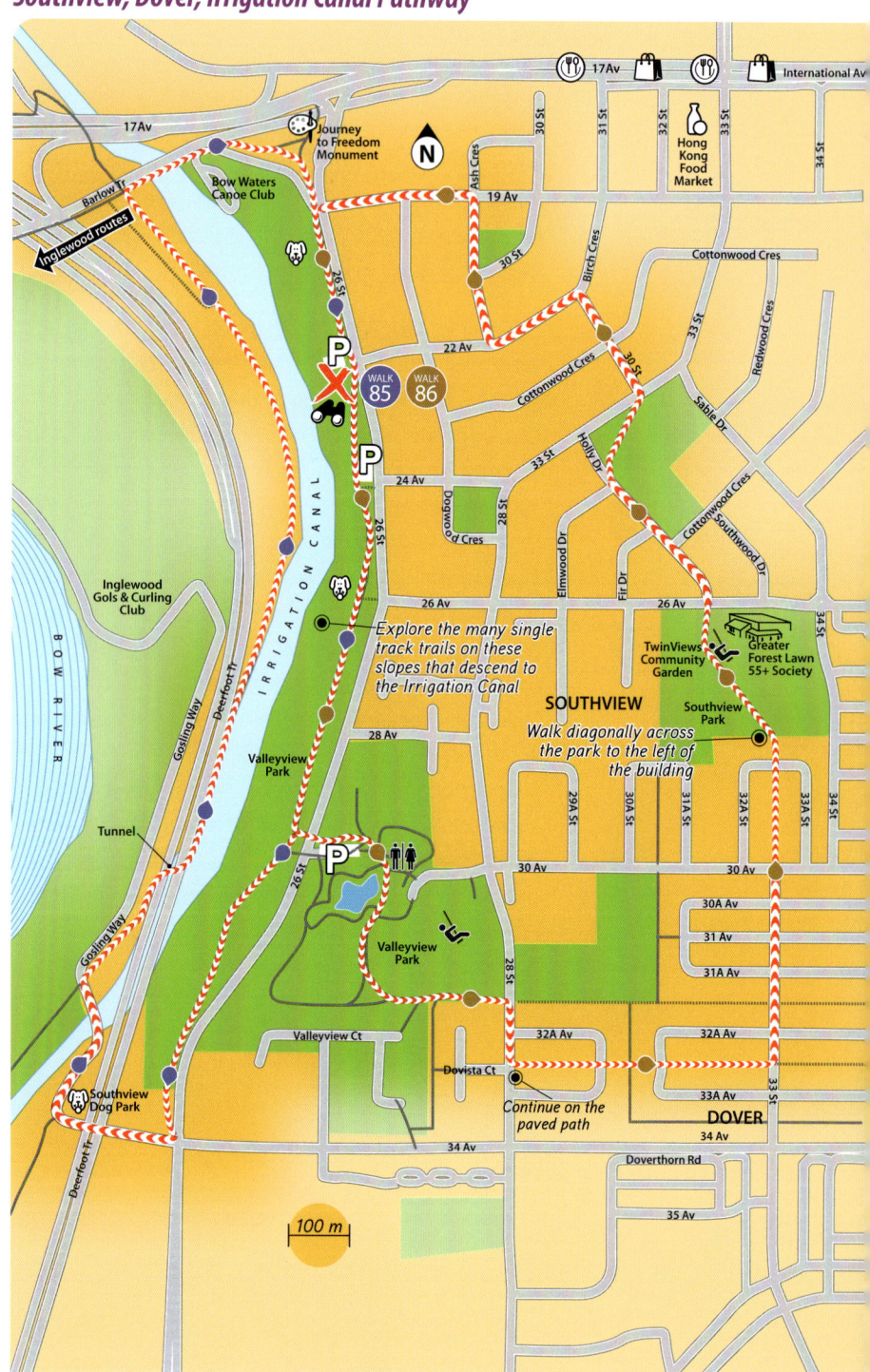

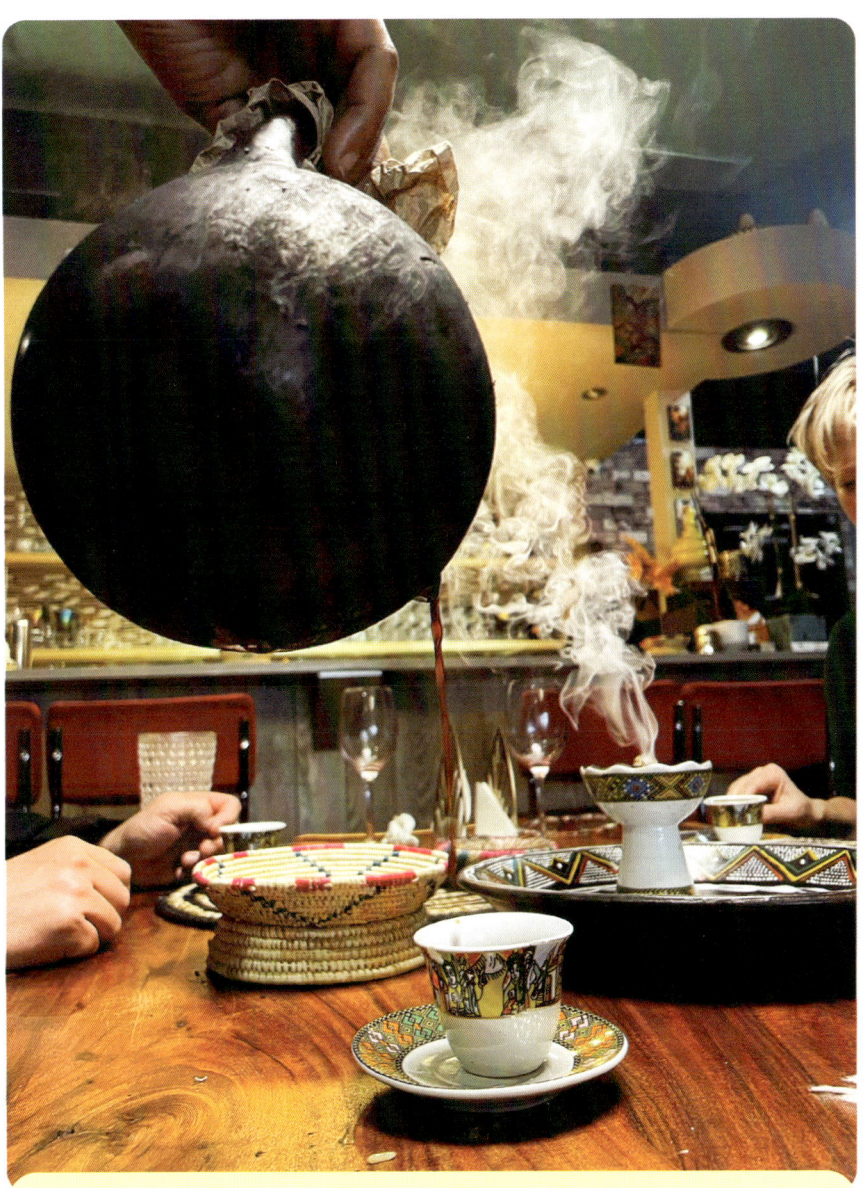

Tasty Pit Stops

Grab lunch or a drink along 17th Avenue, also known as International Avenue, Calgary's most ethnically diverse shopping and eating area. Travel around the world in 35 Blocks with visits to India, Pakistan, Ethiopia, the Mediterranean, Jamaica, Mexico, Nicaragua, Italy, and Germany. Efficient transit and a wide multiuse sidewalk make the area great for walking. Investing in the area to make it nicer while avoiding gentrification is a delicate balance. When walking into Inglewood, plan to stop at Blackfoot Truckstop Diner to refuel. Or sit on the patio at Good News Coffee, a little house turned café tucked into the neighbourhood.

Elliston Park, International Avenue, Forest Lawn

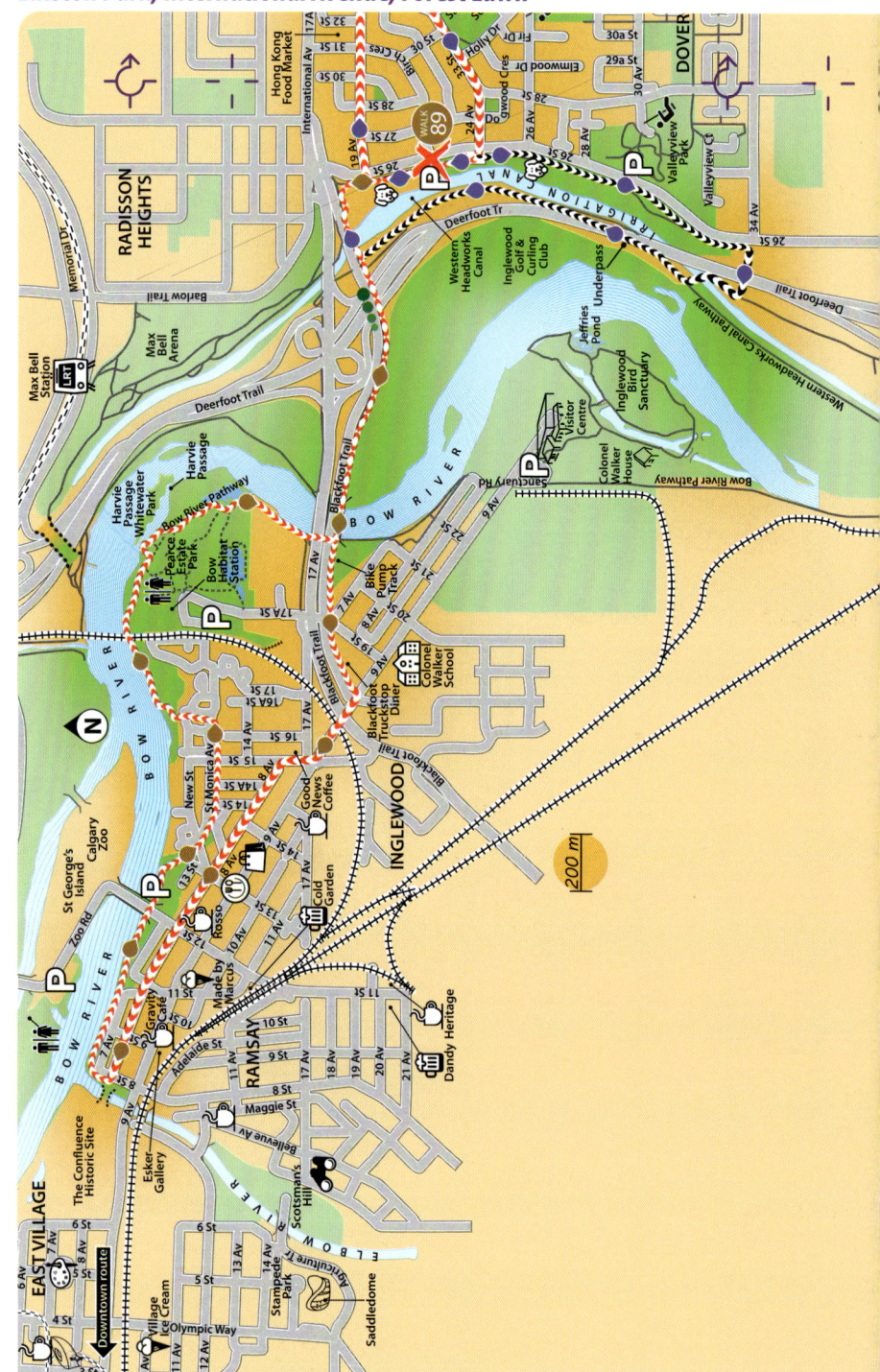

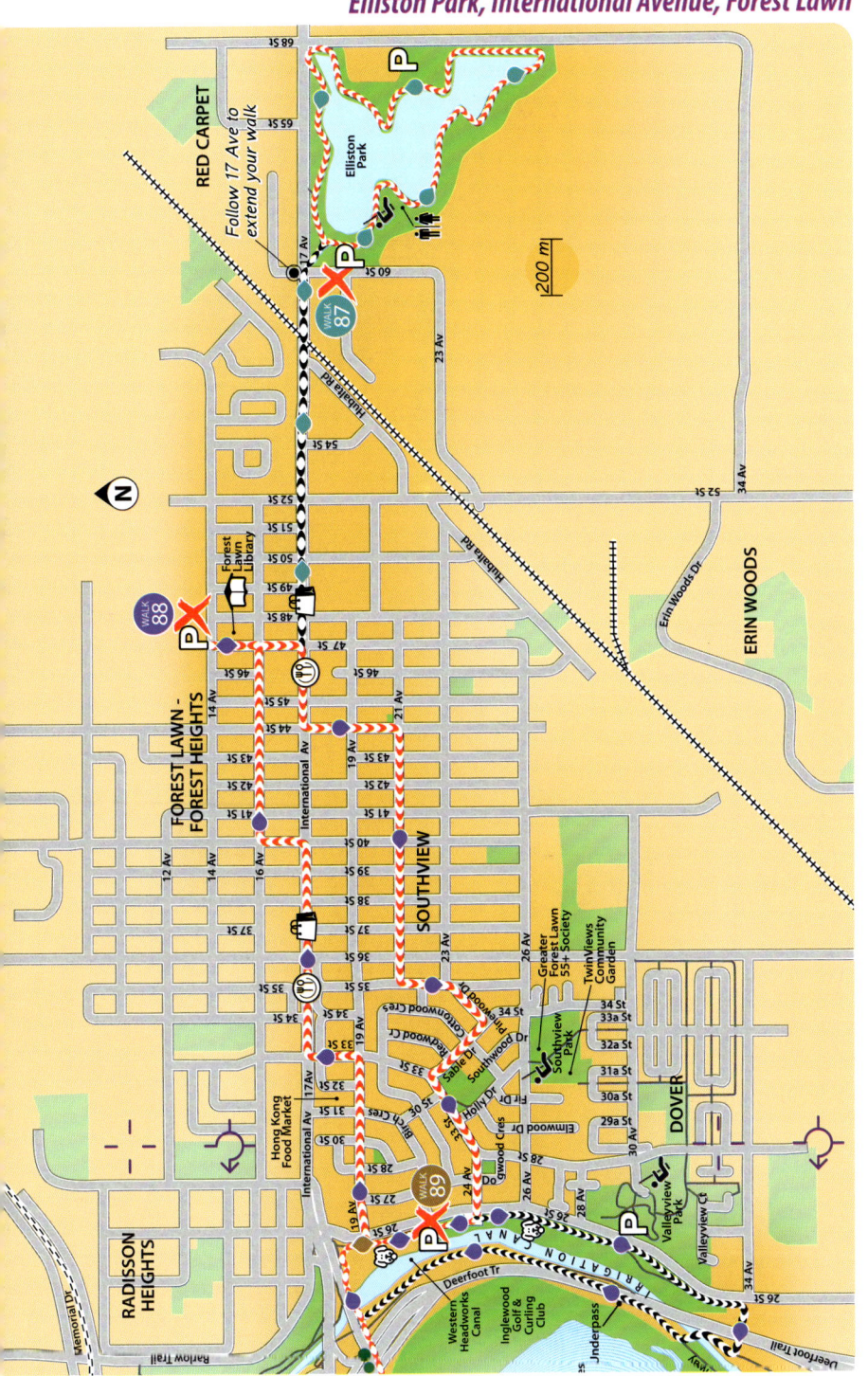

Irrigating Southern Alberta

As you walk along the Irrigation canal you might think to yourself, where does all the canal water go? Since 1904, water has been diverted from the Bow River near Inglewood into the Western Headworks Canal. The water flows to Chestermere Lake and is then funneled north and south. The Western Headworks Canal runs all the way to Brooks and provides irrigation to over 96,000 acres on 400 farms. Four different communities, with a total of 12,000 residents, also get municipal water from the irrigation district canal system. Across southern Alberta, 42,000 people source their household water from irrigation districts. To ensure that contaminants such as salt, phosphorus, and nitrogen do not flow east, Calgary and Alberta Environment created the Shepard Wetland at Ralph Klein Park to clean the stormwater before it washes into the Bow River. The wetland is 385 acres, making it Canada's biggest constructed stormwater treatment wetland.

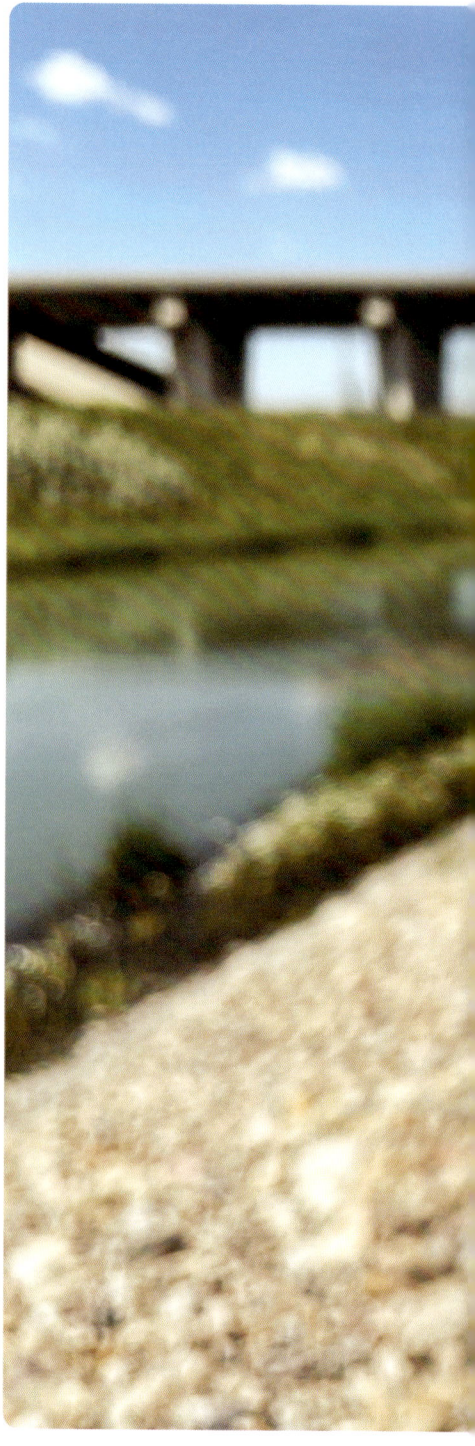

Irrigation Canal Pathway

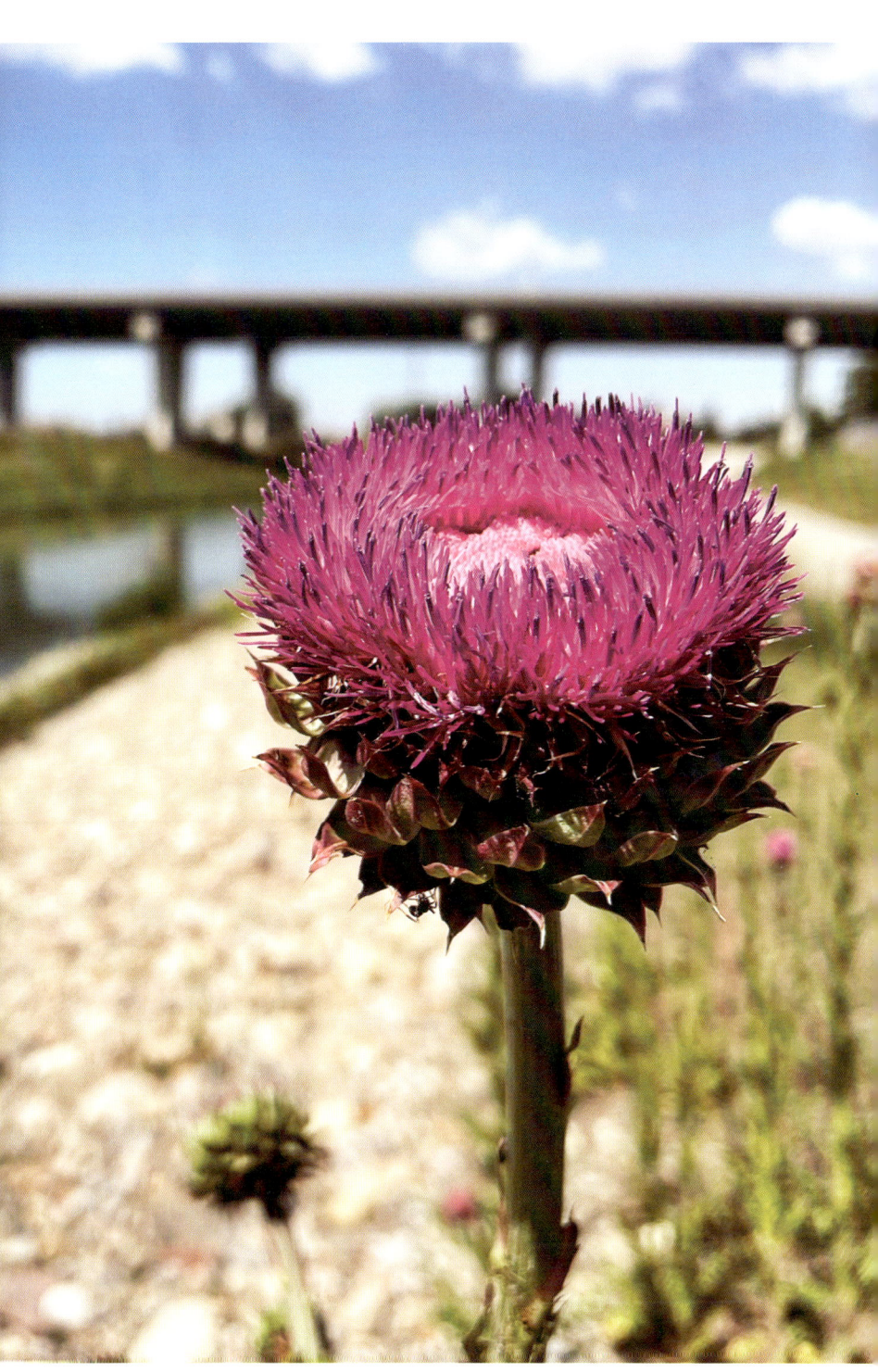

ELLISTON PARK, INTERNATIONAL AVENUE, FOREST LAWN, SOUTHVIEW, DOVER, IRRIGATION CANAL PATHWAY

Pearce Estate Park - Inglewood Bird Sanctuary - Ramsay - St. Patrick's Island

Walks 90-93

SE

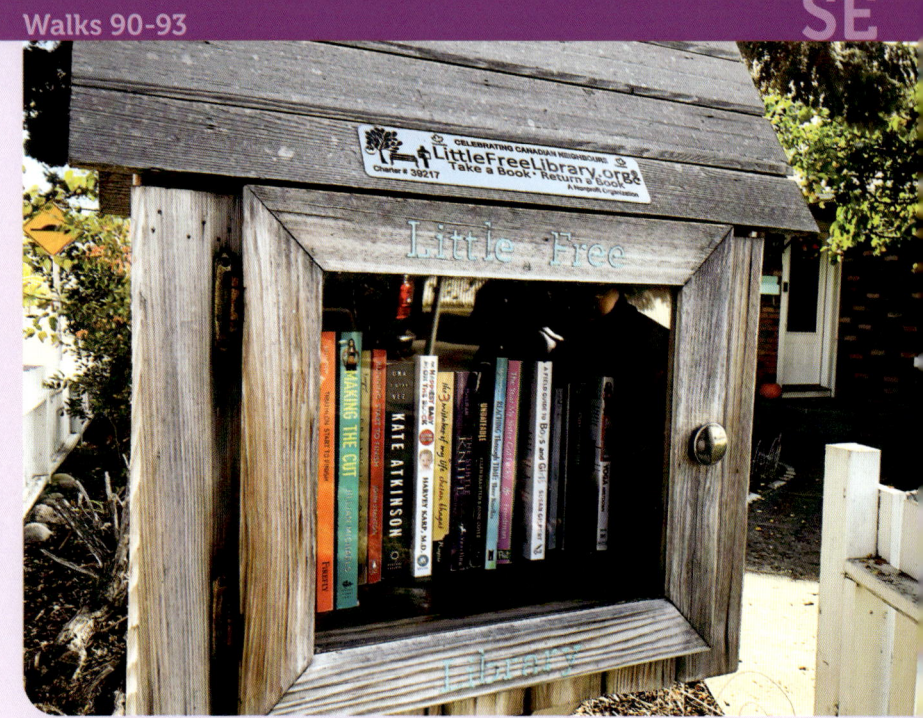

Walks at a Glance:

Eclectic, sometimes gritty, neighbourhoods make for the best urban hikes. Ramsay and Bridgeland are home to old-fashioned corner stores, historic homes and buildings from the early 1900s - some renovated and fantastic, some handyman delights. Ramsay is not polished and perfect, and that is what makes walking here so enjoyable, so unpredictable.

Red, bright yellow, violet blue, chartreuse, forest green, and turquoise: these are just some of the house colours you will see on this trek. And the gardens here are creative, personalized, and fun. Inglewood and Ramsay's

Details

Categories: LRT, Café, Dog (except Inglewood Bird Sanctuary), Nature, Neighbourhood & Parks, People watch & shop, Hilly, Stroller, Historic, Vistas, River, Birds

Start: Walks 90 and 91: Pearce Estate Park, 1440 17 A Street SE; Walk 91: Inglewood Bird Sanctuary, end of 9 Avenue SE; Walks 92 and 93: 17 Avenue and 9 Street SE

LRT: Bridgeland Station

Facilities: Bathrooms at Inglewood Bird Sanctuary Visitor Centre and Pearce Estate Wetland. Many cafés, craft breweries and restaurants along, or a short detour from, 9 Avenue

Distance & Difficulty

Walk 90: Pearce Estate Park- Inglewood- Ramsay: 8.7 km (paved paths, sidewalks)

Walk 91: Inglewood Bird Sanctuary - Pearce Estate Park: 6 km (paved and gravel paths, sidewalks)

Walk 92: Ramsay - St. Patrick's - East Village: 6.5 km (paved paths, sidewalks)

Walk 93: Ramsay - Bridgeland: 7 km (paved paths, sidewalks, stairs)

Highlights, Detours & Destinations

Dog are not allowed in the Inglewood Bird Sanctuary. A variety of waterfowl begin to arrive in March, shorebirds fly in around May, and the songbirds add music to your hike in May and June. Watch for pelicans and cormorants throughout July and August. Colourful Baltimore orioles, yellow warblers, fly catchers, and eastern king birds are a common sight in the warm months. August and September see a variety of species of warblers

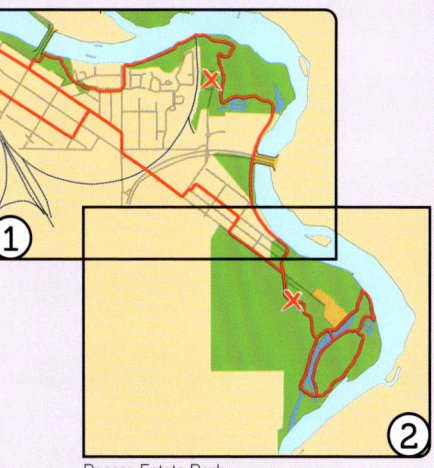

Pearce Estate Park - Inglewood Bird Sanctuary

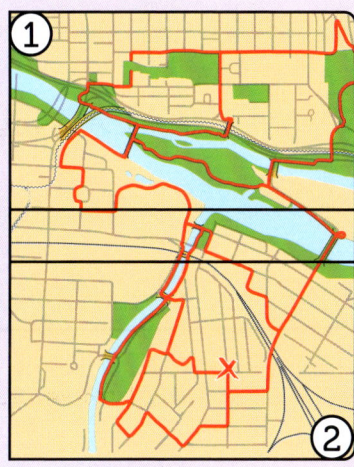

Ramsay - St. Patrick's Island

warm microclimate and rich, flood-plain soil makes green thumbs of everyone. The flowers bloom earlier in the season and last longer here than anywhere else in Calgary, and the pear trees hang heavy with fruit in the fall.

Both Walks 90 and 91 start along the Bow River Pathway and pass by Harvie Passage, the whitewater park that replaces the weir. Once known as the drowning machine, the weir was a serious hazard for all watercraft, but the Harvey passage redesign has made it a destination for river kayakers, recreational rafters and spectators throughout the warmer months. Continue along the pathway and soon you are at the Inglewood Bird Sanctuary. This wildlife reserve was designated a Federal Migratory Bird Sanctuary in 1929. Walk the paved and shale paths that follow the Bow River while keeping a keen eye out for rare birds. Stop by the visitor

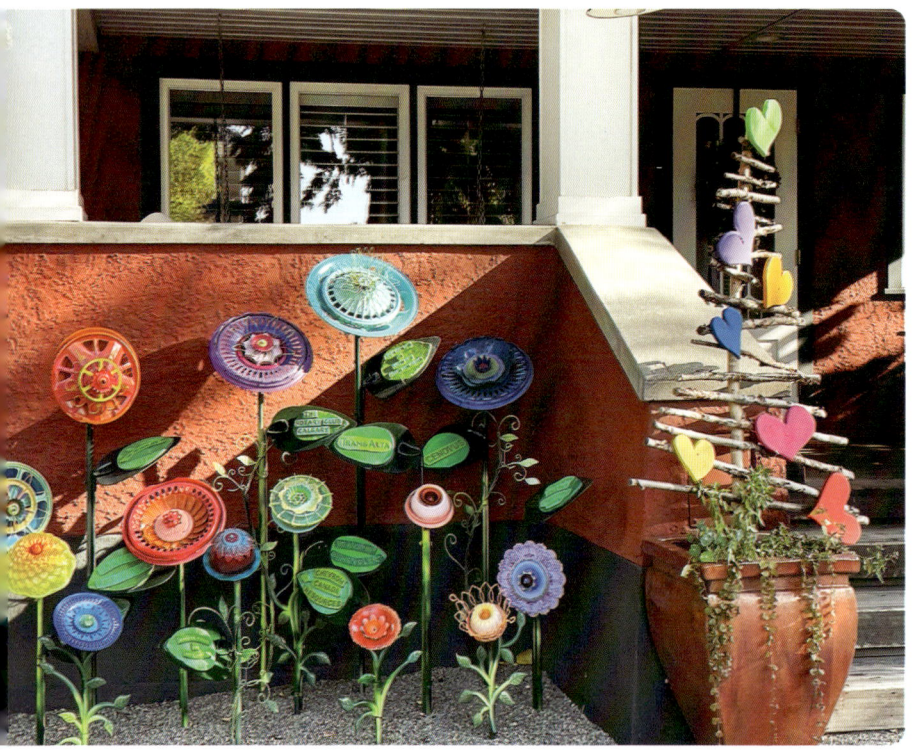

centre to see which feathered friends are frequently flying and nesting in the area. More than 270 species of birds have been seen here, 53 of which nest on site while the rest are migratory. As well, 21 species of mammals and 347 species of plants have been recorded at the sanctuary. Even if you aren't a birder, the sanctuary is a great place to unwind.

Walks 92 and 93 travel Ramsay side streets to the top of Scotsman's Hill. The high point offers a bird's eye view of Stampede Park and is the best place to watch the Stampede fireworks. Look beyond the hardworking core to the Rocky Mountain peaks before descending the staircase to RiverWalk which continues north along the Elbow River to the Bow River and into the East Village. RiverWalk is a beautiful pathway development that connects, or will connect, the East Village, Stampede Park, Lindsay Park, and the community of Mission. With separate pathways for walkers and cyclists, pull-offs with benches, comfy chairs, art installations, and lush landscaping, this walkway is not to be missed. Walk 93 connects to Bridgeland on the north side of the Bow River while Walk 92 explores St. Patrick's Island, at the confluence of the Bow and Elbow Rivers. With waterparks, a playground, sledding hill, picnic tables, wetlands and forests, it is a perfect stop for families.

The variety on these walks is due to the uniqueness of the people who choose to live in Inglewood, Ramsay, and Bridgeland - people who enjoy diversity and who embrace unique designs and personal touches. The creativity and ingenuity of the residents give the urban walker a sense of the personalities who live here.

Pearce Estate Park - Inglewood Bird Sanctuary

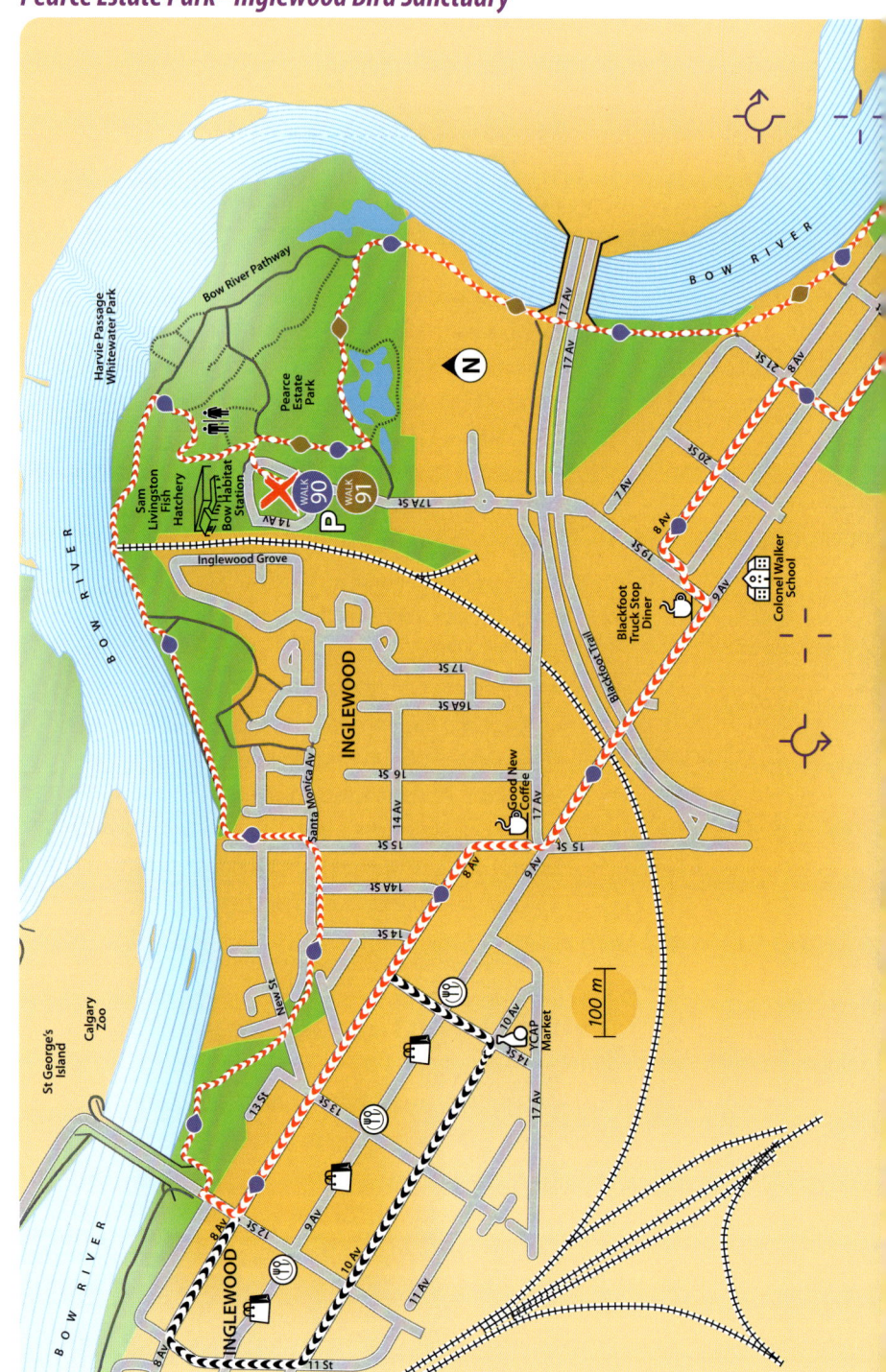

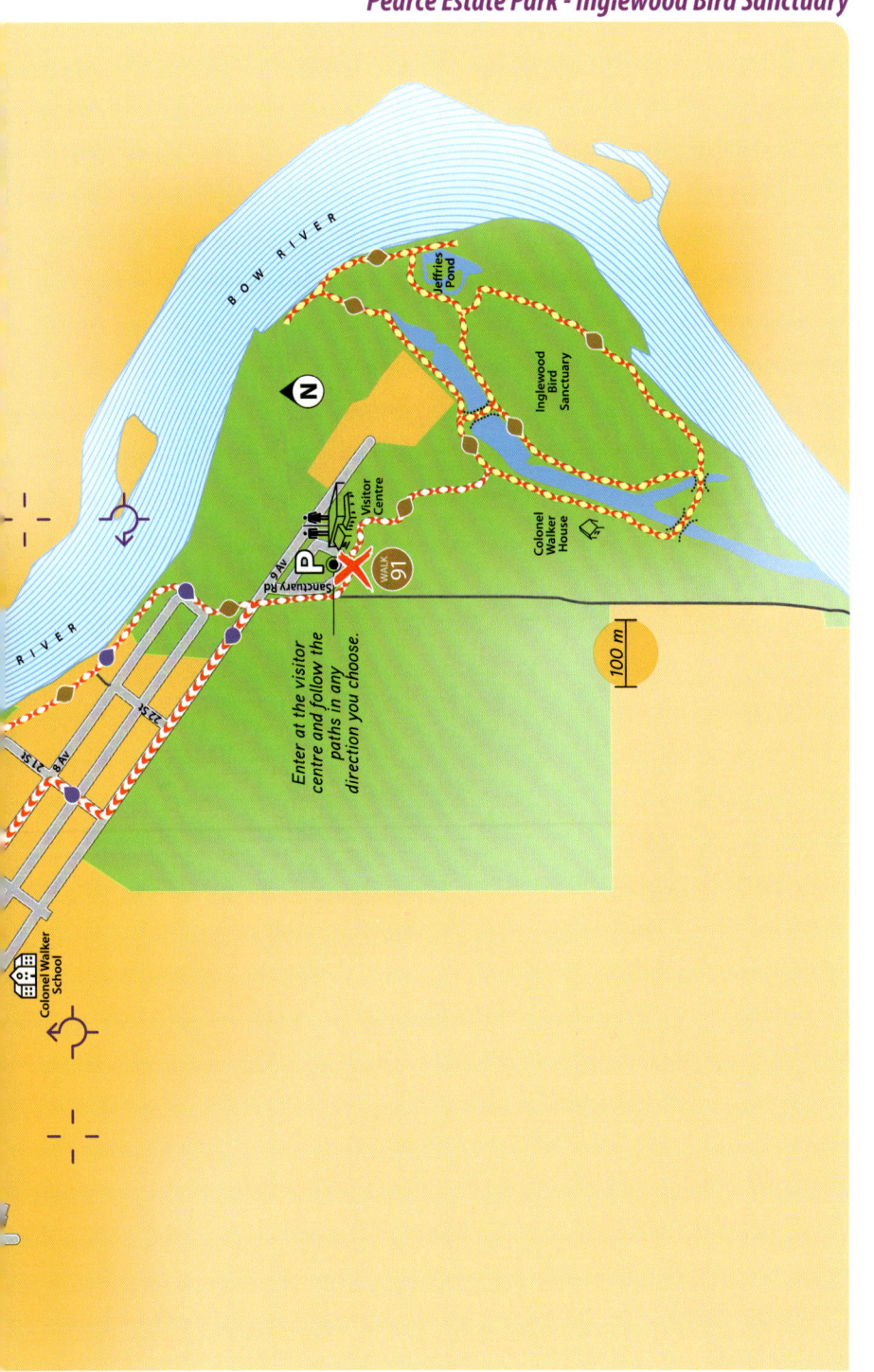

Ramsay - St. Patrick's Island

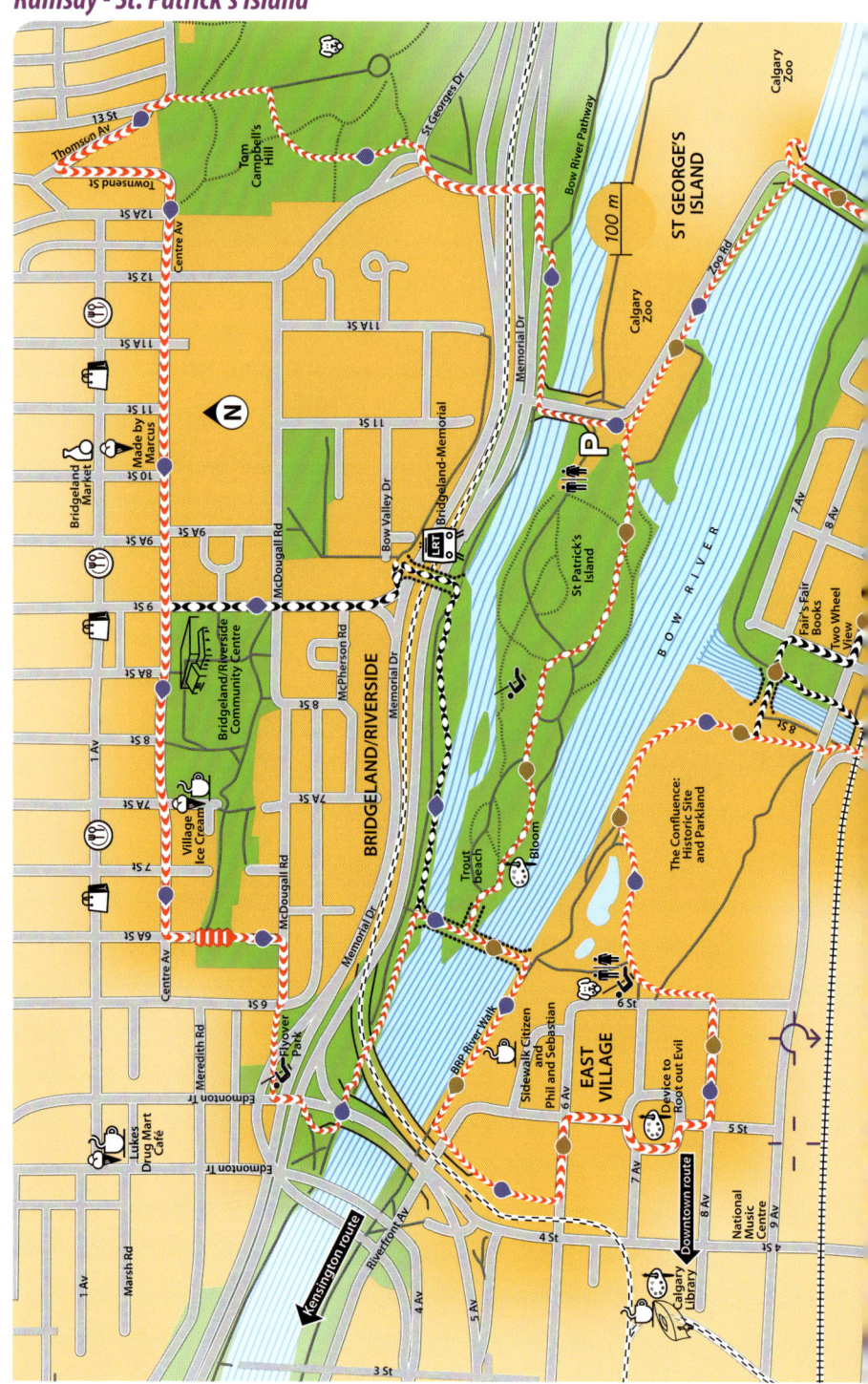

Ramsay - St. Patrick's Island

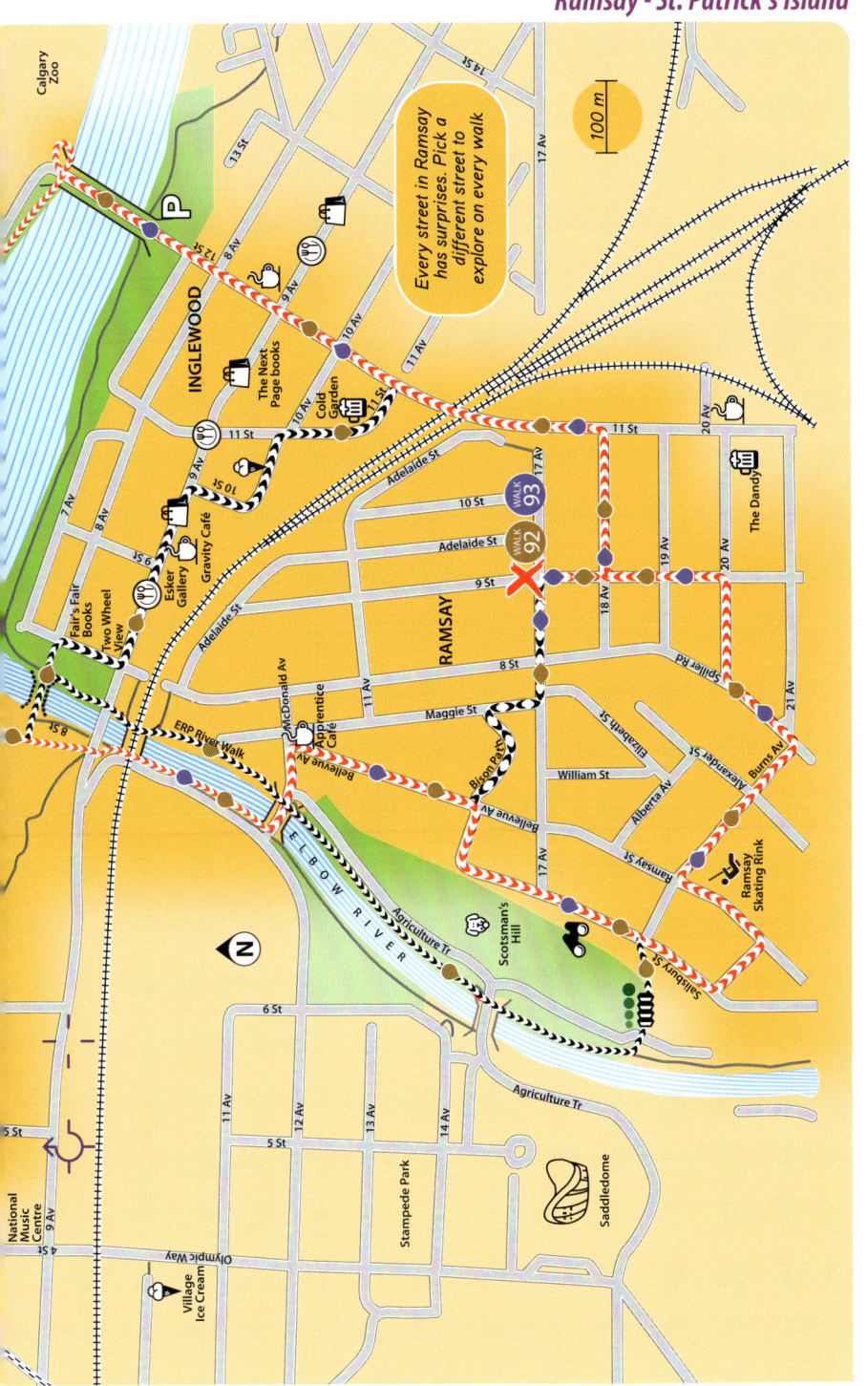

PEARCE ESTATE PARK - INGLEWOOD BIRD SANCTUARY - RAMSAY - ST. PATRICK'S ISLAND

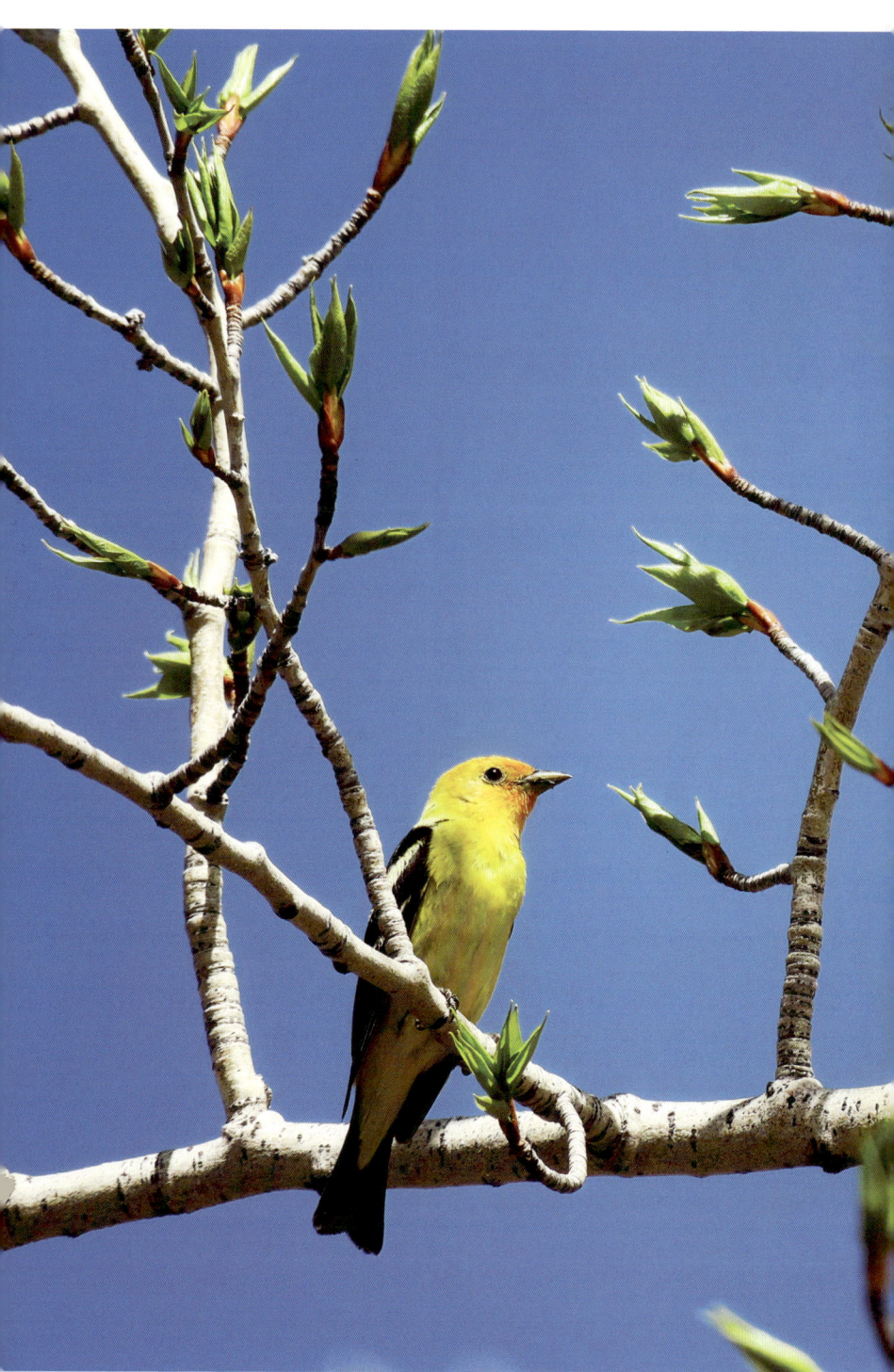

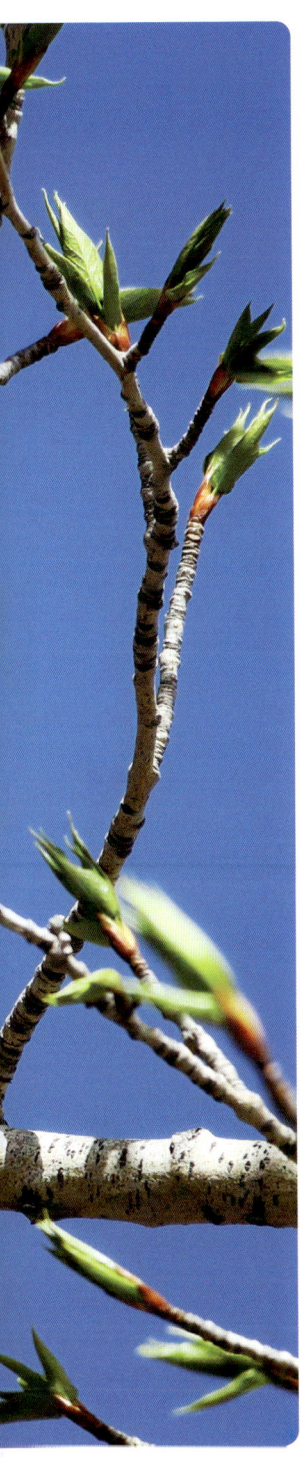

St. Patrick's Island Park

Situated across from the East Village, St. Patrick's Island is one of Calgary's oldest parks. Its development as a public space began in the late 1890s and gained momentum with construction of a bridge to the island in the early 1900s. Redesigned alongside the flood of 2013, the bioliphic design of the park nurtures the bond between people and nature. Some unique features include a restored channel where visitors can wade into the water and venture safely onto a gravel bar; a grassy knoll, nine metres high, that provides a perfect setting for community celebrations, performances, and movies in the park during summer; and tobogganing during winter and a seasonal riparian wetland at the heart of the island, with an elevated boardwalk for no-impact access to the wetland and forest, an important habitat for nesting eagles, owls, and songbirds. And you can't miss Bloom, a 23-metre-tall sculpture made of connected streetlights that represents a towering flower.

Location: 1300 Zoo Road NE

Esker Foundation Contemporary Art Gallery

Detour along Ninth Avenue and drop by the Esker Art Gallery after your walk. This private non-commercial gallery is impressive, and it is free to all. Tour the latest exhibition –there are three shows each year– or register for and take part in one of the gallery's many educational events. Free contemporary art programming, designed to make art accessible to all ages, is offered to anyone who is interested. Tour the birds nest boardroom or settle into the comfy couch sitting area, where visitors are encouraged to relax and enjoy the views or to bring their laptops and write a few inspirational words.

Location: Top floor, 1011 Ninth Avenue SE, www.eskerfoundation.com

Western Tanager by Sara Tehranian

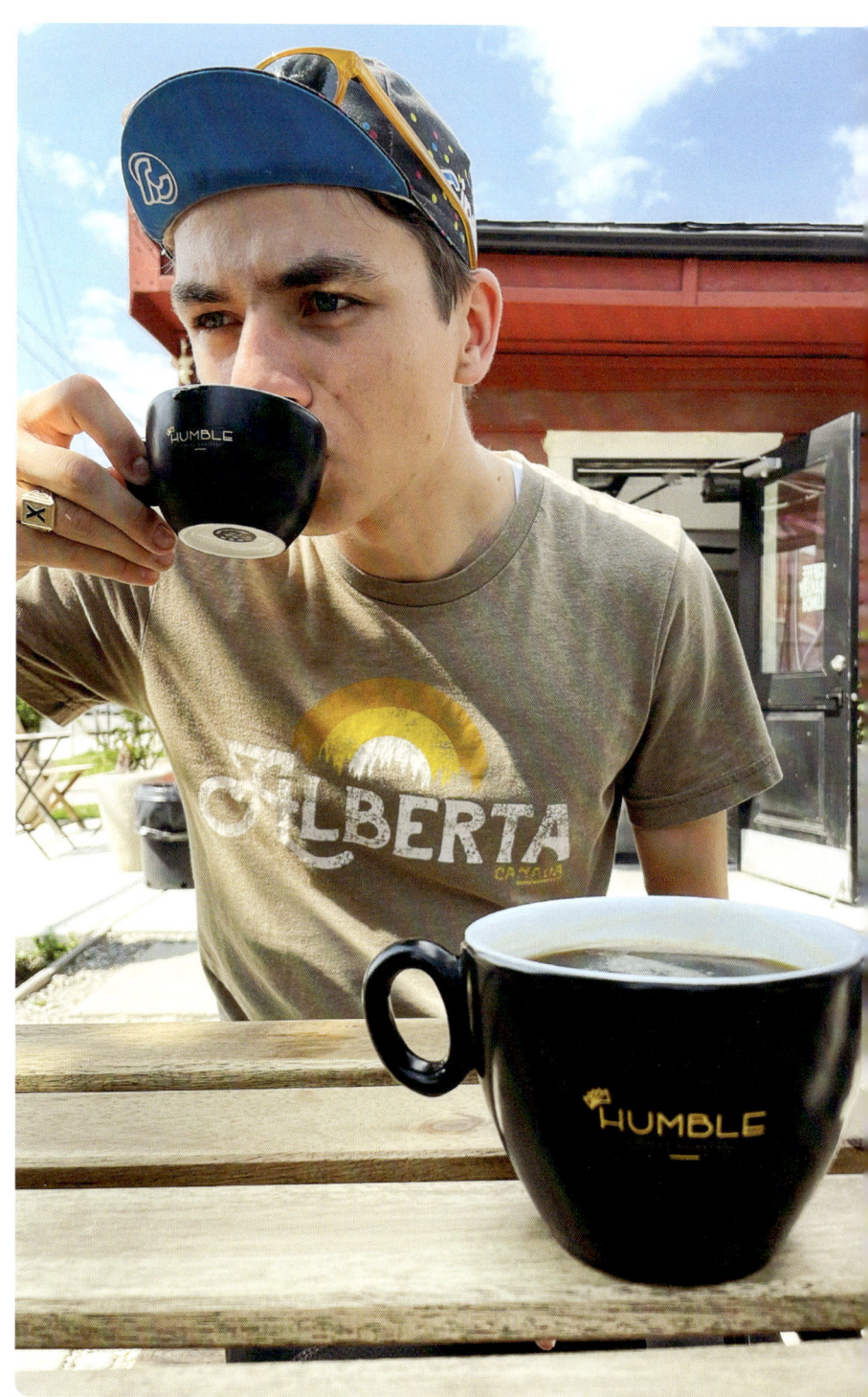

Tasty Pit Stops

Follow the alternate route to 10 Avenue and drop into YCAP Market. The Wood's Homes Youth Culinary Arts Program (YCAP) Market features food and products made by clients who are learning to cook and prepare homemade quality meals under the guidance of Red Seal chefs. A daily special, take away prepared meals, jams and spreads, baked goods and an eclectic little shop make this a stop not to miss. Walk along 9th Avenue, formally Atlantic Avenue, Calgary's first authentic main street. Packed with an eclectic mix of shops selling clothes, spices, knives, books, home decor, quirky collectibles, as well as restaurants, coffee shops, breweries, live music venues, and art galleries, the avenue is a haven for independent businesses. Brewery Flats in Inglewood is home to several craft breweries. While in Inglewood, plan to stop by Cold Garden with your dog, the Dandy or High Line. Walk the area during the Inglewood Night Market, when music, street dancing, and artisans fill the streets with energy and people. Check out www.inglewoodnightmarket.ca for more information. And if it's an authentic truck stop experience that you are craving, with milkshakes that are like drinking cake through a straw and sky-high flapper pie, then stop by the Blackfoot Truckstop Diner to refuel. Burgers, fries, ice cream, fried chicken or a Spolumbo's sausage lunch anyone? Walk to the Inglewood Drive In or Spolumbo's and fuel up. I highly recommend a detour to Gravity for live music, great coffee and house made foods, Good News Coffee for its top-notch coffee and cozy space with patio, or Apprentice Café for home-made ice cream and sandwiches. Check out Canela Vegan Bakery and Cafe, a top-notch family run spot on 9th Avenue where the cinnamon buns take centre stage. Started by Veronica who hails from Mexico, the warm spices of Mexico make their way into their delicious offerings, which also include a selection of gluten free treats. Travel the RiverWalk to the Simmons Building. Built in 1912, the former mattress factory is now a city landmark and the home Sidewalk Citizen Bakery café and Phil and Sebastien Coffee. Heritage Roastery and Coffee Shop on 11 Street is another popular spot that freshly roasted coffee in a wonderfully refurbished 1911 building.

Locations:
Tenth Avenue: YCAP Market (Wed.- Fri.: 12-6 pm, Sat.: 10-3 pm); 9th Avenue: Canela Bakery and Café, Good News Coffee, Gravity, Blackfoot Diner; **12 Street:** Spolumbo's, Inglewood Drive In, Cold Garden; **In Ramsay:** Apprentice Café, Heritage Coffee Shop, High Line, The Dandy; **East Village RiverWalk:** Simmons Building

Good News Coffee

Tour de Calgary, South and North Pathway Loops

Walks 94 and 95

NSEW

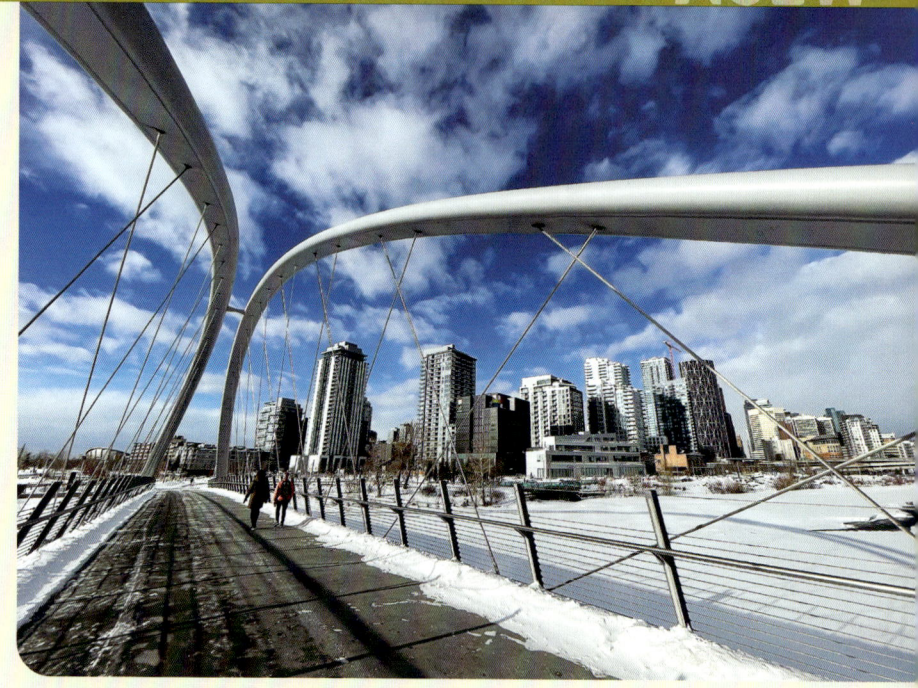

Walks at a Glance:

Explore Calgary's pathway network on foot! Split into bit size segments so you can spread it out over a week, a month or a year, walking the south and north loops is easy to navigate and will give you a unique perspective on Calgary.

The tour of South Calgary travels the Bow and Elbow River Pathways past the Ogden Railyards, through Beaver Dam Flats Park to Rockies viewpoints. Connect to Carburn Park where the deer are abundant and watch for pelicans on the Bow River as you connect to Fish Creek Park. Grasslands soon become a forested canopy of spruce and balsam poplars as you walk west along

Details

Categories: LRT, Café, Dog, Nature, Neighbourhood & Parks, People watch & shop, Hilly, Stroller, Historic, Vistas, River, Birds

Start: Anywhere you want along the pathway network

LRT: South Loop: Fish Creek Park, City Hall, Bridgeland, or Erlton Stations; North Loop: Bridgeland, Sunnyside, Dalhousie, and any downtown station

Facilities: Bathrooms in parks, cafés and libraries along the routes

Distance & Difficulty

Walk 94: South Calgary Pathway Loop: 62 km divided into 4.5- 7 km segments

Walk 95: North Calgary Pathway Loop: 44 km divided into 5- 9 km segments

Highlights, Detours & Destinations

Too many to list!

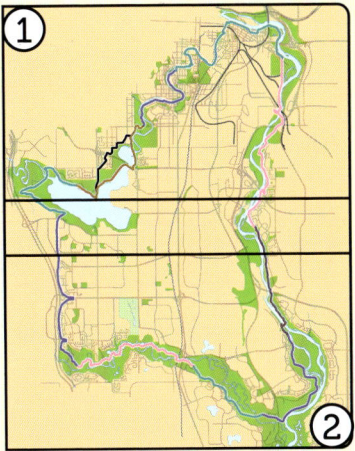

Tour of South Calgary

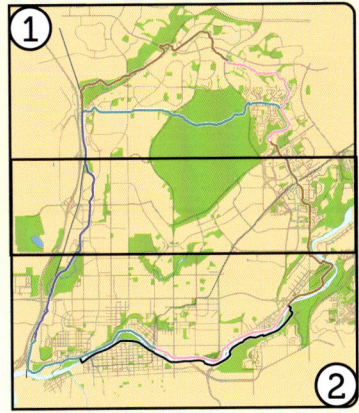

Tour of North Calgary

Fish Creek. Pace north alongside the Tssut'ina Nation to the Glenmore Reservoir, followed by your descent into the wilds of Weaselhead Park.

Keep an eye out for beaver, moose, and deer before climbing to North Glenmore Park where awe-inspiring reservoir and Rockies views are your reward. North Glenmore Park is a popular gathering spot for everything social, from walking to biking to bonfires and picnics. There are paths for both walkers and cyclists here making it a relaxed walk as you enjoy the views along the way to the impressive Glenmore Dam. Rebuilt after the flood of 2013, the pathway is now wider and higher, offering expansive views of the Elbow River valley all the way to the downtown core. Follow the path along the escarpment before walking downhill to Sandy Beach Park.

A mix of paved pathways and pleasant, tree-canopied, side street strolling, the Elbow River Pathway passes by popular swimming holes, rafting and picnic spots as it connects parks and neighbourhoods. Soak up the scents of blossoms in May, the summer gardens through August, and the fall colours well into October as you follow the twists and turns of the river through Rideau, into Mission, and past Stampede Park. At the confluence of the Bow and Elbow rivers the walk loops back through Inglewood, past colourful homes, folk art, little free libraries, and fruit trees. Connect to the pathway again and continue past Pearce Estate Park and Harvey Passage, the white-water park on the Bow. Take a dip and watch the kayakers perfecting their surfing skills before completing the best of the south loop.

Next up, the North Calgary loop. Experience Calgary's world-class pathway network on this walk that is 44 kilometres of pure pathway bliss. You could begin on the Bow River Pathway near Bridgeland where you will walk past the Canadian Wilds enclosure at the Calgary

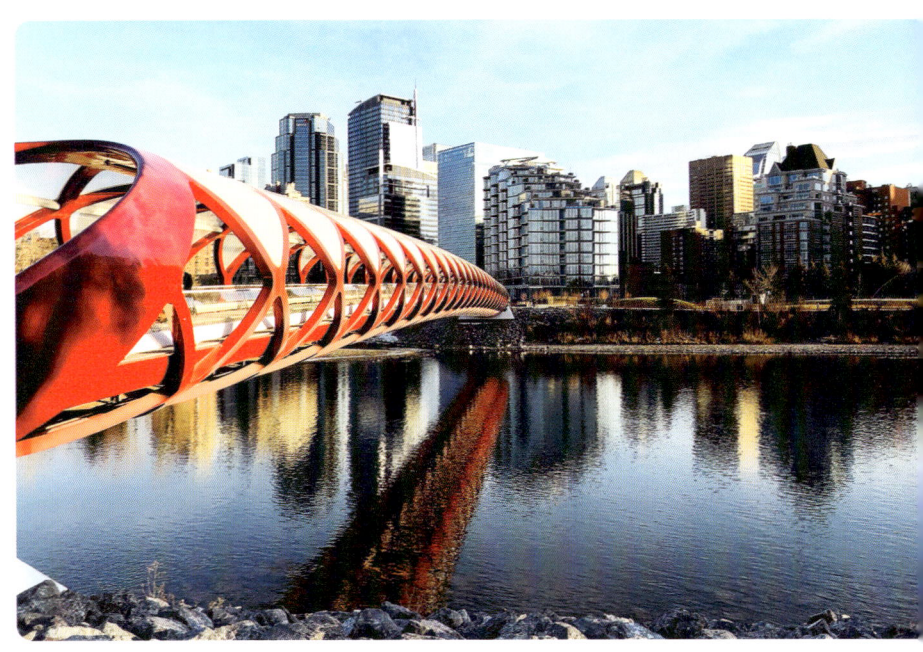

Zoo. Visible from the main pathway, keep an eye out for the moose and grizzly bears that live in the enclosure. The pathway turns north and becomes the quieter Nose Creek Pathway, a pleasant strip of nature that runs parallel to Deerfoot Trail. The climbing is steady and gradual with steeper hills in Nose Hill Park and Edgemont Park Ravines.

Both routes are a mix of paved pathways through neighbourhood green spaces and complete nature immersion in wilderness parks. From Edgemont the walk is all downhill as you connect to the Dalhousie and Varsity Ravine pathway. Pass by Bowmont Park and onto the Bow River Pathway at Shouldice Park where you continue east. At Edworthy Park, choose between the north or south side pathway. A significant ice flow covers the shaded south side in Edworthy Park, below Wildwood, from late fall through late spring and the south side path may be closed at those times. In the summer, the south side route from Edworthy Park is my

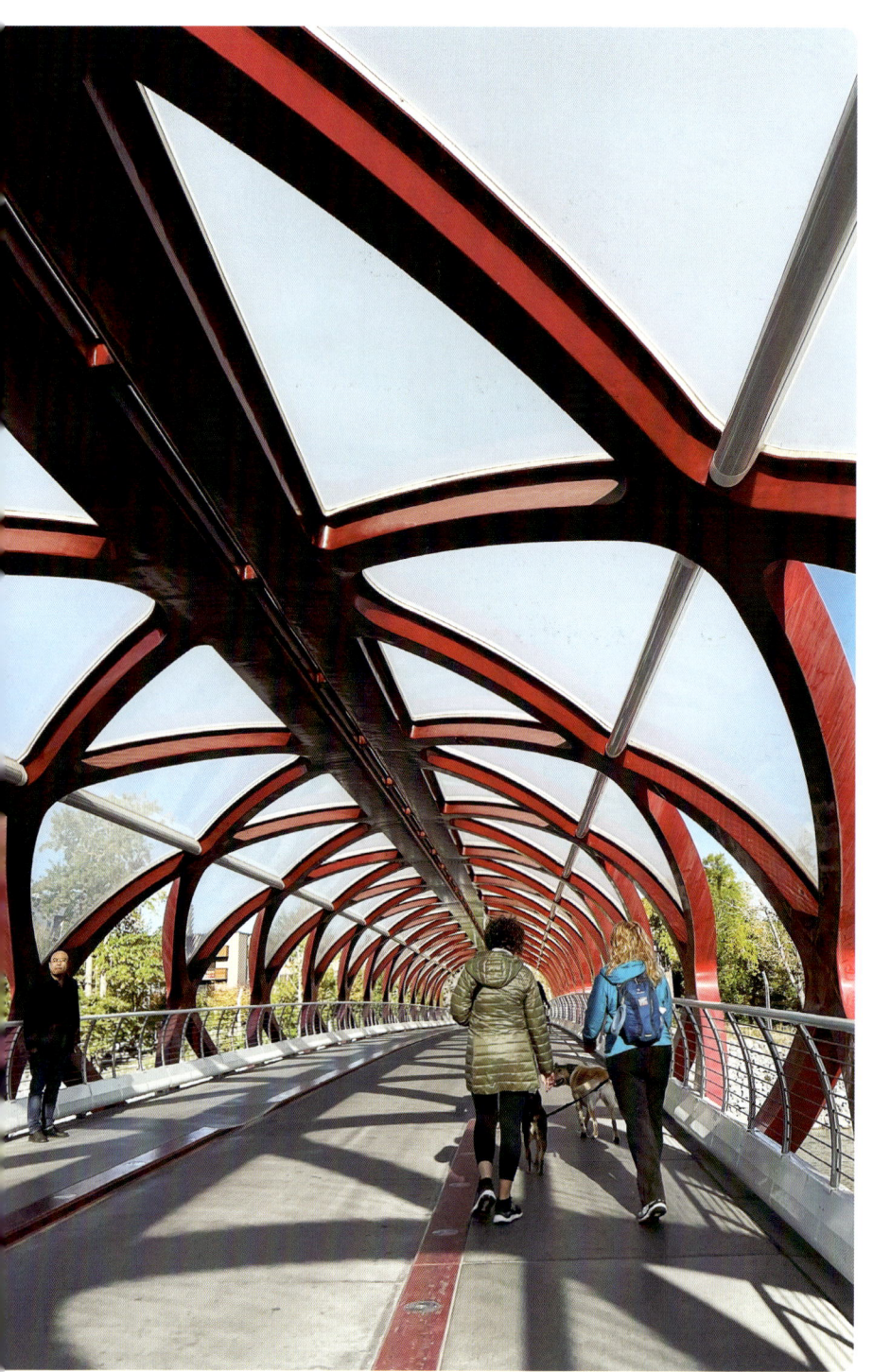

choice as it travels through forests, offering shaded relief and more of a nature immersion. There are many bridges along the way to cross from the north side to south side of the Bow River. Plan a pit stop at one of the many tasty options from Bowness through to East Village. Whether you want to lose yourself in the urban wilds or soak up some urban vibe, this north pathway loop has it all.

Why Walking Makes Us Happy

Joyful, contented, absorbed, satisfied, accomplished, alert, calm and peaceful, confident, powerful, excited— happy. Walking in and around Calgary is enjoyable for so many reasons—big nature, awe-inspiring vistas, peaceful river strolls, fresh air, the physical challenge, and so many destinations to discover along the way. What else is it about walking that makes us feel great?

Focusing on the walk

In our multi-tasking world, it is harder and harder to focus, leaving us feeling scattered and unsatisfied. When we are walking, we are focused, in the moment. This focused state is known as "flow," and some believe it is the secret to happiness. It's your time to think, to observe, and to be in the moment.

Savouring the Beauty

Savouring is what we do when we mentally enlarge or magnify a pleasant experience. Whether it is the quiet appreciation of a stunning view, the calm of the forest, or the post-walk coffee, ice cream or beer and chit-chat with friends, there are many pleasant experiences to be savoured.

Embracing the Challenge

Whether you walk to the top of Nose Hill, navigate and route find through Paskapoo Slopes, trek to the farmers' market and load up on fresh produce, or watch the sunset over the reservoir, these self-propelled moments give a sense of accomplishment, which boosts well-being and improves mood.

Feeling connected

Exploring the city on foot makes the expanse of Calgary more familiar, more like home. As you walk along

pathways, onto hidden stairways, in and out of neighbourhoods, parks and along commercial streets, you'll see how it all fits together. Studies have shown that feeling connected, a part of a place, decreases loneliness and increases wellbeing.

Exercising in the Great Outdoors

Outdoor exercise is good for us, we know that. If you are feeling down, get outside and go for a walk or a bike ride, get your heart rate up, see something new and interact with the world. Find some nature and soak it up as research shows that contact with nature significantly reduces feelings of loneliness. Soaring ravens playing in a chinook wind, blossoming cherry trees along neighbourhood streets, or the calls of the red-winged black birds as you reach the wetland—these experiences, along with the blood-pumping goodness that comes from exercise, help manage anxiety and depression. Exploring, connecting, and discovering Calgary on foot is enjoyable, challenging, and uplifting. Not to mention a lot of fun. And when you have fun, you are happy!

Tour of South Calgary

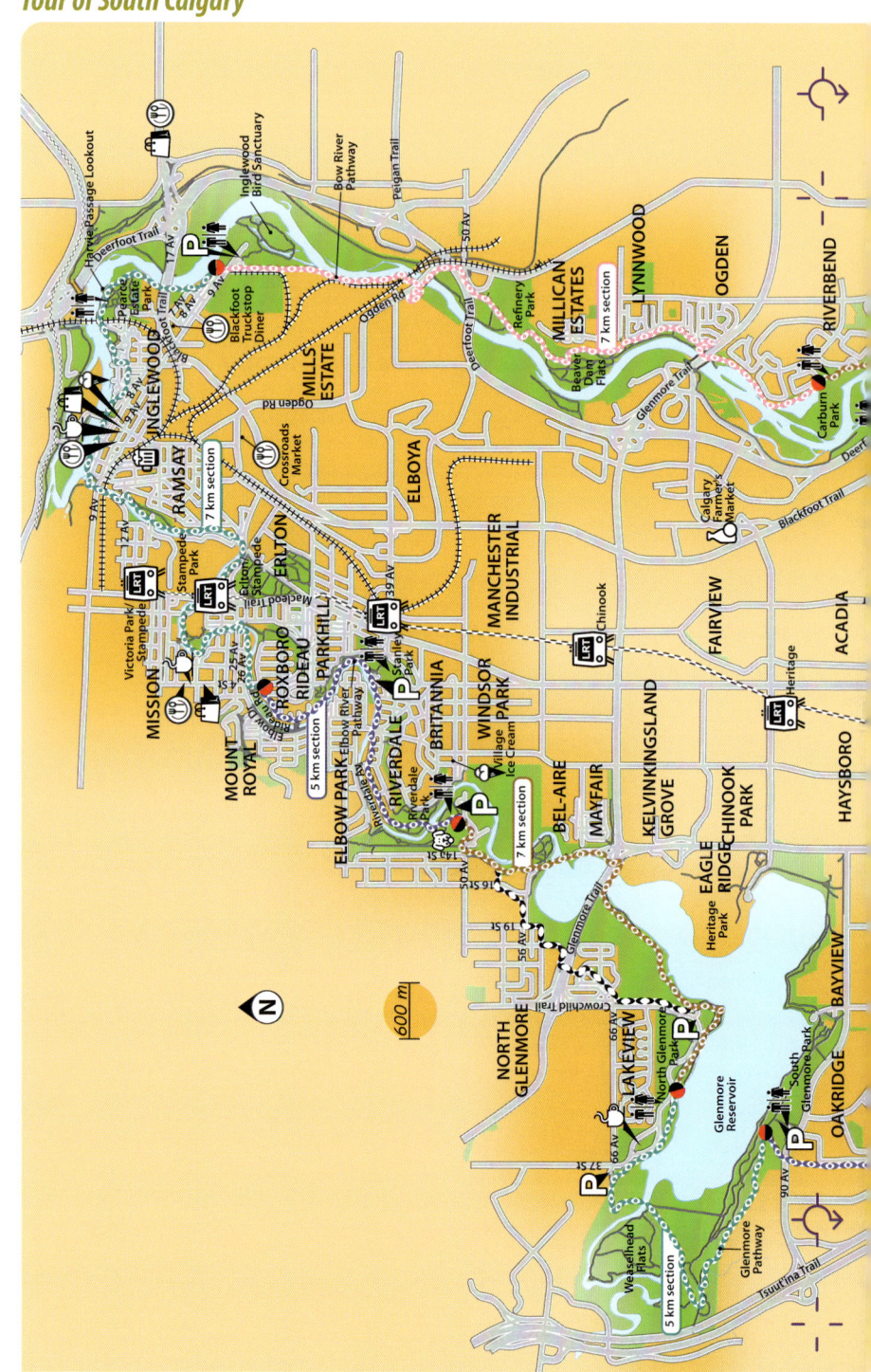

Tour of South Calgary

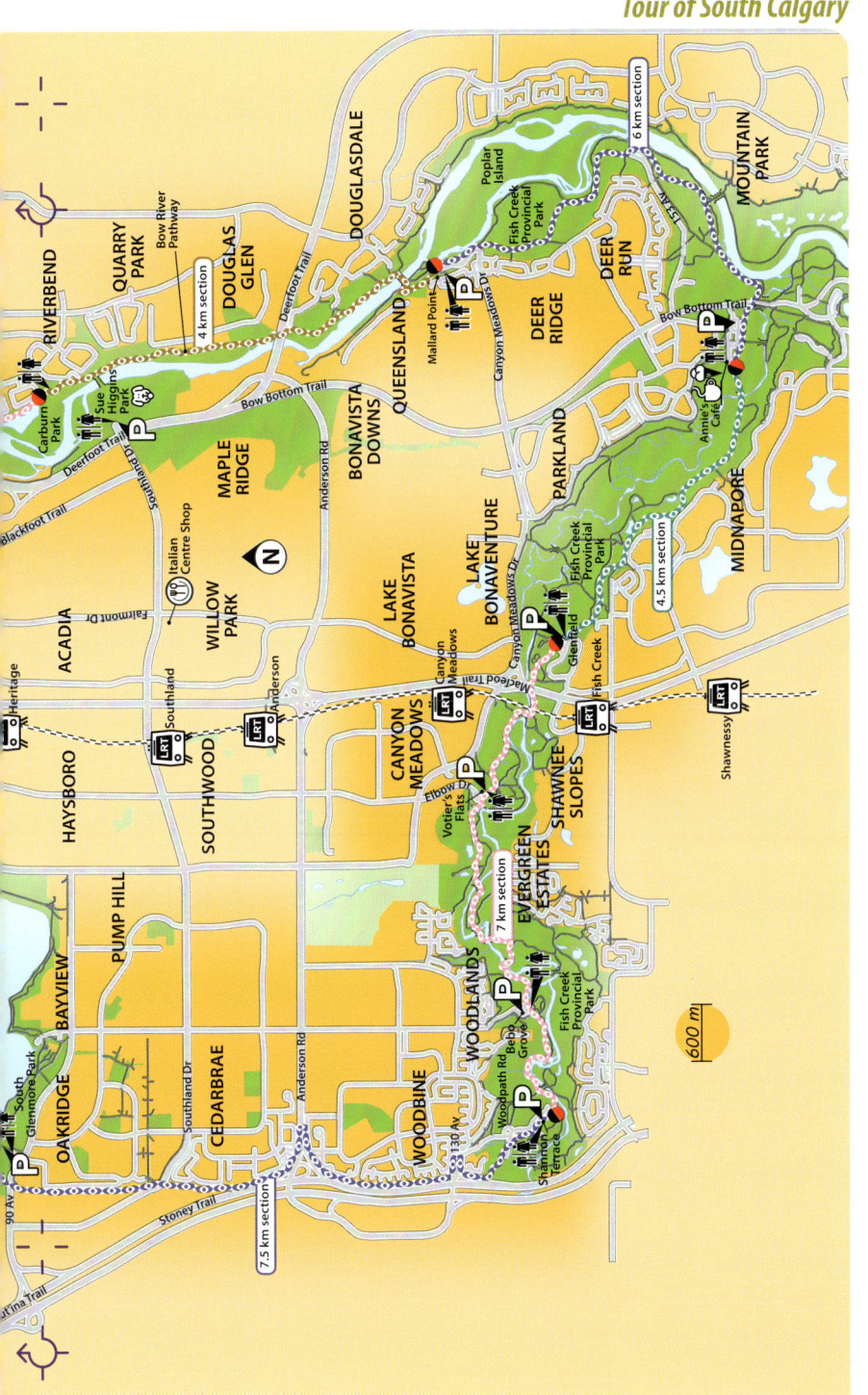

Tour of North Calgary

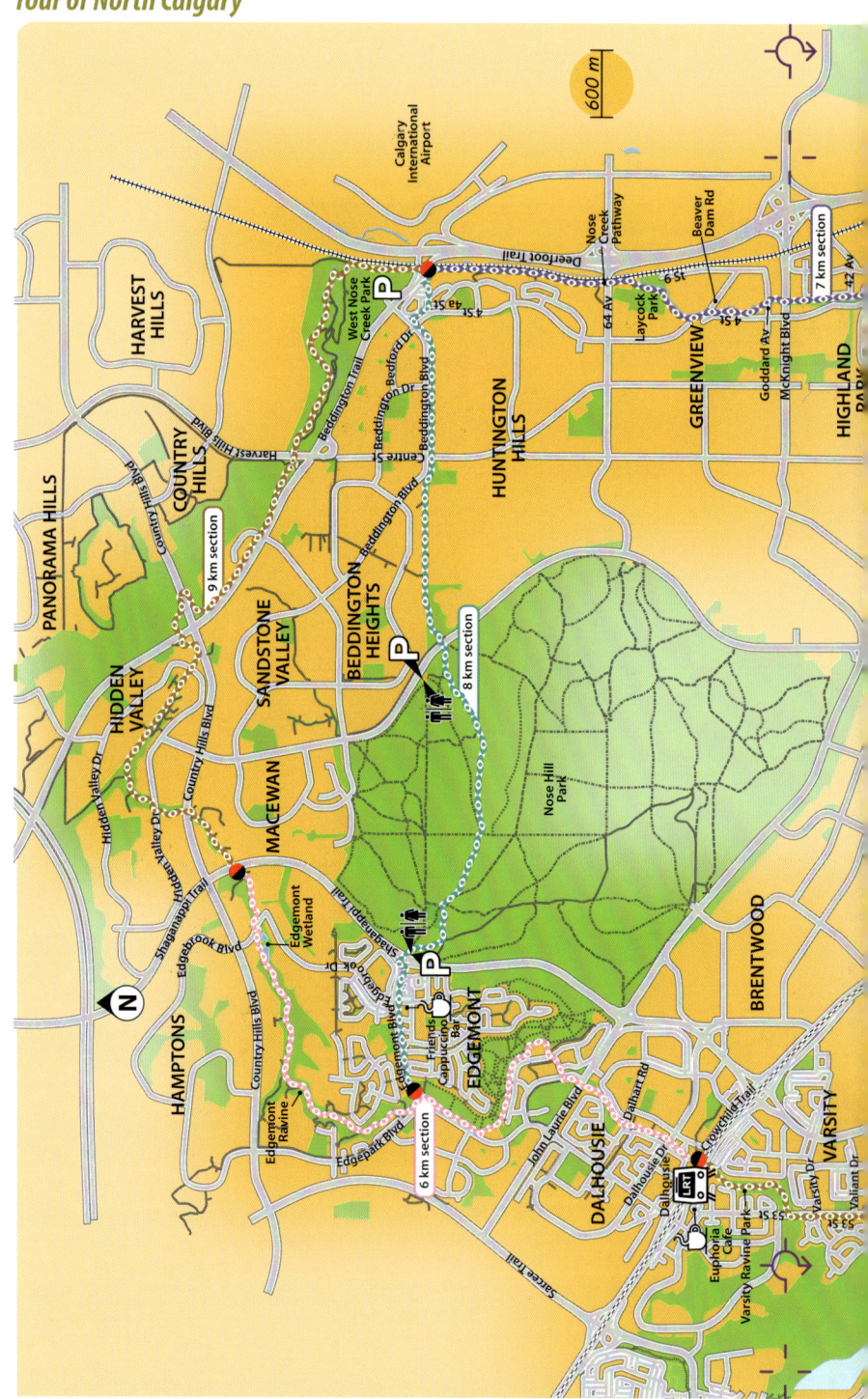

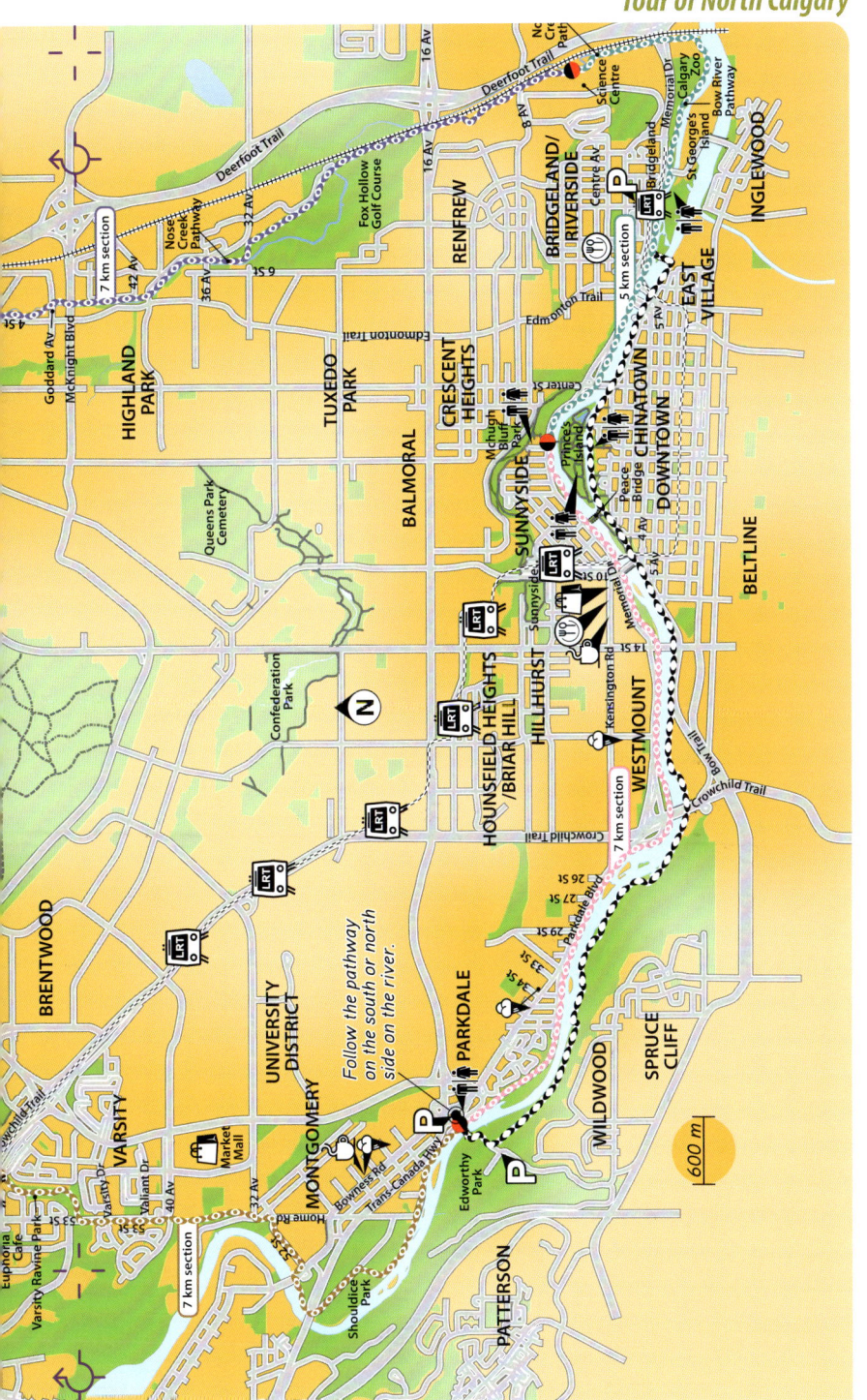

Top 6 Best of Calgary's Best Walks

Dog Favourite (with lots off leash)!

Walks #	
17	Bowmont Park West, NW
28-30	Nose Hill Park, NW
35	Bridgeland-Tom Campbell's Hill Off Leash -Bow River-Nose Creek, NE
48	Edworthy Off Leash - West Trails- Wildwood, SW
60	Sandy Beach-Elbow Park-River Park Off Leash- Britannia, SW
82	Legacy Environmental Reserve, SE

Best Birding

Walks #	
19	Dale Hodges Park and Bowmont Park East, NW
65-66	Weaselhead Flats Park & Jackrabbit Trail, SW
67	Griffith Woods Park, SW
76-81	Fish Creek Provincial Park, SE-SW
83	Carburn and Beaverdam Flats Parks, SE
91	Inglewood Bird Sanctuary- Pearce Estate Park, SE

Bakery Treks

Walks #	
32	Cambrian Heights- Highland Park- Queens Park, NW (Ola Luna Bakeshop)
35	Bridgeland, NE (Mari Bakeshop)
51	Aspen Landing- Aspen Woods, SW (Ladybug Bakery Café)
53	Sunalta- Beltline- Mount Royal- Bankview- Scarboro, SW (Black Sheep, Butterblock, Begonia Bakehouse)
56	Downtown and Beltline Murals and Art, SW (Manuel Latruwe, Yann Haute Patisserie)
92	Ramsay- St. Patrick's - East Village, SE (Sidewalk Citizen, Canela Vegan Bakery)

Amazing views

Walks #	
28-30	Nose Hill Park, NW
18-20	Bowmont Park, NW
40	Kensington- McHugh Bluff- Crescent Heights, NW
58	Roxboro-Erlton-Ramsay, SW-SE
68	Glenmore Reservoir Circumnavigation, SW
84	Ogden- Lynnwood Loop, SE
86, 88	Forest Lawn- International Avenue- Southview, SE

Café Strolls

Walks #	
34	Winston Heights- Nose Creek- Tuxedo, NE
42	Sunnyside - Bow River Pathway- East Village- Inglewood, NW
43	Briar Hill-Hounsfield Heights-West Hillhurst-Westmount, NW
56	Downtown and Beltline Murals and Art, SW
58	Roxboro-Erlton-Ramsay, SW-SE
93	Ramsay- Bridgeland, SE-NE

Neighbourhood Ice Cream Strolls

Walks #	
35	Bridgeland (Lukes, Village and Made by Marcus)
43	Hillhurst- Briar Hill (Made by Marcus and Amato Gelato)
53	Sunalta- Beltline- Mount Royal- Bankview- Scarboro (Made by Marcus, Amato Gelato)
60	Sandy Beach-Elbow Park-Britannia (Village Ice Cream)
63	Garrison- Altadore (Village and My Favourite Ice Cream Shop)
92	Ramsay – Inglewood (Apprentice Café (Affogato!) and Made by Marcus)
93	Lukes, Village and Made by Marcus

Local Shops and Diverse Foods

Walks #	
34	Tuxedo, Centre Street North
35	Bridgeland, 1 Avenue NE
40	Kensington Road and 10 Street NW
53, 56	Beltline, 17 Avenue, 11 Avenue and 4 Street SW
88	Forest Lawn, International Avenue, SE
92	Inglewood, 9 Ave SE

Pub Walks & Craft Breweries

Walks #	
18	Bowness- Bowmont Park, NW
53	Sunalta- Beltline- Mount Royal- Bankview- Scarboro, SW
56	Downtown and Beltline Murals and Art, SW
63	Garrison-Currie-Altadore, SW
92	Ramsay- St. Patrick's - East Village, SE

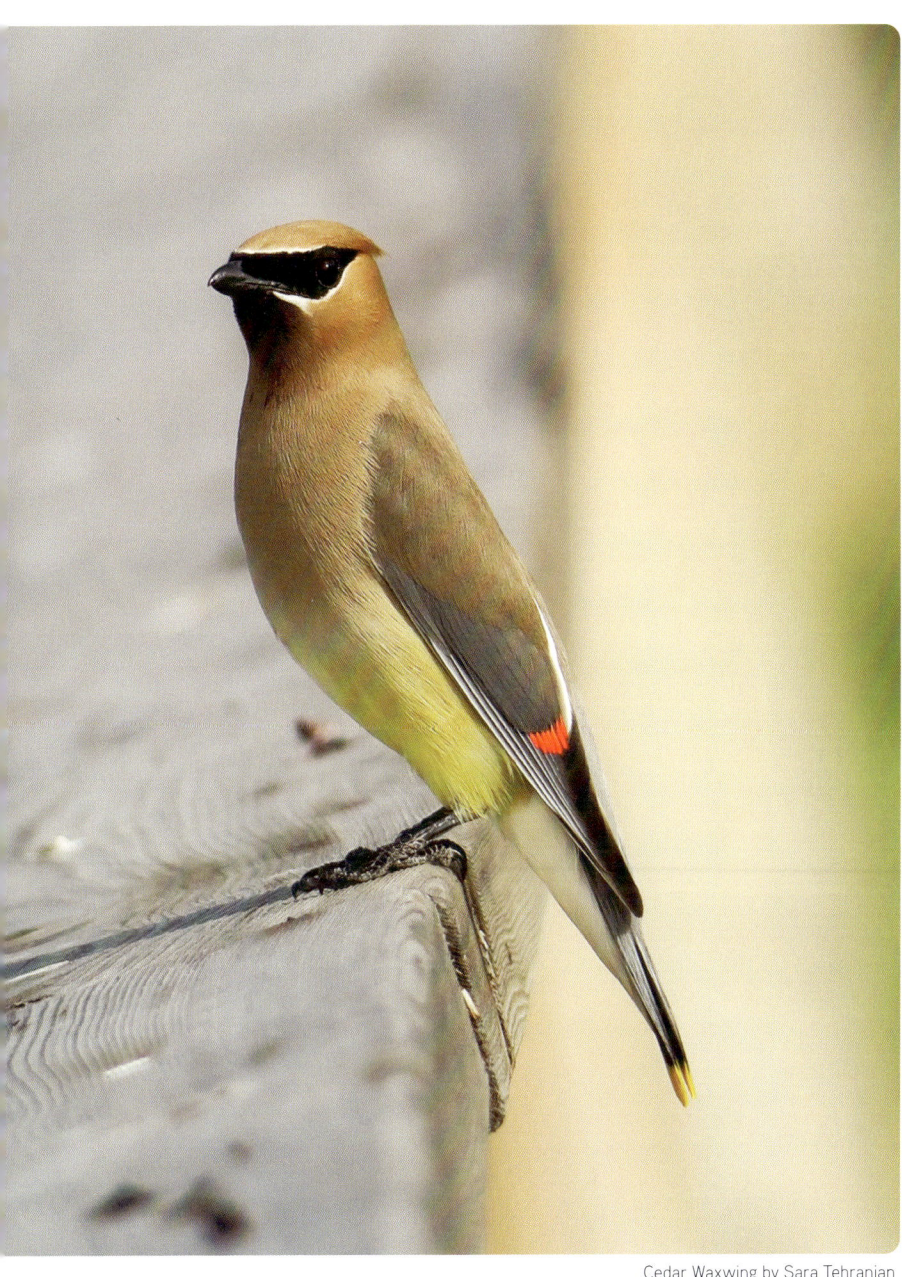
Cedar Waxwing by Sara Tehranian

Best Hikes and Walks Beyond Calgary

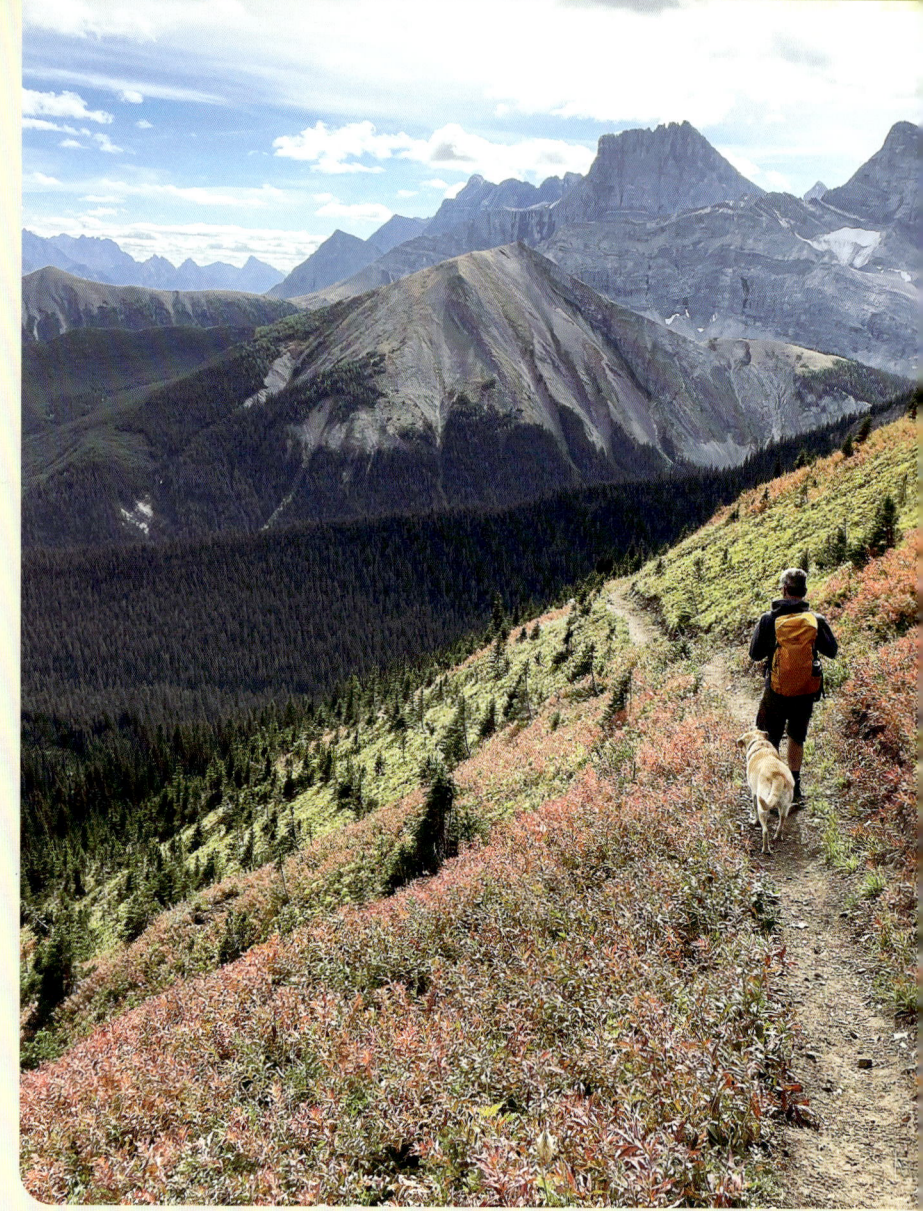

Guinn's Pass, Kananaskis

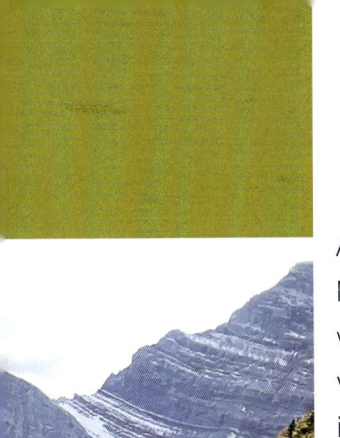
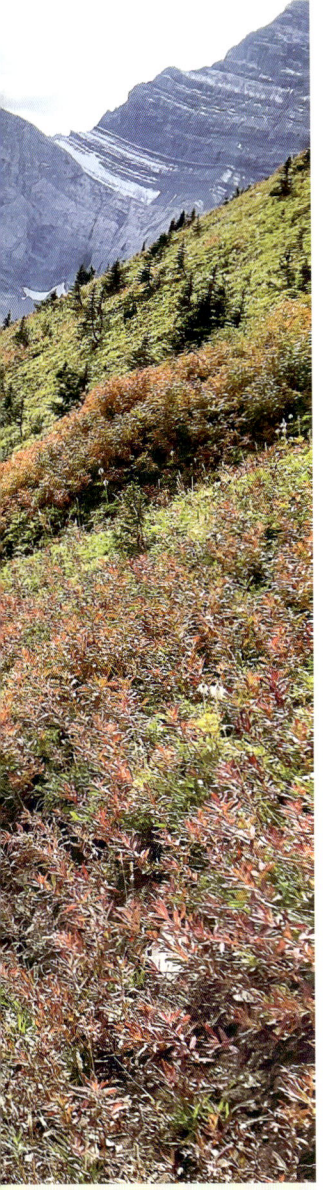

All around Calgary are foothills and Rocky Mountain hikes and walks that lead to waterfalls, wildflower meadows, and stunning views. Here are a few of my favourites including the essential tasty pit stop ending. I recommend you use the Gemtrek trail and topographical maps in conjunction with maps loaded onto your phone. Batteries never die on paper maps, and the Gemtrek maps help you see the entire area, the big picture, so you stay found.

Canmore & Banff walks

I have created some walk and hike routes in Canmore and Banff that get you off the tourist trails and lead you through neighbourhoods, along river paths and onto hiking trails. You will find links to these Google route maps in my Instagram bio link @lorifitfrog and on the book page on www.fitfrog.ca in the tabs at the bottom. Keep checking back as more beyond Calgary routes will be added.

Elbow Valley, Kananaskis near Bragg Creek

Fullerton Loop or Sulpher Springs - Riverview Loop are perfect year-round foothills starter hikes. **Distance & Difficulty:** Fullerton, 6.5 km loop, height gain 220 m, easy; Sulpher Spring-Riverview, 10.5 km, height gain 370 m, easy.

Prairie Mountain is a favourite summit hike that is so close to Calgary. I like to loop from the top to the Prairie Creek Trail to make it a longer day. **Distance & Difficulty:** 8.5 km return, height gain 710 m, difficult; with **Prairie Creek loop:** 12 km return, height gain 800 m, difficult.

Nihahi Ridge leads to stunning Elbow River and Valley views. Experienced hikers can route find up rocky steep terrain to the top of the mountain for a longer and more challenging day. **Distance & Difficulty:** To end of hiking trail: 5 km return, height gain 400 m, moderate; summit and ridge walk: 11 km return, height gain 800 m, difficult.

Jumpingpound Summit is a stunning hike that is my favourite foothills wildflower hike in June and July. All ages will love this hike for its big views for minimal effort. I love to go beyond the summit and follow the rolling hills that dip and climb through the forests and open meadows. **Distance & Difficulty:** 6.5 km return, height gain 400 m, moderate.

Tasty Pit Stops - Canmore & Banff

There are many locally owned cafés to visit in the Canmore area. Just east of downtown Canmore on Hwy 1A is **EPICanmore**, a bakery café that is known for its crèpes and sourdough breads, along with pastries, sandwiches and great coffee. Also along Hwy 1A is **Le Fournil Bakery** that specializes in pastries, breads and gourmet sandwiches. Sounds Continue into Canmore, park in the neighbourhood and walk to any of these spots. **Communitea** is a local favourite for made from scratch meals and baked goods, and often live music in the evenings. **Eclipse Coffee Roasters** has a few locations including one in Deadman's Flats. I love the main street location where I can settle in after a Canmore walk, sit outside by the fire in the winter, and watch the world go by. When in Banff I always stop at the **Wild Flour Bakery** for a hot drink, pastry, muffin or hiking lunch to go. Everything is made in house.

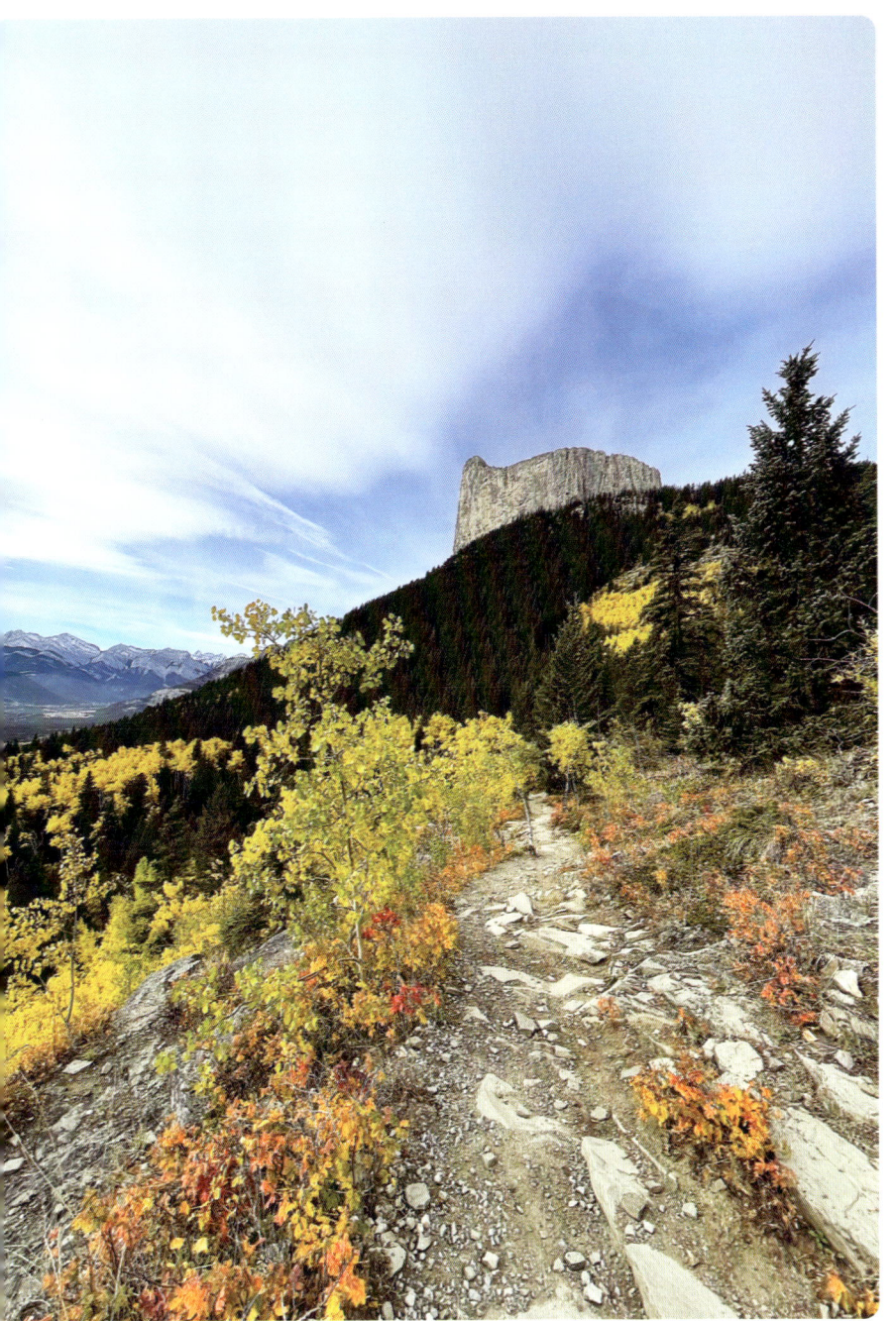

Raven's End trail, Mount Yamnuska

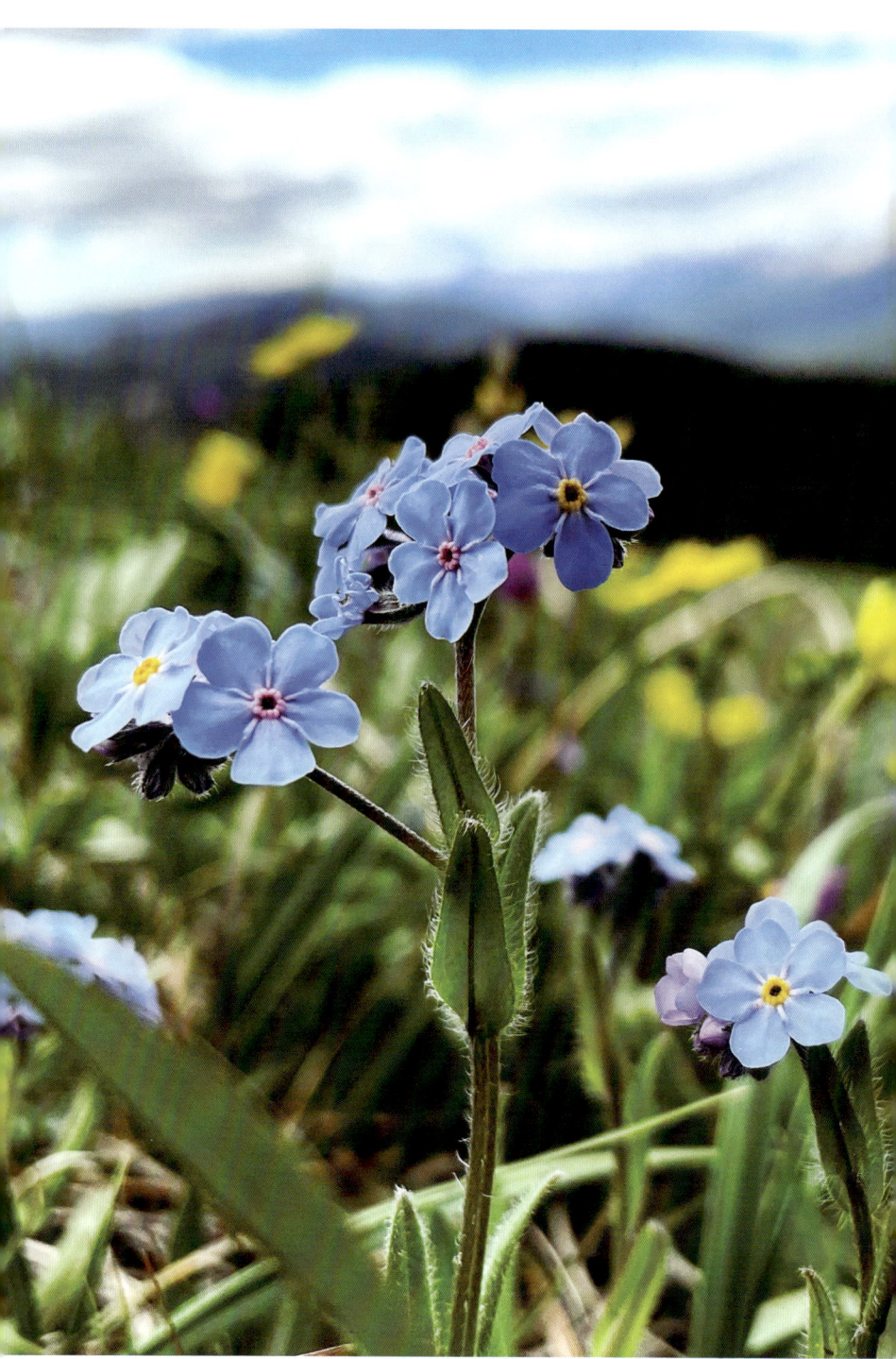
Forgetmenots on Jumpinpound Summit, Kananaskis

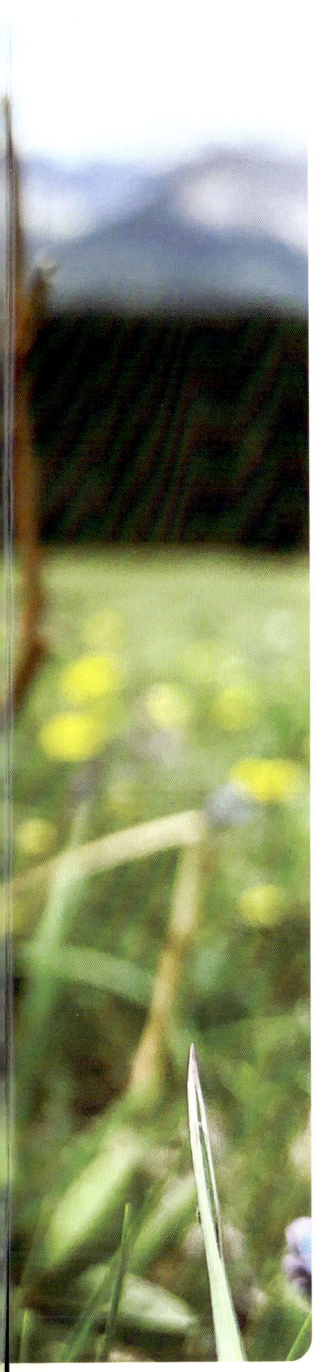

Bow Valley, Kananaskis

The **Raven's End** hiking trail is a great hike most of the year, but especially beautiful late June through fall when wildflowers bloom and foliage and aspens turn golden, orange and red in October. **Distance & difficulty:** 7.6 km return, height gain 550 m, easy.

Mount Yamnuska Traverse is a scramble, not a hike, where you will need proper gear, route finding experience and good physical fitness. There is exposure on this scramble. **Distance & difficulty:** 9.5 km loop return, height gain 880 m, difficult.

Grotto Canyon is perfect for families in all seasons. The winter ice walk is a fun time to go; bring your cleats. In the summer you can creek hop up the canyon. **Distance & difficulty:** 4 km return, height gain 100 m, easy. You can make it a longer hike by continuing up the canyon.

Bow Valley Provincial Park has six interpretive trails that meander alongside the river, lakes and amongst pine forest and meadows. Flowers are in full bloom in late June-early July. **Distance & difficulty:** 8.5 km return, height gain 156 m, easy.

Tasty Pit Stops - Bragg Creek

The Heart of Bragg Creek, a vegan café, offers so many delicious lunches and baked goods. There is a forested patio area for the warmer months and a cozy indoor space year-round.
Location: 12 Balsam Avenue, Bragg Creek towns

Kananaskis Valley, Hwy 40

Elbow Lake, Edworthy Falls, Rae Lake and Piper Pass. There are so many hikes beyond Elbow Lake, from easy valley walking to Edworthy Falls, to single track trails to Rae Lake and Piper Pass. Route finding skills, some creek hoping and steep climbing are on the final two routes. I love them all! **Distance & Difficulty:** Hikes range from 4 km -20 km return, height gain 175 m - 1000 m, easy - difficult.

Jewell Pass & Prairie View Loop. From Barrier Dam this loop hike leads to a waterfall along Jewell Pass and panoramic views. And optional climb to the fire lookout adds even bigger views. One challenging descent from the top of Prairie View may be icy in the cooler months. Brings cleats! **Distance & Difficulty:** 15 km return, height gain 800-900 m, moderate.

Lillian Lake, Galatea Lake and Guinn's Pass. One trail to many beautiful destinations makes. This shaded hike is so nice on a hot summers day as you cross-cross the creek to Lillian Lake before a steep rocky≈climb to Galatea Lakes. Continue to Guinn's Pass for the big finish! **Distance & Difficulty:** Hikes range from 12 km - 17 km return, height gain 570 m- 1000 m, moderate - difficult.

Highwood Pass, Ptarmigan Cirque or Pocaterra Ridge. Starting from the highest paved pass in Canada, both hikes lead to alpine meadows and spectacular views. Ptarmigan Cirque is a short interpretive loop that is wonderful for families while Pocaterra Ridge is a challenging unofficial trail that requires route finding skills, gear for all conditions and excellent fitness. **Distance & Difficulty:** Hikes range from 4.5 km – 18 km return, height gain 210 m - 700 m, moderate - difficult.

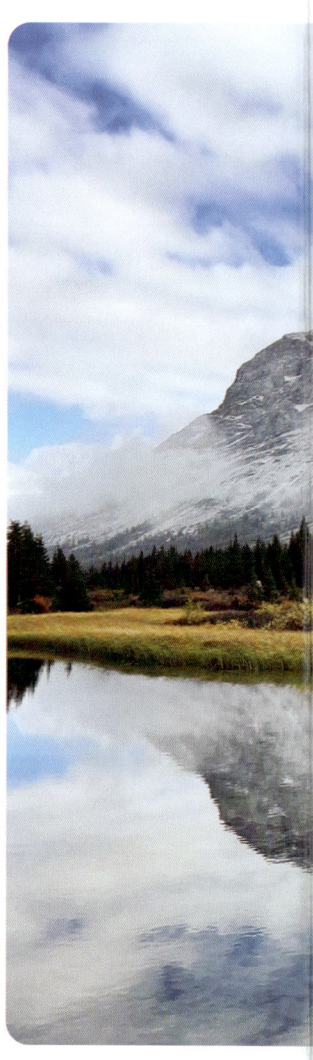

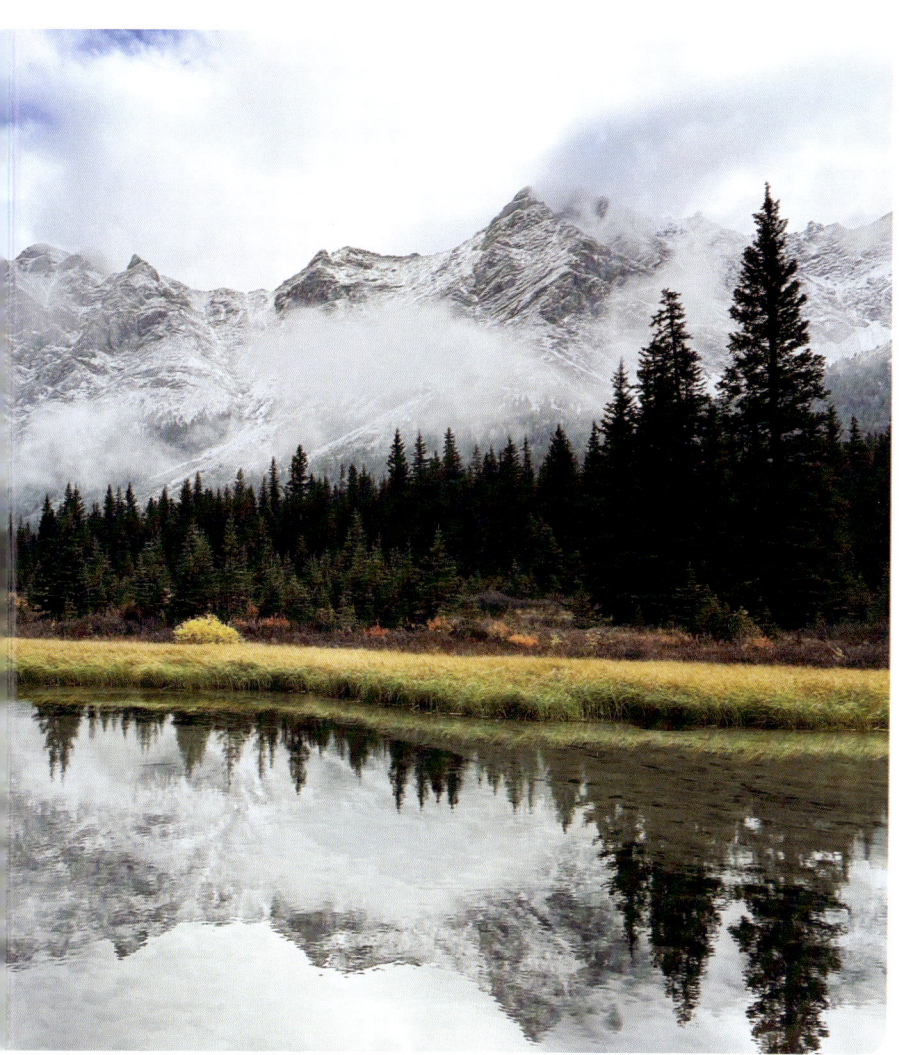
Elbow Lake reflection

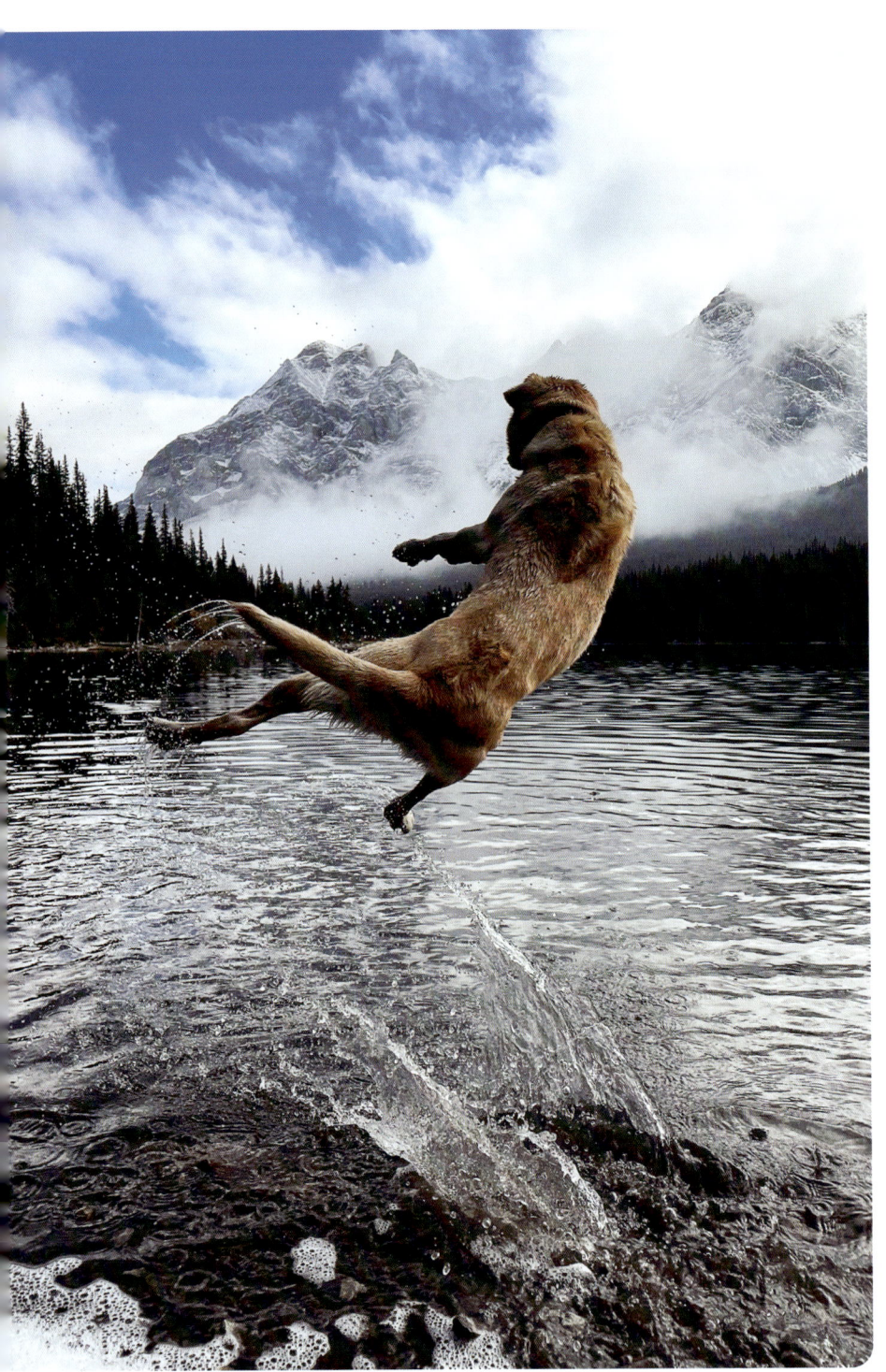

Millarville, Diamond Valley and Sheep River, Kananaskis

Mesa Butte & Grind, Hwy 549. The best half day summit hike close to Calgary! Start from the Mesa Butte Campground to extend the hike on the Curley Connector Trail. There are many interconnected trails with no signs in this area so be sure to have a map. **Distance & Difficulty:** 4 km, height gain 236 m, easy

Foran Grade and Windy Point Loop, Sheep River, Hwy 546. Soak up excellent views of the Sheep Valley on this foothills loop hike. In the winter start from the road closure gate to add another 2 km. **Distance & Difficulty:** 7 km return, height gain 300 m, easy.

Tiger Jaw Falls and Mount Hoffmann, Sheep River, Hwy. 546. Follow a zig-zag trail to stupendous panoramic views that include Junction Mountain, Gibraltar to Bluerock Mountain and beyond. Plan a picnic by the Sheep River near the waterfalls post summit hike. **Distance & Difficulty:** 9 km return, height gain 470 m, moderate. Access this hike from May 15- Nov. 30 when the road is open.

Tasty pit stop

Black Sheep Coffee Co. roast their own coffee and have made in house baked goods. I love to sit on their patio where my hiking pup can join me. **The Chuckwagon Café** hosts all day breakfast and lunch (open until 2:30 midweek and 3:30 on weekends). Continue to the town formally known as Black Diamond for more shops and places to grab a bite.

Jumping for joy! Elbow Lake

Contributors

Jill Thomson

Jill Thomson's artwork evokes her personal history of a small town/prairie childhood, an urban Montreal young adulthood and a settled life as artist, mother and grandmother in Alberta. Her rich colourful palette and complex compositions celebrate a creative life in cities with walking and bicycle paths, generous front porches, cafes, bookstores, gardens and green space.

Connect with Jill at www.jillthomson.ca, on Instagram @jillthomsonart and at Gibson Fine Art in Calgary

Sara Tehranian

Born in Tehran, a city at the foothills of the Alborz Mountains in Iran, Sara was always fascinated with nature. After moving to Calgary to pursue her graduate studies in Engineering, the Rocky Mountains made her feel close to home. She soon started capturing Alberta's stunning sceneries, hoping to turn the fleeting moments she experienced in nature into lasting memories. Sara lives in Calgary with her husband Majid Saeedi.

Connect with Sara on Instagram: @sara.tehranian

Cody Stuart

When he's not out riding his bike (which is often), Cody is likely exploring the city with his family. With twin boys who share his boundless energy, he's on a constant quest to discover Calgary's best forts, swimming holes, and hidden vistas. Whether it's winter or summer, the adventure never stops in the city's expansive park system.

Connect with Cody on Instagram @betamanic

Pam Weber

Harmonious landscapes, playful buildings, whimsical wildlife and florals with personality describe the paintings by local artist Pam Weber. Her small studio is filled with colourful pots of acrylic paint; and if she is lucky one of her cats may decide to curl up on her worktable to provide comfort, distraction or be the muse of the hour. Pam's signature style is bright and bold, a celebration of colour and subject matter.

Connect with Pam at www.pamweber.com and on FB and IG as @pamweberart

Sergio Gaytán

Sergio is an experienced designer; his commitment to a passionate project like this has its roots on his love of nature, adventure, art and design. With proficient knowledge of his craft and a proactive attitude, he fosters a collaborative environment to shape the author's vision and goals through team-work synergy. Creativity, aesthetics and functionality come together to produce books of high quality and value, reliable accomplices to many adventures and discoveries.

Connect with Sergio at gaytan07@yahoo.com and www.sgaytan.art

Author

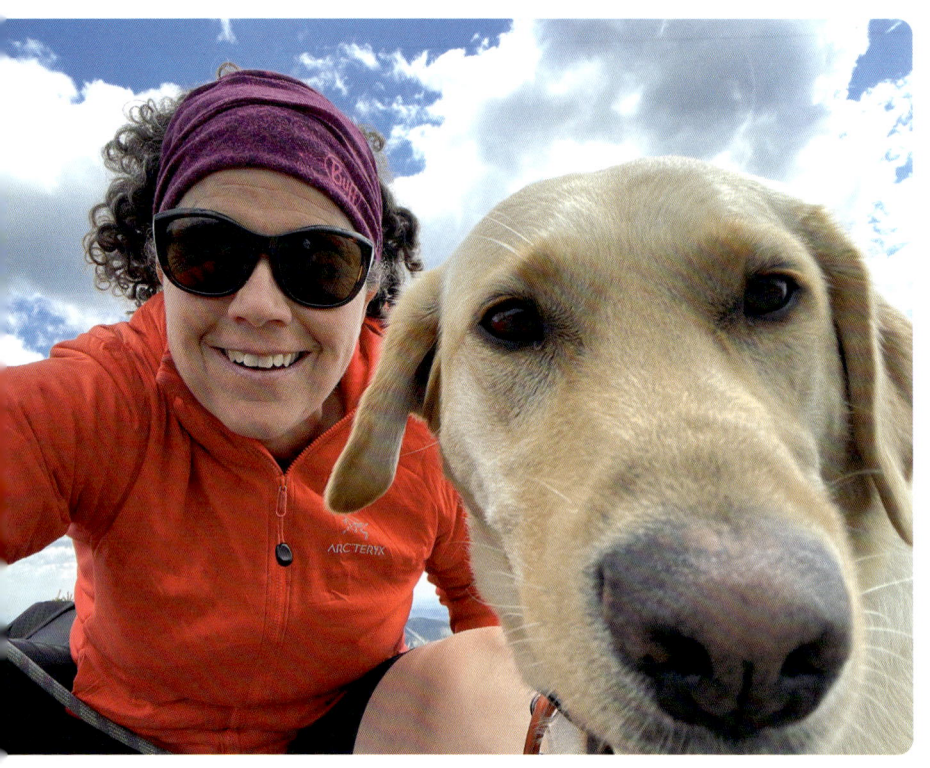

Lori Beattie

A passionate urban explorer, Lori loves getting outside and moving through Calgary and beyond under her own steam, discovering new views and perspectives along the way. She walks and bikes in search of big nature, hidden pathways, farmers' markets and shops, gardens, cafés, folk art, and conversations. She is also the author of Calgary's Best Bike Rides, writes about walking and biking in various publications and she presents to groups about the pleasures of exploring Calgary and beyond on foot and by bike, building community through walking and making Calgary feel like home, one step and pedal at a time. Lori leads Calgarians and visitors on walks, hikes and snowshoe days with her company Fit Frog Adventures. She lives in Calgary and enjoys daily self-propelled exploring in Calgary and throughout Canada with enthusiastic Fit Frog walkers, superb friends and her fantastic family - Keith, Oscar, Eve in NS, Margaret Beattie in NB, and with super dog Wall-E.

Connect with Lori at
lorib@fitfrog.ca or on Instagram @lorifitfrog

Keep watch on www.fitfrog.ca and Instagram for upcoming book events and walks.

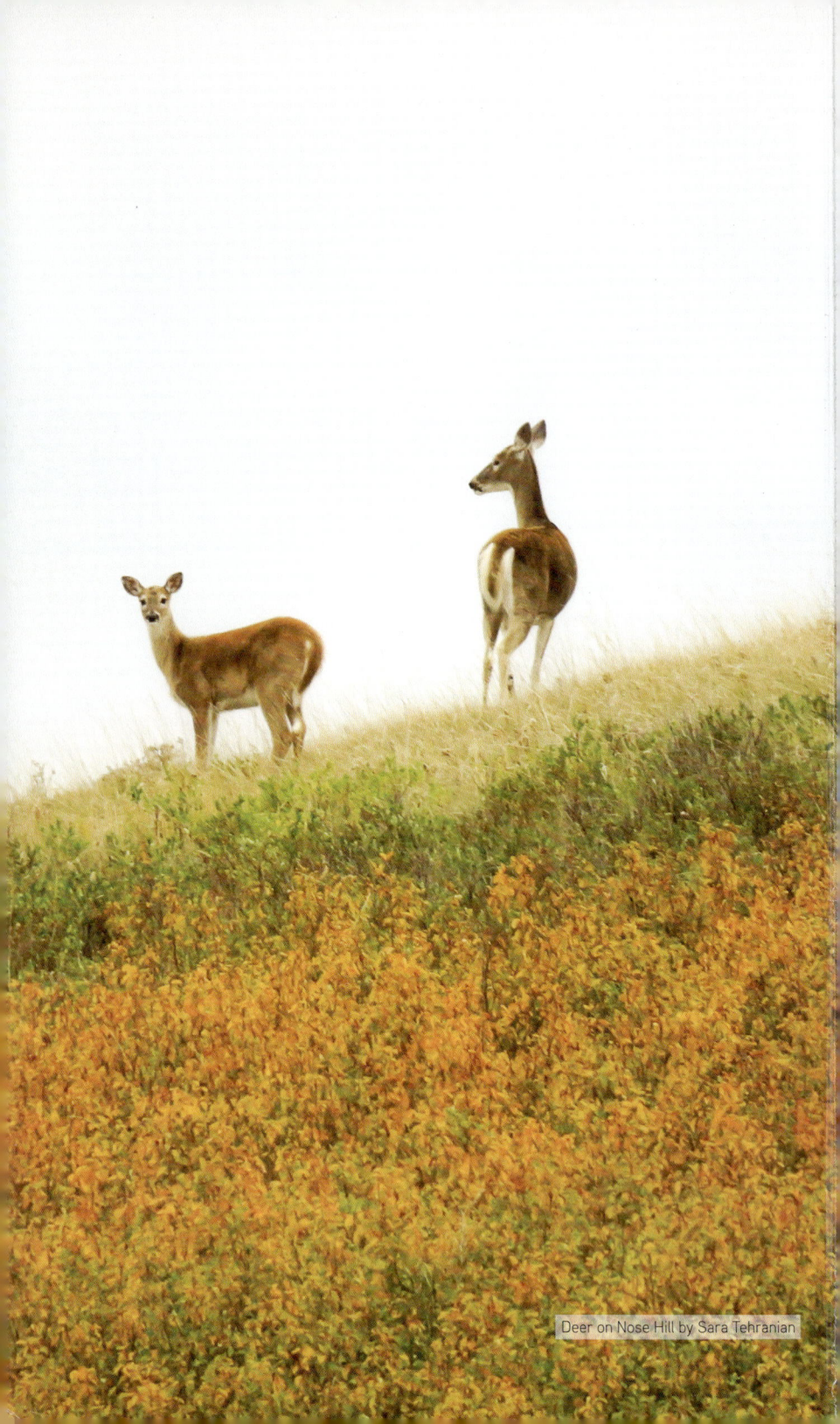

Deer on Nose Hill by Sara Tehranian